CLINICAL
CALCULATIONS

Fourth Edition

CLINICAL CALCULATIONS

WITH APPLICATIONS TO GENERAL AND SPECIALTY AREAS

Joyce LeFever Kee, RN, MS
Associate Professor Emerita
College of Health and Nursing Sciences
University of Delaware
Newark, Delaware

Sally M. Marshall, RN, MSN
Nursing Service
Department of Veterans Affairs
Regional Office and Medical Center
Wilmington, Delaware

W.B. SAUNDERS COMPANY
A Harcourt Health Sciences Company
Philadelphia London Montreal Sydney Tokyo

W.B. SAUNDERS COMPANY
A Harcourt Health Sciences Company

The Curtis Center
Independence Square West
Philadelphia, Pennsylvania 19106

Library of Congress Cataloging-in-Publication Data

Kee, Joyce LeFever.
Clinical calculations: with applications to general and specialty areas /
Joyce L. Kee, Sally M. Marshall.—4th ed.

p. cm.

Includes bibliographical references and index.

ISBN 0-7216-8304-5

1. Pharmaceutical arithmetic. 2. Nursing—Mathematics. I. Marshall, Sally M.
  II. Title.   [DNLM: 1. Pharmaceutical Preparations—administration &
  dosage Nurses' Instruction. 2. Mathematics Nurses' Instruction.
  QV 748 K26c 2000]

RS57.K44 2000   615'.14—dc21

DNLM/DLC   99-35200

CLINICAL CALCULATIONS:
With Applications to General and Specialty Areas   ISBN 0-7216-8304-5

Printed in the United States of America

Last digit is the print number: 9   8   7   6   5   4   3   2

preface

• •

This text arose from the need to bridge the learning gap between education and practice. We believe that this bridge is needed in order for the student to understand the wide range of clinical calculations used in nursing practice. This book provides a comprehensive application of calculations in nursing practice.

The last edition of *Clinical Calculations: With Applications to General and Specialty Areas* has been expanded in this fourth edition on topics in several areas to show the interrelationship between calculation and drug administration, such as in the use of the latest equipment (insulin pump, patient-controlled analgesia pumps, multichannel infusion pumps), various new syringes (prefilled syringes, insulin and tuberculin syringes), various methods to determine body surface area, and more. A Post-Test was developed for students to determine their competency in oral, injectable, intravenous, and pediatric drug calculations. This text also provides the six methods for calculating drug dosages: basic formula, ratio and proportion, fractional equation, dimensional analysis, body weight, and body surface area.

Other changes and additions in the fourth edition include some of the following, along with still useful material from the third edition.

• Problems using the newest drug labels in most chapters
• Further drug problems in Chapters 5, 6, 7, 8, 9, 10, 11, and 13
• Post-Test Drug Calculations (Part Five) for students to test their competency in calculation of drug dosages. The Post-Test has 50 questions and is divided into four sections: oral, injectable, intravenous, and pediatric topics.
• Use of the slide rule and square root for determination of the body surface area. The nomograms are still widely used.
• Use of fingertip units for cream applications
• Use of military time for drug administration and charting
• Explanations for the use of the insulin pump and the patient-controlled analgesic pump
• Illustrations of new types of syringes: safety needle shield, various insulin and tuberculin syringes, needleless syringes
• Illustrations of pumps: insulin, enteral infusion, various intravenous infusion pumps (single and multichannel, patient-controlled analgesia, and syringe)
• Direct intravenous injection (IV push or IV bolus) and with practice problems added to Chapter 8.
• Overview of home infusion therapy
• Additional topics, such as the *Check List of the "5 Rights" in Drug Administration,* are included at the end of the text.
• Testbank questions, in booklet form for instructors, are available.

Clinical Calculations is unique in that it has problems not only for the general patient care areas but also for the specialty units: pediatrics, critical care, pediatric critical care, labor and delivery, and community. The book is useful for nurses in all levels of nursing education who are learning for the first time how to calculate dosage problems and for beginning practitioners in specialty areas. It also can be used in nursing refresher courses, inservice programs, hospital units, home health care, and other places of nursing practice.

The book is divided into five parts. Part One is the basic math review, written concisely for nursing students to review Roman numerals, fractions, decimals, percentages, and ratio and proportion. A post-math review test follows. The math test can be taken first, and if the student has a score of 90% or higher, the basic review section can be omitted. Part Two covers metric, apothecary, and household systems used in drug calculations; conversion of units; reading drug labels, drug orders, and abbreviations; and methods of calculations. Part Three covers calculation of drug and fluid dosages for oral, injectable, and intravenous administration. Clinical drug calculations for specialty areas are found in Part Four. This part includes pediatrics, critical care for adults and children, labor and delivery, and community. Part Five contains the Post-Test for students to test their competency in mastering oral, injectable, intravenous, and pediatric drug calculations. A passing grade is 88%.

In the appendix, guidelines for administrations of medications (oral, injectable, and intravenous) are given. The index assists in locating content in the text.

Each chapter has a content list, objectives, introduction, and numerous practice problems. The practice problems are related to clinical drug problems that are currently used in clinical settings. Illustrations such as tablets, capsules, medicine cup, syringes, ampules, vials, intravenous bag and bottle, IV tubing, electronic IV devices, intramuscular injection sites, central venous sites, and many others are provided throughout the text.

Calculators may be used in solving dosage problems. Many institutions have calculators available. It is suggested that the nurse work the problem without a calculator and then check the answer with a calculator.

Joyce LeFever Kee
Sally M. Marshall

TO THE INSTRUCTOR: A suggestion on how this book may be used by the student: Assign Part One and Part Two that cover delivery of medication prior to the class. A testbank of questions is also available for the instructor's use.

TO THE READER

Consult the product information contained in the package insert
of each drug before administering the medication.

acknowledgments

We wish to extend our sincere appreciation to the individuals who have helped with this fourth edition: Adrienne Woods, RN, MSN, for her suggestions and use of her book, *Nurses' Drug Handbook*, by George Spratto and Adrienne Woods; Janice Compton, RN, BSN, and Zach Koshy, PharmD, both from the Veterans Administration Medical Center, Wilmington, Delaware; Gail H. Wade, RN, MSN, Assistant Professor from the University of Delaware; Kim Marie Falk, RN, MSN, Northeastern Hospital, Temple University Health System, Philadelphia; and Drew Marshall for his typing assistance. We also thank Don Passidomo, head librarian at the Veterans Administration Medical Center, for his research assistance.

Our deepest appreciation goes to pharmaceutical companies for permission to use their drug labels. These labels are samples used for educational purposes only. The pharmaceutical companies that extended this courtesy include

Abbott Laboratories
American Regent
  Luitold Pharmaceuticals
Bristol-Myers Squibb
  Apothecon
  Mead Johnson Pharmaceuticals
  Squibb Diagnostic Division
Du Pont Merck Pharmaceutical
Eli Lilly and Company
Elkins-Sinn, Incorporated
  A subsidiary of A.H. Robins, Wyeth-Ayerst Laboratories, Cherry Hill, New Jersey

GlaxoWellcome
Marion Merrell Dow, Incorporated
McNeil Consumer Products Company
Ortho McNeil Pharmaceutical
Merck & Company (labels used with permission of Merck & Company, Inc.)
Mylan Pharmaceuticals
SmithKline Beecham Pharmaceuticals
Warner-Lambert Consumer Health Products
Parke-Davis
Wyeth-Ayerst Laboratories

We extend our sincere thanks to the companies and publishers who gave us permission to use photographs, illustrations, and other materials in the text. These include

American Association of Critical Care Nursing
Appleton & Lange
Baxter Healthcare
Becton Dickinson & Company
Ciba-Geigy Pharmaceuticals

Mosby
F. A. Davis
IMED Corporation
W.B. Saunders
Wyeth-Ayerst Laboratories

Joyce LeFever Kee
Sally M. Marshall

GUIDELINES ON SELF-DIRECTED USE OF THIS TEXT

You may use this text, *Clinical Calculations: With Applications to General and Specialty Areas, Fourth Edition,* as a self-instructional mathematics and dosage calculations review tool.

Part I, *Basic Math Review,* is a review of math concepts usually taught in middle school. Some students may need to review Part I as a refresher of basic math, and they will then take the comprehensive math test at the end of the book. Other students may choose to take the math test first. If your score on this test is 90% or higher, you should proceed to Part II; if your score is less than 90%, you should review Part I.

Part II, *Systems, Conversions, and Methods of Drug Calculation,* should be studied prior to the class related to oral, injectable, and intravenous calculations, which is covered in Part III. In Part II you will learn the various systems of drug administration, conversion within the various systems, charting, drug orders, abbreviations, methods of drug calculations, and alternative methods for drug administration. You can study Part II on your own.

Chapter 5, Methods of Calculation, gives the four methods commonly used to calculate drug dosages. Drug calculations by body weight and body surface area (BSA) are also presented. You or the instructor should select one of the four methods to calculate drug dosages. Use that method in all practice problems starting with Chapter 5. This approach will improve your proficiency in the calculation of drug dosages.

Part III, *Calculations for Oral, Injectable, and Intravenous Drugs,* is usually discussed in class and during a clinical practicum. Prior to class, you should review the three chapters in Part III. Questions may be addressed and answered during class time. During the class or clinical practicum, you may practice drug calculations and the drawing up of drug doses in a syringe.

Part IV, *Calculations for Specialty Areas,* is usually presented when the topics are discussed in class. You should review this content in these chapters—Pediatrics and Pediatric Critical Care, Critical Care, Labor and Delivery, and Community—before the scheduled class. This content may or may not be covered, according to the requirements of your specific nursing program.

brief contents

· ·

contents

basic math review

● bjectives

- Convert Roman numerals to Arabic numerals.
- Multiply and divide fractions and decimals.
- Solve ratio and proportion problems.
- Change percentage to decimals, fractions, and ratio and proportion.
- Demonstrate an understanding of Roman numerals, fractions, decimals, ratio and proportion, and percentage by passing the math test.

● utline

The basic math review assists nurses in converting Roman and Arabic numerals, multiplying and dividing fractions and decimals, and solving ratio and proportion problems and percentage problems. Nurses need to master basic math skills to solve drug problems used in the administration of medication.

A math test, found on page 13, follows the basic math review. The test may be taken first, and if a score of 90% or greater is achieved, the math review, or Part One, can be omitted. If the test score is less than 90%, the nurse should do the basic math review section. Some nurses may choose to start with Part One and then take the test.

Answers to the Practice Problems are at the end of Part One, before the Post-Math Test.

NUMBER SYSTEMS

Two systems of numbers currently used are Arabic and Roman. Both systems are used in drug administration.

Arabic System

The Arabic system is expressed in numbers: 0, 1, 2, 3, 4, 5, 6, 7, 8, 9. These can be written as whole numbers or with fractions and decimals. This system is commonly used today.

Roman System

Numbers used in the Roman system are designated by selected capital letters, i.e., I, V, X. Roman numbers can be changed to Arabic numbers.

Conversion of Systems

ROMAN NUMBER	ARABIC NUMBER
I	1
V	5
X	10
L	50
C	100

The apothecary system of measurement uses Roman numerals for writing drug dosages. The Roman numerals are written in lower case letters, i.e., i, v, x, xii. The lower case letters can be topped by a horizontal line, i.e., ī, v̄, x̄, x̄ī.

Roman numerals can appear together, such as xv and ix. Reading multiple Roman numerals requires the use of addition and subtraction.

METHOD A

If the first Roman numeral is greater than the following numeral(s), then **ADD**.

examples

$$\overline{viii} = 5 + 3 = 8$$
$$\overline{xv} = 10 + 5 = 15$$

METHOD B

If the first Roman numeral is less than the following numeral(s), then **SUBTRACT**. Subtract the first numeral from the second (i.e., the smaller from the larger).

examples

$$\overline{iv} = 5 - 1 = 4$$
$$\overline{ix} = 10 - 1 = 9$$

Some Roman numerals require both addition and subtraction to ascertain their value. Read from left to right.

examples

$$\overline{xix} = 10 + 9 \ (10 - 1) = 19$$
$$\overline{xxxiv} = 30 \ (10 + 10 + 10) + 4 \ (5 - 1) = 34$$

I Practice Problems: Roman Numerals

1. xvi

$10 + 5 + 1 = 16$

2. xii

$10 + 1 + 1 = 12$

3. xxiv

$10 + 10 + (5 - 1) = 24$

4. xxxix

$10 + 10 + 10 + (10 - 1) = 39$

5. XLV

$(50 - 10) + 5 = 45$

6. XC

$100 - 10 = 90$

FRACTIONS

Fractions are expressed as part(s) of a whole or part(s) of a unit. A fraction is composed of two basic numbers: a *numerator* (the top number) and a *denominator* (the bottom number). The denominator indicates the total number of parts

Fraction: <u>3</u> numerator (3 of 4 parts)
       4 denominator (4 of 4 parts, or 4 total parts)

The value of a fraction depends mainly on the denominator. When the denominator increases, for example, from ⅒ to ½₀, the value of the fraction decreases, because it takes more parts to make a whole.

Which fraction has the greater value: ¼ or ⅙? The denominators are 4 and 6.

The larger value is ¼, because four parts make the whole, whereas for ⅙, it takes six parts to make a whole. Therefore, ⅙ has the smaller value.

Proper, Improper, and Mixed Fractions

In a *proper fraction* (simple fraction), the numerator is less than the denominator, i.e., ½, ⅔, ¾, ⅖. When possible, the fraction should be reduced to its lowest term, i.e., ⅔ = ⅓ (2 goes into 2 and 6).

In an *improper fraction*, the numerator is greater than the denominator, i.e., 4/2, 8/5, 14/4. Reduce improper fractions to whole numbers or mixed numbers, i.e., 4/2 = 2 (4/2 means the same as 4 ÷ 2); 8/5 = 1⅗ (8 ÷ 5, 5 goes into 8 one time with 3 left over, or ⅗); and 14/4 = 3²/4 = 3½ (14 ÷ 4, 4 goes into 14 three times with 2 left over, or 2/4, which can then be reduced to ½).

A *mixed number* is a whole number and a fraction, i.e., 1⅗, 3½. Mixed numbers can be changed to improper fractions by multiplying the denominator by the whole number, then adding the numerator, i.e., 1⅗ = 8/5 (5 × 1 = 5, + 3 = 8).

The apothecary system uses fractions to indicate drug dosages. Fractions may be added, subtracted, multiplied, or divided. Multiplying fractions and dividing fractions are the two common methods used in solving dosage problems.

Multiplying Fractions

To multiply fractions, multiply the numerators and then the denominators. Reduce the fraction, if possible, to lowest terms.

examples

1. $$\dfrac{1}{3} \times \dfrac{3}{5} = \dfrac{\overset{1}{\cancel{3}}}{\underset{5}{\cancel{15}}} = \dfrac{1}{5}$$

The answer is ³⁄₁₅, which can be reduced to ⅕. The number that goes into both 3 and 15 is 3. Therefore, 3 goes into 3 one time, and 3 goes into 15 five times.

2. $$\dfrac{1}{3} \times 6 = \dfrac{6}{3} = 2$$

A whole number can also be written as that number over one ($\frac{6}{1}$). Six is divided by 3 (6 ÷ 3); 3 goes into 6 two times.

Dividing Fractions

To divide fractions, invert the *second fraction, or divisor,* and then multiply.

examples

1. $$\dfrac{3}{4} \div \dfrac{3}{8} \text{ (divisor)} = \dfrac{\overset{1}{\cancel{3}}}{\underset{1}{\cancel{4}}} \times \dfrac{\overset{2}{\cancel{8}}}{\underset{1}{\cancel{3}}} = \dfrac{2}{1} = 2$$

When dividing, invert the divisor ⅜ to ⁸⁄₃ and multiply. To reduce the fraction to lowest terms, 3 goes into both 3s one time, and 4 goes into 4 and 8 one time and two times, respectively.

2. $$\dfrac{1}{6} \div \dfrac{4}{18} = \dfrac{1}{\underset{1}{\cancel{6}}} \times \dfrac{\overset{3}{\cancel{18}}}{4} = \dfrac{3}{4}$$

Six and 18 are reduced, or canceled, to 1 and 3.

Decimal Fractions

Fractions can be changed to decimals. Divide the numerator by the denominator, i.e., ¾ = $4\overline{)3.00}$ with 0.75 above. Therefore, ¾ is the same as 0.75.

II Practice Problems: Fractions

1. **a.** Which has the greatest value: ¹⁄₅₀, ¹⁄₁₀₀, or ¹⁄₁₅₀? _____ 1/50

   b. Which has the lowest value: ¹⁄₅₀, ¹⁄₁₀₀, or ¹⁄₁₅₀? _____ 1/150

2. Reduce improper fractions to whole or mixed numbers.

   a. ¹²⁄₄ = 3

   c. ²²⁄₃ = 7⅓

b. $^{20}/_5 =$ _4_

d. $^{32}/_6 =$ _5 $^2/_6$ = 5 $^1/_3$_

3. Multiply fractions.

   a. $^2/_3 \times ^1/_8 =$ _$\frac{2}{24}$ = $\frac{1}{12}$_

   c. $^{500}/_{350} \times 5 =$ _$\frac{50}{7}$ = 7 $^1/_7$_

   b. $2^2/_5 \times 3^3/_4 =$ _$\frac{12^3}{8} \times \frac{15^3}{4}$ = 9_

      $^{12}/_5 \times ^{15}/_4 =$

   d. $^{400,000}/_{200,000} \times 3 =$ _$\frac{4}{2} \times 3$ = 6_

4. Divide fractions.

   a. $^2/_3 \div 6 =$ _$\frac{2}{3} \cdot \frac{1}{6}$ = $\frac{2}{18}$ = $\frac{1}{9}$_

   d. $^1/_{150}/^1/_{100} = (^1/_{150} \div ^1/_{100}) =$ _$\frac{1}{150} \cdot \frac{100}{1}$ = $\frac{10}{15}$ = $\frac{2}{3}$_

   b. $^1/_4 \div ^1/_5 =$ _$\frac{1}{4} \cdot \frac{5}{1}$ = $\frac{5}{4}$ = 1 $\frac{1}{4}$_

   e. $^1/_{200} \div ^1/_{300} =$ _$\frac{1}{200} \cdot \frac{300}{1}$ = $\frac{3}{2}$ = 1 $^1/_2$_

   c. $^1/_6 \div ^1/_8 =$ _$\frac{1}{3} \cdot \frac{4}{1}$ = $\frac{4}{3}$ = 1 $^1/_3$_

   f. $9^3/_5 \div 4 =$ _$\frac{48}{5} \cdot \frac{1}{4}$ = $\frac{12}{5}$ = 2 $^2/_5$_

      $^{48}/_5 \div ^4/_1 =$

5. Change fraction to a decimal.

   a. $^1/_4 =$ _.25_   **b.** $^1/_{10} =$ _.1_   **c.** $^2/_5 =$ _.4_

DECIMALS

Decimals consist of (1) whole numbers (numbers to the left of decimal point) and (2) decimal fractions (numbers to the right of decimal point). The number 2468.8642 is an example of the division of units for a whole number with a decimal fraction.

WHOLE NUMBERS					DECIMAL FRACTIONS			
2	4	6	8	●	8	6	4	2
Thousands	Hundreds	Tens	Units		Tenths	Hundredths	Thousandths	Ten Thousandths

Decimal fractions are written in tenths, hundredths, thousandths, and ten-thousandths. Frequently, decimal fractions are used in drug dosing. The metric system is referred to as the *decimal system.* After decimal problems are solved, decimal fractions are rounded off to tenths. If the hundredth column is 5 or greater, the tenth is increased by 1, i.e., 0.67 is rounded up to 0.7 (tenths).

Decimal fractions are an integral part of the metric system. Tenths mean 0.1 or $\frac{1}{10}$, hundredths mean 0.01 or $\frac{1}{100}$, and thousandths mean 0.001 or $\frac{1}{1000}$. When a decimal is changed to a fraction, the denomination is based on the number of digits to the right of the decimal point (0.8 is $\frac{8}{10}$, 0.86 is $\frac{86}{100}$).

. . . .

examples

1. 0.5 is $\frac{5}{10}$, or 5 tenths.
2. 0.55 is $\frac{55}{100}$, or 55 hundredths.
3. 0.555 is $\frac{555}{1000}$, or 555 thousandths.

Multiplying Decimals

To multiply decimal numbers, multiply the multiplicand by the multiplier. Count how many numbers (spaces) are to the right of the decimals in the problem. Mark off the number of decimal spaces in the answer (right to left) according to the number of decimal spaces in the problem. Round off in tenths.

. . . .

example

$$
\begin{array}{rl}
1.34 & \text{multiplicand} \\
\underline{2.3} & \text{multiplier} \\
402 & \\
\underline{268\emptyset} & \\
3.082 & \text{or} \quad 3.1 \text{ (rounded off in tenths)}
\end{array}
$$

Answer: 3.1. Because 8 is greater than 5, the "tenth" number is increased by 1.

Dividing Decimals

To divide decimal numbers, move the decimal point in the divisor to the right to make a whole number. The decimal point in the dividend is also moved to the right according to the number of decimal spaces in the divisor.

example

Dividend ÷ Divisor

$$2.46 \div 1.2 \quad \text{or} \quad \frac{2.46}{1.2} =$$

$$\begin{array}{r} 2.05 = 2.1 \\ \text{(divisor) } 1.2\,\overline{)2.4\,60} \text{ (dividend)} \\ \underline{2\,4} \\ 60 \\ \underline{60} \\ 0 \end{array}$$

III Practice Problems: Decimals

1. Multiply decimals.

   a. $6.8 \times 0.123 =$ **b.** $52.4 \times 9.345 =$

_____   _____

2. Divide decimals.

   a. $69 \div 3.2 =$ **c.** $100 \div 4.5 =$

_____   _____

   b. $6.63 \div 0.23 =$ **d.** $125 \div 0.75 =$

_____   _____

3. Change decimals to fractions.

   a. $0.46 =$ **b.** $0.05 =$ **c.** $0.012 =$

_____   _____   _____

4. Which has the greatest value: 0.46, 0.05, or 0.012? Which has the smallest value?

_____

RATIO AND PROPORTION

A _ratio_ is the relation between two numbers and is separated by a colon, i.e., 1:2 (1 is to 2). It is another way of expressing a fraction, i.e., $1:2 = \frac{1}{2}$.

    Proportion is the relation between two ratios separated by a double colon (::) or equal sign (=).

    To solve a ratio and proportion problem, the middle numbers _(means)_ are multiplied and the end numbers _(extremes)_ are multiplied. To solve for the unknown, which is X, the X goes to the left side and is followed by an equals sign.

··

e x a m p l e s

1. $1:2::2:X$ (1 is to 2, as 2 is to X)

means

extremes

   $X = 4$ (1 X is the same as X)

Answer: 4 $(1:2::2:4)$

2. $4:8 = X:12$

   $8X = 48$
   $X = {}^{48}\!/_8 = 6$

Answer: 6 $(4:8 = 6:12)$

3. A ratio and proportion problem may be set up as a fraction.

Ratio and Proportion	Fraction
$2:3::4:X$	$\dfrac{2}{3} = \dfrac{4}{X}$ (cross multiply)
$2X = 12$	$2X = 12$
$X = {}^{12}\!/_2 = 6$	$X = 6$

Answer: 6. Remember to cross-multiply when the problem is set up as a
         fraction.

IV Practice Problems: Ratio and Proportion

Solve for X.

1. $2:10::5:X$

_____

2. $0.9:100 = X:1000$

_____

3. Change ratio and proportion to fraction.
   $3:5::X:10$

_____

4. It is 500 miles from Washington, DC, to Boston, MA. Your car averages
   22 miles per 1 gallon of gasoline. How many gallons of gasoline will be
   needed for the trip?

_____

PERCENTAGE

Percent (%) means 100. Two percent (2%) means 2 parts of 100, and 0.9% means 0.9 part (less than 1) of 100. A percent can be expressed as a fraction, a decimal, or a ratio.

example

Percent		Fraction	Decimal	Ratio
60%	=	$^{60}/_{100}$	0.60	60 : 100

Note: To change a percent to a decimal, move the decimal point two places to the left. In the example, the decimal point comes before the whole number 60.

V Practice Problems: Percentage

Change percent to fraction, decimal, and ratio.

Percent	Fraction	Decimal	Ratio
1. 2%			
2. 0.33%			
3. 150%			
4. ½% (0.5%)			
5. 0.9%			

ANSWERS

I. Roman Numerals

1. 10 + 5 + 1 = 16

2. 10 + 2 = 12

3. 20 (10 + 10) + 4 (5 − 1) = 24

4. 30 (10 + 10 + 10) + 9 (10 − 1) = 39

5. 40 (50 − 10) + 5 = 45

6. 100 − 10 = 90

II. Fractions

1. **a.** ⅟₅₀ has the greatest value. **b.** ⅟₁₅₀ has the lowest value.

2. **a.** 3 **c.** 7⅓
   b. 4 **d.** 5⅚ or 5⅓

3. a. $\frac{2}{24} = \frac{1}{12}$

b. $\frac{12}{5} \times \frac{15}{4} = \frac{180}{20} = 9$

c. $\frac{\overset{10}{\cancel{500}}}{\underset{7}{\cancel{350}}} \times 5 = \frac{50}{7} = 7.1$

d. $\frac{\overset{2}{\cancel{400{,}000}}}{\underset{1}{\cancel{200{,}000}}} \times 3 = 6$

4. a. $\frac{2}{3} \div 6 = \frac{2}{3} \times \frac{1}{6}$
    $= \frac{2}{18} = \frac{1}{9}$

b. $\frac{1}{4} \div \frac{1}{5} =$
    $\frac{1}{4} \times \frac{5}{1} = \frac{5}{4} =$
    $1\frac{1}{4}$, or 1.25

c. $\frac{1}{6} \div \frac{1}{8} = \frac{1}{\underset{3}{\cancel{6}}} \times \frac{\overset{4}{\cancel{8}}}{1} = \frac{4}{3} = 1.33$

d. $\frac{1}{150} \div \frac{1}{100} = \frac{1}{\underset{3}{\cancel{150}}} \times \frac{\overset{2}{\cancel{100}}}{1}$
    $= \frac{2}{3}$, or 0.666, or 0.67

e. $\frac{1}{200} \div \frac{1}{300} = \frac{1}{200} \times \frac{300}{1} =$
    $\frac{300}{200} = 1\frac{1}{2}$, or 1.5

f. $\frac{48}{5} \div \frac{4}{1} = \frac{48}{5} \times \frac{1}{4}$
    $= \frac{48}{20} = 2.4$

5. a. $\frac{1}{4} = 4\overline{)1.00}^{\,0.25}$ **b.** $\frac{1}{10} = 10\overline{)1.00}^{\,0.10}$ **c.** $\frac{2}{5} = 5\overline{)2.00}^{\,0.40}$

III. Decimals

1. a. 0.8364, or 0.8
      0.123
      6.8
      984
      738
      0.8364, or 0.8 (round off in tenths: 3 hundredths is less than 5)

b. 489.6780, or 489.7 (7 hundredths is greater than 5)

2. a. 21.56, or 21.6 (6 hundredths is greater than 5, so the tenth is increased by one)

b. 28.826, or 28.8 (2 hundredths is *not* 5 or greater than 5, so the tenth is not changed

c. $100 \div 4.5 = 4.5\overline{)100.0} = 22.2$, or 22

d. $125 \div 0.75 = 0.75\overline{)125.00} = 166.6$, or 167

3. a. $\frac{46}{100}$ **b.** $\frac{5}{100}$ **c.** $\frac{12}{1000}$

4. 0.46 has the greatest value; 0.012 has the lowest value. Forty-six hundredths is greater than 5 hundredths or 12 thousandths.

IV. Ratio and Proportion

1. $2X = 50$
    $X = 25$

2. $100X = 900$
    $X = 9$

3. $\frac{3}{5} = \frac{X}{10} = 5X = 30$
    $X = 6$

4. 1 gal : 22 miles :: X gal : 500
    $22X = 500$
    $X = 22.7$ gal
    22.7 gallons of gasoline are needed

V. Percentage

	Percent	Fraction	Decimal	Ratio
1.	2	$^2\!/_{100}$	0.02	2 : 100
2.	0.33	$^{0.33}\!/_{100}$, or $^{33}\!/_{10,000}$	0.0033	0.33 : 100, or 33 : 10,000
3.	150	$^{150}\!/_{100}$	1.50	150 : 100
4.	0.5	$^{0.5}\!/_{100}$, or $^5\!/_{1000}$	0.005	0.5 : 100, or 5 : 1000
5.	0.9	$^{0.9}\!/_{100}$, or $^9\!/_{1000}$	0.009	0.9 : 100, or 9 : 1000

POST-MATH TEST

The math test is composed of five sections: Roman and Arabic numerals, fractions, decimals, ratios and proportions, and percentages. There are 60 questions. A passing score is 54 or more correct answers (90%). A nonpassing score is 7 or more incorrect answers.

Roman and Arabic Numerals

Convert Roman numerals to Arabic numerals.

1. vii

$5 + 1 + 1 = 7$

2. xi

$10 + 1 = 11$

3. xvi

$10 + 5 + 1 = 16$

4. xiv

$10 + (5 - 1) = 14$

5. xliii, or XLIII

$(50 - 10) + 1 + 1 + 1 = 43$

Convert Arabic numerals to Roman numerals.

6. 4

IV

7. 18

XVIII

8. 29

XXIX

9. 37

XXXVII

10. 62

LXII

Fractions

Which fraction has the larger value?

11. $^1\!/_{100}$ or $^1\!/_{150}$?

12. $^1\!/_3$ or $^1\!/_2$?

Reduce improper fractions to whole or mixed numbers.

13. $^{45}\!/_9 =$ **14.** $^{74}\!/_3 =$

_____   _____

Change a mixed number to an improper fraction.

15. $5^2\!/_3 =$

_____

Change fractions to decimals.

16. $^2\!/_3 =$ **17.** $^1\!/_{12} =$

_____   _____

Multiply fractions.

18. $^7\!/_8 \times ^4\!/_6 =$ **19.** $2^3\!/_5 \times ^5\!/_8 =$

_____   _____

Divide fractions.

20. $^1\!/_2 \div ^1\!/_3 =$ **22.** $^1\!/_8 \div ^1\!/_{12} =$

_____   _____

21. $6^3\!/_4 \div 3 =$ **23.** $20^3\!/_4 \div ^1\!/_6 =$

_____   _____

Decimals

Round off decimal numbers to tenths.

24. $0.87 =$ **26.** $0.42 =$

_____   _____

25. $2.56 =$

_____

Change decimals to fractions.

27. $0.68 =$ **29.** $0.012 =$

_____   _____

28. $0.9 =$ **30.** $0.33 =$

_____   _____

Multiply decimals.

31. $0.34 \times 0.6 =$

_____

32. $2.123 \times 0.45 =$

_____

Divide decimals.

33. $3.24 \div 0.3 =$

_____

34. $69.4 \div 0.23 =$

_____

Ratio and Proportion

Change ratios to fractions.

35. $3:4 =$ **37.** $65:90 =$

_____   _____

36. $1:175 =$ **38.** $0.9:100 =$

_____   _____

Solve ratio and proportion problems.

39. $2:3::8:X$

_____

40. $0.5:20::X:100$

_____

41. $3:100 = X:1000$

_____

42. $5:25 = 10:X$

_____

Change ratios and proportions to fractions and solve.

43. $1:2::4:X$

_____

44. $5:50::X:300$

_____

45. $0.9:10 = X:100$

_____

Percentage

Change percents to fractions.

46. 3% =   **47.** 27% =   **48.** 1.2% =   **49.** 5.75% =

Change percents to decimals.

50. 8% =   **52.** 0.9% =   **54.** 0.25% =
51. 15% =   **53.** 3.5% =   **55.** 0.45% =

Change percents to ratios.

56. 35% =   **58.** 4% =   **60.** 0.45% =
57. 12.5% =   **59.** 0.9% =

ANSWERS

Roman and Arabic Numerals

1. 7   **3.** 16   **5.** 43   **7.** xviii   **9.** xxxvii
2. 11   **4.** 14   **6.** iv   **8.** xxix   **10.** LXII

Fractions

11. $^1/_{100}$ **17.** 0.08

12. ½   **18.** $\frac{28}{48}$ or $\frac{7}{12}$

13. 5

14. 24⅔   **20.** ½ × ³⁄₁ =   **22.** $\frac{1}{\cancel{8}_{2}} \times \frac{\cancel{12}^{3}}{1} =$

15. $^{17}/_3$ ³⁄₂ = 1½

16. 0.66, or 0.7   **19.** $\frac{13}{\cancel{5}_1} \times \frac{\cancel{5}^1}{8} =$ ³⁄₂ = 1½

                          $^{13}/_8 = 1^5/_8$ **21.** $\frac{\cancel{27}^9}{4} \times \frac{1}{\cancel{3}_1} =$ **23.** $\frac{83}{\cancel{4}_2} \times \frac{\cancel{6}^3}{1} =$

                                        $\frac{9}{4} = 2\frac{1}{4}$ $^{249}/_2 = 124.5$

Decimals

24. 0.9   **27.** $^{68}/_{100}$ **30.** $^{33}/_{100}$ **33.** 10.8
25. 2.6   **28.** $^9/_{10}$ **31.** 0.204   **34.** 301.739, or
26. 0.4   **29.** $^{12}/_{1000}$ **32.** 0.95535, or   301.7
                                   0.96, or 1.0

Ratio and Proportion

35. ¾   **41.** 30   **44.** $\frac{\cancel{5}^1}{\cancel{50}_{10}} = \frac{X}{300}$
36. $^1/_{175}$ **42.** 50
37. $^{65}/_{90}$ **43.** ½ × ⁴⁄x =   10X = 300
38. $^9/_{1000}$ (cross-multiply)   X = 30
39. 12   X = 8   **45.** $^{0.9}/_{10} = ^X/_{100}$
40. 2.5   10X = 90
                                            X = 9

Percentage

46. $^3/_{100}$ **51.** 0.15   **56.** 35:100
47. $^{27}/_{100}$ **52.** 0.009   **57.** 12.5:100, or 125:1000
48. $^{12}/_{1000}$ **53.** 0.035   **58.** 4:100
49. $^{575}/_{10,000}$ **54.** 0.0025   **59.** 0.9:100, or 9:1000
50. 0.08   **55.** 0.0045   **60.** 0.45:100, or 45:10,000

part

two

systems, conversion, and methods of drug calculation

systems used for drug administration

chapter 1

The three systems used for measuring drugs and solutions are the metric, apothecary, and household. The metric system, developed in 1799 in France, is the chosen system for measurements in the majority of European countries. The metric system, also referred to as the decimal system, is based on units of 10. Since the enactment of the Metric Conversion Act of 1975, the United States has been moving toward the use of this system. The intention of the act is to adopt the International Metric System worldwide.

The apothecary system dates back to the Middle Ages and has been the system of weights and measurements used in England since the seventeenth century. This system is also referred to as the fractional system because anything less than one is expressed in fractions. In the United States, the apothecary system is rapidly being phased out and is being replaced with the metric system.

Standard household measurements are used primarily in home settings. With the trend toward home care, conversions to household measurements may gain importance.

METRIC SYSTEM

The metric system is a decimal system based on multiples of 10 and fractions of 10. There are three basic units of measurements. These basic units are:

Gram (g, gm, G, Gm): unit for weight

Liter (l, L): unit for volume or capacity

Meter (m, M): unit for linear measurement or length

Prefixes are used with the basic units to describe whether the units are larger or smaller than the basic unit. The prefixes indicate the size of the unit in multiples of 10. The prefixes for basic units are:

PREFIX FOR LARGER UNIT		PREFIX FOR SMALLER UNIT	
Kilo	1000 (one thousand)	Deci	0.1 (one-tenth)
Hecto	100 (one hundred)	Centi	0.01 (one-hundredth)
Deka	10 (ten)	Milli	0.001 (one-thousandth)
		Micro	0.000001 (one-millionth)
		Nano	0.000000001 (one-billionth)

Abbreviations of metric units that are frequently written in drug orders are listed in Table 1–1. Lowercase letters are usually used for abbreviations rather than capital letters.

The metric units of weight, volume, and length are given in Table 1–2. Meanings of the prefixes are stated next to the units of weight. Note that the larger units are 1000, 100, and 10 times the basic units (in bold type), and the smaller units differ by factors of 0.1, 0.01, 0.001, 0.000001, and 0.000000001. The size of a basic unit can be changed by multiplying or dividing by 10. Micrograms and nanograms are the exceptions: one (1) milligram = 1000 micrograms, and one (1) microgram = 1000 nanograms. Micrograms and nanograms are changed by 1000 instead of by 10.

table 1•1
METRIC UNITS AND ABBREVIATIONS

	NAMES	ABBREVIATIONS
Weight	Kilogram	kg, Kg
	Gram	g, gm, G, Gm
	Milligram	mg, mgm
	Microgram	mcg, μg
	Nanogram	ng
Volume	Kiloliter	kl, kL
	Liter	l, L
	Deciliter	dl, dL
	Milliliter	ml, mL
Length	Kilometer	km, Km
	Meter	m, M
	Centimeter	cm
	Millimeter	mm

Conversion Within the Metric System

Drug administration often requires conversion within the metric system to prepare the correct dosage. Two basic methods are given for changing larger to smaller units and smaller to larger units.

METHOD A

To change from a **larger** unit to a **smaller** unit, multiply by 10 for each unit decreased or move the decimal point one space to the right for each unit changed.

table 1•2
UNITS OF MEASUREMENT IN THE METRIC SYSTEM WITH THEIR PREFIXES

WEIGHT PER GRAM	MEANING
1 kilogram (kg) = 1000 grams	One thousand
1 hectogram (hg) = 100 grams	One hundred
1 dekagram (dag) = 10 grams	Ten
1 gram (g) = 1 gram	One
1 decigram (dg) = 0.1 gram ($\frac{1}{10}$)	One-tenth
1 centigram (cg) = 0.01 gram ($\frac{1}{100}$)	One-hundredth
1 milligram (mg) = 0.001 gram ($\frac{1}{1,000}$)	One-thousandth
1 microgram (mcg) = 0.000001 gram ($\frac{1}{1,000,000}$)	One-millionth
1 nanogram (ng) = 0.000000001 gram ($\frac{1}{1,000,000,000}$)	One-billionth

VOLUME PER LITER	LENGTH PER METER
1 kiloliter (kL) = 1000 liters	1 kilometer (km) = 1000 meters
1 hectoliter (hL) = 100 liters	1 hectometer (hm) = 100 meters
1 dekaliter (daL) = 10 liters	1 dekameter (dam) = 10 meters
1 liter (l, L) = 1 liter	**1 meter (m) = 1 meter**
1 deciliter (dL) = 0.1 liter	1 decimeter (dm) = 0.1 meter
1 centiliter (cL) = 0.01 liter	1 centimeter (cm) = 0.01 meter
1 milliliter (mL) = 0.001 liter	1 millimeter (mm) = 0.001 meter

When changing three units from larger to smaller, such as from gram to milligram (a change of three units), multiply by 10 three times (or by 1000) or move the decimal point three spaces to the right.

Change 1 gram (g) to milligrams (mg):

a. $1 \times 10 \qquad \times 10 \qquad \times 10 \qquad = 1000$ mg

b. $1 \text{ g} \times 1000 = 1000$ mg

or

c. $1 \text{ g} = 1.000 \text{ mg } (1000 \text{ mg})$

When changing two units, such as kilogram to dekagram (a change of two units from larger to smaller), multiply by 10 twice (or by 100) or move the decimal point two spaces to the right.

Change 2 kilograms (kg) to dekagrams (dag):

a. $2 \times 10 \qquad \times 10 \qquad = 200$ dag

b. $2 \text{ kg} \times 100 = 200$ dag

or

c. $2 \text{ kg} = 2.00 \text{ dag } (200 \text{ dag})$

When changing one unit, such as liter to deciliter (a change of one unit from larger to smaller), multiply by 10 or move the decimal point one space to the right.

Change 3 liters (L) to deciliters (dL):

a. $3 \times 10 = 30$ dL

b. $3 \text{ L} \times 10 = 30$ dL

or

c. $3 \text{ L} = 3.0 \text{ dL } (30 \text{ dL})$

A micro unit is one-thousandth of a milli unit, and a nano unit is one-thousandth of a micro unit. Unit change of micro and nano to its nearest unit is done by multiplying by 1000 instead of by 10. When changing milli units to micro units, multiply by 1000 or move the decimal point three spaces to the right; the same procedure is used to change micro units to nano units.

· ·

examples

PROBLEM 1: Change 2 grams (g) to milligrams (mg).

$$2 \text{ g} \times 1000 = 2000 \text{ mg}$$

or

$$2 \text{ g} = 2.000 \text{ mg } (2,000 \text{ mg})$$

PROBLEM 2: Change 10 milligrams (mg) to micrograms (mcg).

$$10 \text{ mg} \times 1000 = 10,000 \text{ mcg } (\mu g)$$

or

$$10 \text{ mg} = 10.000 \text{ mcg } (10,000 \text{ mcg})$$

PROBLEM 3: Change 4 liters (L) to milliliters (mL).

$$4 \text{ L} \times 1000 = 4000 \text{ mL}$$

or

$$4 \text{ L} = 4.000 \text{ mL } (4000 \text{ mL})$$

PROBLEM 4: Change 2 kilometers (km) to hectometers (hm).

$$2 \text{ km} \times 10 = 20 \text{ hm}$$

or

$$2 \text{ km} = 2.0 \text{ hm } (20 \text{ hm})$$

METHOD B

To change from a **smaller** unit to a **larger** unit, divide by 10 for each unit increased or move the decimal point one space to the left for each unit changed.

When changing three units from smaller to larger, divide by 1000 or move the decimal point three spaces to the left.

Change 1500 milliliters (mL) to liters (L):

a. $1500 \text{ mL} \div 1000 = 1.5 \text{ L}$

or

b. $1500 \text{ mL} = 1\,500.\text{ L } (1.5 \text{ L})$

When changing two units from smaller to larger, divide by 100 or move the decimal point two spaces to the left.

Change 400 centimeters (cm) to meters (m):

a. $400 \text{ cm} \div 100 = 4 \text{ m}$

or

b. $400 \text{ cm} = 4\,00.\text{ m } (4 \text{ m})$

When changing one unit from smaller to larger, divide by 10 or move the decimal point one space to the left.

Change 150 decigrams (dg) to grams (g):

a. $150 \text{ dg} \div 10 = 15 \text{ g}$

or

b. $150 \text{ dg} = 15\,0.\text{ g } (15 \text{ g})$

examples

PROBLEM 1: Change 8 grams to kilograms (kg).

$$8 \text{ g} \div 1000 = 0.008 \text{ kg}$$

or

$$8 \text{ g} = 008. \text{ kg } (0.008 \text{ kg})$$

PROBLEM 2: Change 1500 milligrams (mg) to decigrams (dg).

$$1500 \text{ mg} \div 100 = 15 \text{ dg}$$

or

$$1500 \text{ mg} = 15\,00. \text{ dg } (15 \text{ dg})$$

PROBLEM 3: Change 750 micrograms (mcg) to milligrams (mg).

$$750 \text{ mcg} \div 1000 = 0.75 \text{ mg}$$

or

$$750 \text{ mcg} = 750. \text{ mg } (0.75 \text{ mg})$$

PROBLEM 4: Change 2400 milliliters (mL) to liters (L).

$$2400 \text{ ml} \div 1000 = 2.4 \text{ L}$$

or

$$2400 \text{ ml} = 2\,400. \text{ L } (2.4 \text{ L})$$

I Practice Problems: Metric Conversions

Answers can be found on page 31.

1. Conversion from larger units to smaller units: *multiply* by 10 for each unit changed (multiply by 10, 100, 1000) or move the decimal point one space to the *right* for each unit changed (move one, two, or three spaces), Method A.

   a. 7.5 grams to milligrams

   _____

   b. 10 milligrams to micrograms

   _____

   c. 35 kilograms to grams

   _____

   d. 2.5 liters to milliliters

   _____

   e. 1.25 liters to milliliters

   _____

f. 20 centiliters to milliliters

_____

g. 18 decigrams to milligrams

_____

h. 0.5 kilograms to grams

_____

2. Conversion from smaller units to larger units: _divide_ by 10 for each unit changed (divide by 10, 100, 1000) or move the decimal point one space to the _left_ for each unit changed (move one, two, or three spaces), Method B.

a. 500 milligrams to grams

_____

b. 7500 micrograms to milligrams

_____

c. 250 grams to kilograms

_____

d. 4000 milliliters to liters

_____

e. 325 milligrams to grams

_____

f. 100 milliliters to deciliters

_____

g. 2800 milliliters to liters

_____

h. 75 millimeters to centimeters

_____

APOTHECARY SYSTEM

The basic unit of weight in the apothecary system is the grain (gr), and the basic unit of fluid volume is the minim (ℳ); these are the smaller units in the apothecary system. Larger units of measurements for weight and fluid volume are the dram (dr or ʒ) and the ounce (oz or ℥). In the apothecary system, Roman numerals are written in lower case letters, e.g., gr x, to express numbers.

Table 1–3 gives the equivalents of units of dry weight (grain, dram, ounce) and units of liquid volume (minim, fluid dram, fluid ounce). The apothecary system uses fluid ounces and fluid drams to differentiate between liquid volume and dry weight. In clinical practice, units of liquid

table 1•3

ABBREVIATIONS AND UNITS OF MEASUREMENT IN THE APOTHECARY SYSTEM

ABBREVIATIONS

Weight		Liquid Volume	
grain	gr	quart	qt
ounce	oz, ℥	pint	pt
dram*	dr, ℨ	fluid ounce	fl oz, fl ℥
		fluid dram	ℨ
		minim†	♏

BASIC EQUIVALENT UNITS

Weight		Liquid Volume†	
Larger units	*Smaller units*	*Larger units*	*Smaller units*
1 ounce	= 480 grains	1 quart	= 2 pints
1 ounce	= 8 drams	1 pint	= 16 fluid ounces
1 dram†	= 60 grains	1 fluid ounce	= 8 fluid drams
		1 fluid dram	= 60 minims
		1 minim†	= 1 drop (gt)

* Drams and minims are rarely used for drug administration; however, know their symbols.
† Liquid volume of basic units is frequently used.
Note: Constant values are the numbers of the smaller equivalent units.

volume are commonly seen as dram and ounce. Often, the term "fluid," which is the correct labeling of liquid volume, is dropped. However, the proper names for units of dry weight and units of liquid volume are used in this text.

The apothecary system is being phased out, and in the near future, all measurements will be in the metric system. Because there are physicians who still write medication orders using apothecary units, and probably will be for the next several decades, nurses need to know and to be able to interpret the apothecary system.

Conversion Within the Apothecary System

It is often necessary to change units within the apothecary system. The method applied when changing larger units to smaller units is:

METHOD C

To change a **larger** unit to a **smaller** unit, multiply the constant value found in Table 1–3 by the number of the larger unit.

NOTE   The constant values are the basic equivalent numbers of the smaller units given in Table 1–3. You might want to memorize these equivalents or refer to the table as needed.

examples

PROBLEM 1: 2 drams (dr) = _____ grains (gr).

      1 dr = 60 gr (60 is the constant value, dry weight)

    $2 \times 60 = 120$ gr

PROBLEM 2: 3 pints (pt) = _____ fluid ounces (fl oz or fl ℥).

      1 pt = 16 fl oz (16 is the constant value)

    $3 \times 16 = 48$ fl oz, fl ℥

PROBLEM 3: 3 fluid ounces (fl ℥) = _____ fluid drams (fl ℨ).

      1 fl oz = 8 fl dr (8 is the constant value)

    $3 \times 8 = 24$ fl dr, fl ℨ

PROBLEM 4: 4 fluid drams (fl dr, fl ℨ) = _____ minims (♏).

      1 fl dr = 60 minims (60 is the constant value)

    $4 \times 60 = 240$ ♏

The method applied when changing smaller units to larger units is:

METHOD D

To change a **smaller** unit to a **larger** unit, divide the constant value found in Table 1–3 into the number of the smaller unit.

examples

PROBLEM 1: 30 grains (gr) = _____ dram (dr or ℨ).

      1 dr = 60 gr (60 is the constant value)

    $30 \div 60 = \frac{1}{2}$ dr

PROBLEM 2: 80 fluid ounces (fl oz, fl ℥) = _____ pints (pt).

      1 pt = 16 fl oz (16 is the constant value)

    $80 \div 16 = 5$ pts

PROBLEM 3: 2 fluid drams (fl dr, fl ℨ) = _____ fluid ounces (fl oz, fl ℥).

      1 fl oz = 8 fl dr (8 is the constant value)

    $2 \div 8 = \frac{1}{4}$ fl oz

PROBLEM 4: 180 minims (♏) = _____ fluid drams (fl dr, fl ℨ).

      1 fl dr = 60 minims (60 is the constant value)

    $180 \div 60 = 3$ fl dr

II Practice Problems: Apothecary System

Answers can be found on page 31.

1. Give the abbreviations for:

   a. grain = _____

   b. dram = _____

   c. fluid dram = _____

   d. minim = _____

   e. drop = _____

   f. fluid ounce = _____

   g. pint = _____

   h. quart = _____

2. Give the equivalent using Method C, changing larger units to smaller units.

   a. ʒ v = _____ gr

   b. fl ʒ (fl oz) v = _____ fl ʒ (fl dr)

   c. qt iii, = _____ pt

   d. pt ii, = _____ fl ʒ (fl oz)

   e. fl ʒ (fl dr) iiss (2½) = _____ ♏

3. Give the equivalent using Method D, changing smaller units to larger units.

   a. gr 240 = _____ dr or ʒ

   b. ʒ xvi = _____ oz or ʒ

   c. fl ʒ (fl dr) xxiv = _____ fl ʒ (fl oz)

   d. ♏ xxx = _____ fl ʒ (fl dr)

   e. ♏ xv = _____ gtt

HOUSEHOLD SYSTEM

The use of household measurements is on the increase because more patients/clients are being cared for in the home. The household system of measurement is not as accurate as the metric system because of a lack of standardization of spoons, cups, and glasses. A teaspoon (t) is considered 5 mL, although it could be anywhere from 4 to 6 mL. Three household teaspoons are equal to one tablespoon (T). A drop size can vary with the size of the lumen of the dropper. Basically, a drop and a minim are considered equal. Again, household measurements must be considered approximate measurements. Some of the household units are the same as the apothecary units, because there is a blend of these two systems.

table 1•4
UNITS OF MEASUREMENT IN THE HOUSEHOLD SYSTEM

1 drop (gt)	= 1 minim (♏)
1 teaspoon (t)	= 60 drops (gtt), 5 mL
1 tablespoon (T)	= 3 teaspoons (t)
1 ounce (oz)	= 2 tablespoons (T)
1 coffee cup (c)	= 6 ounces (oz)
1 medium size glass	= 8 ounces (oz)
1 measuring cup	= 8 ounces (oz)

Note: Constant values are the numbers of the smaller equivalent units.

The community health nurse may use and teach the household units of measurements to patients / clients.

Table 1–4 gives the commonly used units of measurement in the household system. You might want to memorize the equivalents in Table 1–4 or refer to the table as needed.

Conversion Within the Household System

For changing larger units to smaller units and smaller units to larger units within the household system, the same methods that applied to the apothecary system can be used. With household measurements, a fluid ounce is usually indicated as ounce.

METHOD E

To change a **larger** unit to a **smaller** unit, multiply the constant value found in Table 1–4 by the number of the larger unit.

> The constant values are the basic equivalent numbers of the smaller units in Table 1–4. **NOTE**

examples

PROBLEM 1: 2 medium size glasses = _____ ounces (oz).

$$1 \text{ medium glass} = 8 \text{ fl oz (8 is the constant value)}$$

$$2 \times 8 = 16 \text{ oz}$$

PROBLEM 2: 3 tablespoons (T) = _____ teaspoons (t).

$$1 \text{ T} = 3 \text{ t (3 is the constant value)}$$

$$3 \times 3 = 9 \text{ t}$$

PROBLEM 3: 5 ounces (oz or ℥) = _____ tablespoons (T).

1 oz = 2 T (2 is the constant value)

5 × 2 = 10 T

PROBLEM 4: 2 teaspoons (t) = _____ drops (gtt).

1 t = 60 gtt (60 is the constant value)

2 × 60 = 120 gtt

METHOD F

To change a **smaller** unit to a **larger** unit, divide the constant value found in Table 1–4 into the number of the smaller unit.

examples

PROBLEM 1: 120 drops (gtt) = _____ teaspoons (t).

1 t = 60 gtt (60 is the constant value)

120 ÷ 60 = 2 t

PROBLEM 2: 6 teaspoons (t) = _____ tablespoons (T).

1 T = 3 t (3 is the constant value)

6 ÷ 3 = 2 T

PROBLEM 3: 18 ounces (oz) = _____ coffee cups (c).

1 c = 6 oz (6 is the constant value)

18 ÷ 6 = 3 c

PROBLEM 4: 4 tablespoons (T) = _____ ounces (oz).

1 oz = 2 T (2 is the constant value)

4 ÷ 2 = 2 oz

III Practice Problems: Household System

Answers can be found on page 31.

1. Give the equivalents using Method E, changing larger units to smaller units.

    a. 2 glasses = _____16_____ oz

    b. 3 ounces = _____6_____ T

    c. 4 tablespoons = _____12_____ t

    d. 1½ cups = _____12_____ oz

    e. ½ teaspoon = _____30_____ gtt

2. Give the equivalents using Method F, changing smaller units to larger units.

a. 9 teaspoons = _____ T

b. 6 tablespoons = _____ oz

c. 90 drops = _____ t

d. 12 ounces = _____ c

e. 24 ounces = _____ medium size glasses

ANSWERS

I. Metric Conversions

1. a. 7.5 g to mg
   7.5 g × 1000 = 7500 mg
   or
   7.500 mg (7500 mg)

   b. 10,000 mcg
   c. 35,000 g
   d. 2500 mL
   e. 1250 mL
   f. 200 mL
   g. 1800 mg
   h. 500 g

2. a. 500 mg to g
   500 ÷ 1000 = 0.5 g
   or
   500 mg = 500. g (0.5 g)

   b. 7.5 mg
   c. 0.25 kg
   d. 4 L
   e. 0.325 g
   f. 1 dL
   g. 2.8 L
   h. 7.5 cm

II. Apothecary System

Abbreviations

1. a. grain = gr
   b. dram = dr of ʒ
   c. fluid dram = fl
      ʒ, fl dr
   d. minim = ♏
   e. drop = gt
   f. fluid ounce =
      fl ℥, fl oz
   g. pint = pt
   h. quart = qt

Equivalents

2. a. ʒ v = _____ gr
      5 × 60 = 300 gr
   b. 40 fl ʒ, fl dr
   c. 6 pt
   d. 32 fl ℥, fl oz
   e. 150 ♏

Equivalents

3. a. gr 240 = _____ dr
      240 ÷ 60 = 4 dr or ʒ
   b. 2 oz or ℥
   c. 3 fl ℥, fl oz
   d. ½ fl ʒ, fl dr
   e. 15 gtt

III. Household System

1. a. 2 glasses = _____ oz
      2 × 8 = 16 oz
   b. 6 T
   c. 12 t
   d. 9 oz
   e. 30 gtt

2. a. 9 teaspoons = _____ T
      9 ÷ 3 = 3 T
   b. 3 oz
   c. 1½ t
   d. 2 c
   e. 3 glasses

SUMMARY PRACTICE PROBLEMS

1. Metric system.
   a. 30 mg = _____ mcg (μg)

   b. 3 g = _____ mg

   c. 6 L = _____ mL

   d. 1.5 kg = _____ g

   e. 10,000 mcg = _____ mg

   f. 500 mg = _____ g

   g. 2500 mL = _____ L

   h. 125 g = _____ kg

   i. 120 mm = _____ cm

   j. 5 m = _____ cm

2. Apothecary system.
   a. 90 gr = _____ dr

   b. fl ʒ (fl dr) iv = _____ fl ℥ (fl oz)

   c. fl ℥ (fl oz) iiss = _____ fl ʒ (fl dr)

   d. ♏ xxx = _____ fl ʒ (fl dr)

   e. 8 pt = _____ qt

   f. fl ʒ (fl dr) ii = _____ ♏

3. Household system.
   a. 12 t = _____ T

   b. 5 glasses = _____ oz

   c. 3 T = _____ t

   d. 2 c = _____ oz

   e. 30 oz = _____ c

   f. 4 oz = _____ T

   g. 12 gtt = _____ ♏

ANSWERS: SUMMARY PRACTICE PROBLEMS

1. a. 30,000 mcg
   b. 3000 mg
   c. 6000 mL
   d. 1500 g
   e. 10 mg
   f. 0.5 g
   g. 2.5 L
   h. 0.125 kg
   i. 12 cm
   j. 500 cm

2. a. 1.5 ʒ
   b. ½ or ss fl ℥ (fl oz)
   c. 20 fl ʒ (fl dr)
   d. ½ or ss fl ʒ (fl dr)
   e. 4 qt
   f. 120 ♏

3. a. 4 T
   b. 40 oz
   c. 9 t
   d. 12 oz
   e. 5 c
   f. 8 T
   g. 12 ♏

conversion within the metric, apothecary, and household systems

objectives

- State rules for converting drug dosage by weight between the apothecary and metric systems.
- Convert grams/milligrams to grains and grains to grams/milligrams.
- Convert drug dosage by weight from one system to another system using the ratio method.
- State rules for converting drug dosage by volume among the metric, apothecary, and household systems.
- Convert liters/milliliters to ounces/pints and milliliters to drams, tablespoons, and teaspoons.

outline

Drug doses are usually ordered in metric units (grams, milligrams, liters, and milliliters). Although the apothecary system is being phased out, there are some physicians who still order drug doses by apothecary units. To calculate a drug dose, the same unit of measurement must be used. Therefore, the nurse must know the metric and apothecary equivalents either by memorizing a conversion table or by using methods for converting from one system to the other. After the conversion is made, the dosage problem can be solved. Some authorities state it is easier to *convert to the unit used on the container (bottle).* If the physician ordered phenobarbital gr ½ and the bottle is labeled 30 mg, then the conversion would be from grains to milligrams.

Metric and apothecary equivalents are approximations, e.g., 1 gram equals 15.432 grains. When values are unequal, they should be rounded off to the nearest whole number (1 gram = 15 grains).

Dosage conversion tables are available in many institutions; however, when you need a conversion table, one might not be available. Nurses should either memorize metric and apothecary equivalents or be able to convert from one system to the other by using calculation methods.

UNITS, MILLIEQUIVALENTS, AND PERCENTS

Units, milliequivalents, and percents are measurements used to indicate the strength or potency of certain drugs. When all drugs are developed, their strength is based on either chemical assay or biological assay. Chemical assay denotes strength by weight, e.g., milligrams or grains. Biological assays are used for drugs in which the chemical composition is difficult to determine. Biological assays assess potency by the effect that one unit of the drug can have on a laboratory animal. Units mainly measure the potency of hormones, vitamins, anticoagulants, and some antibiotics. Drugs that were once standardized by units and later synthesized to their chemical composition may still retain units as an indication of potency, e.g., insulin.

Milliequivalents measure the strength of an ion concentration. Ions are given primarily for electrolyte replacement. They are measured in milliequivalents, mEq, one of which is $\frac{1}{1000}$ of the equivalent weight of an ion. Potassium chloride, KCl, is a common electrolyte replacement and is ordered in mEq.

Percents are the concentrations of weight dissolved in a volume and are always expressed as units of mass per units of volume. Common concentrations are g/mL, g/L, and mg/mL. These concentrations, expressed as percentages, are based on the definition of a 1% solution as 1 g of a drug in 100 mL of solution. Dextrose 50% in a 50-mL pre-filled syringe is a concentration of 50 g of dextrose in 100 mL of water. Calcium gluconate 10% in a 30-mL bottle is a concentration of 10 g of calcium gluconate in 100 mL of solution. Proportions can also express concentrations. A solution that is 1:100 has the same concentration as a 1% solution. Epinephrine 1:1000 means that 1 g of epinephrine was dissolved in a 1000-mL solution.

Units, milliequivalents, and percents cannot be directly converted into the metric, apothecary, or household system.

table 2•1
APPROXIMATE METRIC, APOTHECARY, AND HOUSEHOLD EQUIVALENTS

	METRIC SYSTEM	APOTHECARY SYSTEM	HOUSEHOLD SYSTEM
Weight	1 kg; 1000 g	2.2 lb	2.2 lb
	30 g	1 oz	
	15 g	4 dr	
	1 g; 1000 mg*	15 (16) gr	
	0.5 g; 500 mg	7½ gr	
	0.3 g; 300 mg	5 gr	
	0.1 g; 100 mg	1½ gr	
	0.06 g; 60 (65) mg*	1 gr	
	0.03 g; 30 (32) mg	½ gr	
	0.01 g; 10 mg	⅙ gr	
	0.6 mg	¹⁄₁₀₀ gr	
	0.4 mg	¹⁄₁₅₀ gr	
	0.3 mg	¹⁄₂₀₀ gr	
Volume	1 L; 1000 mL (cc)	1 qt; 32 fl oz (fl ℨ)	1 qt
	0.5 L; 500 mL	1 pt; 16 fl oz	1 pt
	0.24 L; 240 mL	8 oz	1 glass
	0.18 L; 180 mL	6 oz	1 c
	30 mL*	1 oz or 8 dr (fl ℨ)	2 T or 6 t
	15 mL	½ oz or 4 dr	1 T
	4–5 mL		1 t
	4 mL	1 dr or 60 minims (℧)	1 t
	1 mL	15 (16) ℧	15–16 gtt
Height	2.54 cm	1 inch	1 inch
Distance	25.4 mm	1 inch	1 inch

* Equivalents commonly used for computing conversion problems by ratio.

Note: ½ may be written as ss̄.

METRIC, APOTHECARY, AND HOUSEHOLD EQUIVALENTS

Knowing how to convert drug doses among the systems of measurement is essential in the clinical setting. In discharge teaching for individuals receiving liquid medication, converting metric to household measurement may be important.

Table 2–1 gives the metric and apothecary equivalents by weight and the metric, apothecary, and household equivalents by volume.

Remember, conversion from one system to another is an approximate equivalent. Either memorize Table 2–1 or use the methods that follow in the text for system conversion.

Conversion in Metric and Apothecary Systems by WEIGHT

GRAMS AND GRAINS   1 g = 15 gr

a. To convert grams to grains, *multiply* the number of grams by 15, the constant value.

b. To convert grains to grams, *divide* the number of grains by 15, the constant value.

examples

PROBLEM 1: Change 2 grams to grains.

$$2 \times 15 = 30 \text{ gr (grains)}$$

PROBLEM 2: Change 60 grains to grams.

$$60 \div 15 = 4 \text{ g (grams)}$$

GRAINS AND MILLIGRAMS   1 gr = 60 mg

a. To convert grains to milligrams, *multiply* the number of grains by 60, the constant value.

b. To convert milligrams to grains, *divide* the number of milligrams by 60, the constant value.

examples

PROBLEM 1: Change 3 grains to milligrams.

$$3 \times 60 = 180 \text{ mg (milligrams)}$$

PROBLEM 2: Change 300 milligrams to grains.

NOTE: 325 milligrams may be ordered instead of 300. Round off to the whole number. One grain is equivalent to 60, 64, or 65 milligrams. In this situation, you may want to divide by 65 instead of rounding off to the whole number.

$$300 \div 60 = 5 \text{ gr (grains)}$$

or

$$325 \div 65 = 5 \text{ gr}$$

or

$$325 \div 60 = 5.43 \text{ gr, or 5 gr (0.43 is less than 0.5)}$$

RATIO AND PROPORTION

Multiply the means (numbers that are closest to each other) by the extremes (numbers that are farthest from each other). You are solving for X, so it goes first.

If it is difficult for you to recall these methods, then use the ratio and proportion method to convert from one system to another.

You must MEMORIZE:

1 gram = 1000 milligrams

1 gram = 15 grains

1 grain = 60 milligrams

examples

PROBLEM 1: Convert 2.5 grams to grains.

$$Known \quad Desired$$
$$g : gr : : g : gr$$
$$1 : 15 : : 2.5 : X$$

means

extremes

$$X = 37.5 \text{ gr}$$

PROBLEM 2: Convert 10 grains to milligrams.

$$Known \quad Desired$$
$$gr : mg : : gr : mg$$
$$1 : 60(65) : : 10 : X$$

$$X = 600 \text{ mg or } 650 \text{ mg}$$

NOTE: Because conversion gives approximate values, the answer could be 600 mg or 650 mg. If the problem uses 1 gr = 60 mg, the answer is 600 mg. However, the bottle may be labeled 10 gr = 650 mg. Both 600 mg and 650 mg are correct.

I Practice Problems: Conversion by Weight

Answers can be found on page 40.

Grams and Grains

1. 10 g = _____ gr

2. 0.5 g = _____ gr

3. 0.1 g = _____ gr

4. 0.03 g = _____ gr

5. 3 gr = _____ g

6. 1½ gr = _____ g

Grains and Milligrams

1. 4 gr = _____ mg

2. 1½ gr = _____ mg

3. 7½ gr = _____ mg

4. ½ gr = _____ mg

5. 150 mg = _____ gr

6. 30 mg = _____ gr

7. 15 mg = _____ gr

8. 0.6 mg = _____ gr

Ratio and Proportion: Grams, Milligrams, and Grains

1. 2.5 g = _____ mg

2. 0.5 g = _____ gr

3. 100 mg = _____ g

4. 500 mg = _____ g

5. 1 gr = _____ g

6. ¼ gr = _____ mg

Conversion in Metric, Apothecary, and Household Systems by LIQUID VOLUME

LITERS AND OUNCES 1 L = 32 oz

a. To convert liters and quarts to ounces, *multiply* the number of liters by 32, the constant value.

b. To convert ounces to liters or quarts, *divide* the number of ounces by 32, the constant value.

----

examples

PROBLEM 1: Change 3 liters to ounces.

$$3 \text{ L} \times 32 = 96 \text{ oz, or fl } ʒ \text{ (ounces)}$$

PROBLEM 2: Change 64 ounces to liters.

$$64 \text{ oz} \div 32 = 2 \text{ L (liters)}$$

OUNCES AND MILLILITERS 1 oz = 30 mL

a. To convert ounces to milliliters, *multiply* the number of ounces by 30, the constant value.

b. To convert milliliters to ounces, *divide* the number of milliliters by 30, the constant value.

----

examples

PROBLEM 1: Change 5 ounces to milliliters.

$$5 \text{ oz} \times 30 = 150 \text{ mL (milliliters)}$$

PROBLEM 2: Change 120 milliliters to ounces.

$$120 \text{ mL} \div 30 = 4 \text{ oz or fl } ʒ \text{ (ounces)}$$

MILLILITERS AND DROPS 1 mL = 15 drops (gtt) or 15 minims (℥) (number of drops may vary according to the size of the dropper)

a. To convert milliliters to minims or drops, *multiply* the number of milliliters by 15, the constant value.

b. To convert minims and drops to milliliters, *divide* the number of minims or drops by 15, the constant value.

examples

PROBLEM 1: Change 4 milliliters to minims or drops.

$$4 \text{ mL} \times 15 = 60 \text{ minims or } 60 \text{ drops}$$

PROBLEM 2: Change 10 drops (gtt) to milliliters.

$$10 \ \text{℥} \ \text{or gtt} \div 15 = \text{⅔ mL or } 0.667 \text{ mL or } 0.7 \text{ mL}$$

RATIO AND PROPORTION

The ratio method is useful when converting smaller units within the three systems.

If it is difficult for you to recall these methods, then use the ratio and proportion method to convert from one system to the other.

You must MEMORIZE:

$$30 \text{ mL} = 1 \text{ oz} = 8 \text{ dr} = 2 \text{ T} = 6\text{t}$$

These are equivalent values.

examples

PROBLEM 1: Change 20 mL to teaspoons.

$$\begin{array}{cc} Known & Desired \\ \text{mL}:\text{t}::\text{mL}:\text{t} \\ 30:6::20:\text{X} \end{array}$$

$$30 \text{ X} = 120$$
$$\text{X} = 4 \text{ t (teaspoons)}$$

PROBLEM 2: Change 15 mL to tablespoons.

$$\begin{array}{cc} Known & Desired \\ \text{mL}:\text{T}::\text{mL}:\text{T} \\ 30:2::15:\text{X} \\ 30 \text{ X} = 30 \\ \text{X} = 1 \text{ T (tablespoon)} \end{array}$$

PROBLEM 3: Change 5 oz to tablespoons.

$$\begin{array}{cc} Known & Desired \\ \text{oz}:\text{T}::\text{oz}:\text{T} \\ 1:2::5:\text{X} \\ \text{X} = 10 \text{ T (tablespoons)} \end{array}$$

II Practice Problems: Conversion by Liquid Volume

Answers can be found on page 41.

Liters and Ounces

1. 2.5 L = _____ oz (fl oz, fl ℥)

2. 0.25 L = _____ oz

3. 40 oz (fl oz, fl ℥) = _____ L

4. 24 oz = _____ L

Ounces and Milliliters

1. 4 oz (fl oz, fl ℥) = _____ mL

2. 6½ oz = _____ mL

3. ½ oz = _____ mL

4. 45 mL = _____ oz

5. 150 ml = _____ oz

6. 15 mL = _____ oz

Milliliters and Drops

1. 1.5 mL = _____ gtt

2. 12 mL = _____ gtt

3. 20 gtt = _____ mL

4. 8 gtt = _____ mL

ANSWERS

I. Conversion by Weight

Grams and Grains

1. $10 \times 15 = 150$ gr
2. $0.5 \times 15 = 7.5$ or $7\frac{1}{2}$ gr
3. $0.1 \times 15 = 1.5$ or $1\frac{1}{2}$ gr

4. $0.03 \times 15 = 0.45$ or 0.5 gr
5. $3 \div 15 = 0.2$ g
6. $1.5 \div 15 = 0.1$ g

Grains and Milligrams

1. $4 \times 60 = 240$ mg
2. $1.5 \times 60 = 90$ (100) mg
3. $7.5 \times 60 = 450$ mg
4. $0.5 \times 60 = 30$ mg
5. $150 \div 60 = 2.5$ or $2\frac{1}{2}$ gr

6. $30 \div 60 = 0.5$ or ½ gr
7. $15 \div 60 = \frac{1}{4}$ gr
8. $0.6 \div 60 =$

$$60\overline{)0.60} \;\; ^{.01} = 0.01 \text{ or } \tfrac{1}{100} \text{ gr}$$

Ratio and Proportion: Grams, Milligrams, and Grains

1. g: mg :: g :mg
1 : 1000 : : 2.5 : X
    X = 2500 mg

or

Move decimal point three spaces to the right (conversion within the metric system)

$$2.5 \text{ g} = 2.500 \text{ mg}$$

2. g: gr ::   g: gr
1 : 15 : : 0.5 : X
    X = 7.5 or 7½ gr

3. mg :g: : mg : g
1000 : 1 : : 100 : X
1000 X = 100
    X = 0.1 g
4. mg :g: : mg : g
1000 : 1 : : 500 : X
1000 X = 500
    X = 0.5 g
5. g: gr : : g: gr
1 : 15 : : X : 1
15 X = 1
    X = 0.06 g
6. gr:mg: : gr :mg
1 : 60 : : 0.25 : X
    X = 60 × 0.25
    X = 15 mg

II. Conversion by Liquid Volume

Liters and Ounces

1. 2.5 L × 32 = 80 oz
2. 0.25 L × 32 = 8 oz

3. 40 oz ÷ 32 = 1.25 L
4. 24 oz ÷ 32 = 0.75 L

Ounces and Milliliters

1. 4 oz × 30 = 120 mL
2. 6.5 oz × 30 = 195 mL
3. 0.5 oz × 30 = 15 mL

4. 45 mL ÷ 30 = 1½ oz
5. 150 mL ÷ 30 = 5 oz
6. 15 mL ÷ 30 = ½ oz

Milliliters and Drops

1. 1.5 mL × 15 = 22.5 or 23 gtt
2. 12 ℳ × 1 = 12 gtt (1 ℳ = 1 gt)

3. 20 gtt ÷ 15 = 1.3 mL
4. 8 gtt ÷ 15 = 0.5 mL

SUMMARY PRACTICE PROBLEMS

Before dosage problems can be completed, one system of measurement must be selected. If a medication is ordered in one system and the drug label is in another system, then conversion to one of the systems is necessary. As previously stated, it may be easier to convert to the system used on the drug label.

There are three methods of conversion for the three systems: (1) memorization of a conversion table, (2) conversion methods, and (3) ratio method. You need to convert not only within three systems, but also within the same system if units are not the same, e.g., grams and milligrams. Again, units of measurement *must* be the same to solve problems.

> *Multiply* when converting from larger to smaller units, and *divide* when converting from *smaller to larger units.*   **REMEMBER**

Weight: Metric and Apothecary Conversion

1. To convert grams to grains, _____ the number of grams

   by _____; to convert grains to grams, _____

   the number of grains by _____.

   a. 2 g = _____ gr

   b. 7½ gr (gr viiss) = _____ g

   c. 3 gr = _____ g

   d. 0.02 g = _____ gr

   e. 150 gr = _____ g

   f. 0.06 g = _____ gr

2. To convert grains to milligrams, _____ the number of

   grains by _____; to convert milligrams to grains,

   _____ the number of milligrams by _____.

a. 3 gr (gr ⅲ) = _____ mg   **d.** 5 gr = _____ mg

b. 10 mg = _____ gr   **e.** 7½ gr = _____ mg

c. ¼ gr = _____ mg   **f.** 0.4 mg = _____ gr

3. Ratio and proportion.
   Remember: 1 g or 1000 mg = 15 gr; 60 (65) mg = 1 gr
   a. Change 5 g to gr

   _____

   b. Change 120 mg to gr

   _____

Volume: Metric, Apothecary, and Household Conversion

4. To convert liters and quarts to ounces, _____ the number

   of liters by _____; to convert ounces to liters and quarts,

   _____ the number of ounces by _____ .

   a. 3 L = _____ oz (fl ℥)   **d.** ½ L = _____ oz

   b. 1½ qt = _____ oz   **e.** 8 oz = _____ L or qt

   c. 64 oz (fl ℥) = _____ qt   **f.** 24 oz = _____ qt

5. To convert ounces to milliliters, _____ the number of

   ounces by _____; to convert milliliters to ounces,

   _____ the number of milliliters by _____ .

   a. 1½ oz = _____ mL   **d.** 75 mL = _____ oz (fl ℥)

   b. 15 mL = _____ oz (fl ℥)   **e.** 3 oz (fl ℥) = _____ mL

   c. 60 mL = _____ oz   **f.** 8 oz = _____ mL

6. To convert milliliters to minims or drops, _____ the number

   of milliliters by _____; to convert minims or drops to millili-

   ters, _____ the number of minims or drops

   by _____ .

   a. 15 mL = _____ ℳ or gtt   **d.** 4 mL = _____ ℳ or gtt

   b. 10 gtt = _____ mL   **e.** 30 ℳ or gtt = _____ mL

   c. 18 ℳ or gtt = _____ mL   **f.** ½ mL = _____ gtt

7. Ratio and proportion.
   Remember: 30 mL = 1 oz = 8 dr = 2 T = 6 t

a. Change 16 oz (fl ʒ) to L or qt

_____

b. Change 1½ oz to T

_____

c. Change 1 T to t

_____

d. Change 20 mL to t

_____

e. Change 2½ oz to mL

_____

f. Change 4 oz to mL

_____

8. Client intake for lunch included a carton of milk (8 oz), cup of coffee (6 oz), small glass of apple juice (4 oz), and jello (4 oz). How many milliliters (mL) did the client consume?

ANSWERS: SUMMARY PRACTICE PROBLEMS

1. multiply, 15; divide, 15
  a. 2 g × 15 = 30 gr
  b. 7.5 gr ÷ 15 = ½ or 0.5 g
  c. 3 gr ÷ 15 = 0.2 g
  d. 0.02 g × 15 = 0.3 or ⅓ gr
  e. 150 gr ÷ 15 = 10 g
  f. 0.06 g × 15 = 0.9 or 1 gr
    (round off to 1)

2. multiply, 60; divide, 60
  a. 3 gr × 60 = 180 mg
  b. 10 mg ÷ 60 = ¹⁰⁄₆₀ = ⅙ gr
  c. 0.25 gr × 60 = 15 mg
  d. 5 gr × 60 = 300 mg
  e. 7.5 gr × 60 = 450 mg
  f. 0.4 mg ÷ 60 = ⁴⁄₆₀₀ = ¹⁄₁₅₀ gr

3. Ratio and proportion

  Known   Desired

  a.   g : gr : : g : gr
       1 : 15 : : 5 : X
           X = 75 gr
  b. gr : mg : : gr : mg
       1 : 60 : : X : 120
       60 X = 120
           X = 2 gr

           or

    mg : gr : : mg : gr
    60 : 1 : : 120 : X
    60 X = 120
        X = 2 gr

4. multiply, 32; divide, 32
   a. 3 L × 32 = 96 oz
   b. 1.5 qt × 32 = 48 oz
   c. 64 oz ÷ 32 = 2 qt
   d. 0.5 L × 32 = 16 oz
   e. 8 oz ÷ 32 = $\frac{8}{32}$ = ¼ L or ¼ qt
   f. 24 oz ÷ 32 = $\frac{24}{32}$ = ¾ qt

5. multiply, 30; divide, 30
   a. 1½ oz × 30 = 45 mL
   b. 15 mL ÷ 30 = $\frac{15}{30}$ = ½ oz
   c. 60 mL ÷ 30 = 2 oz
   d. 75 mL ÷ 30 = 2½ oz
   e. 3 oz × 30 = 90 mL
   f. 8 oz × 30 = 240 mL

6. multiply, 15; divide, 15
   a. 15 mL × 15 = 225 ♏ or gtt
   b. 10 gtt ÷ 15 = $\frac{10}{15}$ = ⅔ mL
   c. 18 ♏ or gtt ÷ 15 = 1⅕ mL
   d. 4 ml × 15 = 60 ♏ or gtt
   e. 30 ♏ or gtt ÷ 15 = 2 mL
   f. ½ mL × 15 = 7.5 gtt

7. Ratio and proportion

   Known   *Desired*

   a.   L : oz : : L : oz
        1 : 32 : : X : 16
        32 X = 16
        X = ½ L
   b.   oz : T : : oz : T
        1 : 2 : : 1½ : X
        X = 3 T
   c.   T : t : : T : t
        2 : 6 : : 1 : X
        2 X = 6
        X = 3 t
   d.   mL : t : : mL : t
        30 : 6 : : 20 : X
        30 X = 120
        X = 4 t
   e. oz : mL : : oz : mL
        1 : 30 : : 2½ : X
        X = 75 mL
   f. oz : mL : : oz : mL
        1 : 30 : : 4 : X
        X = 120 mL

8.   (1 ounce = 30 mL)

            milk = 240 mL
          coffee = 180 mL
     apple juice = 120 mL
            jello = <u>120 mL</u>
                    660 mL

   The client's intake for lunch is 660 mL.

interpretation of drug labels, drug orders, charting, "5 rights," and abbreviations

objectives

- Identify brand names, generic names, drug forms, dosages, expiration dates, and lot numbers on drug labels.
- Give examples of drugs with "look-alike" drug names.
- Recognize the components of a drug order.
- Identify the drug information for charting.
- Name the "5 rights" in drug administration and give examples of each.
- Utilize the chart related to the "5 rights."
- Provide meanings of abbreviations: drug form, drug measurement, and routes and times of drug administration.

outline

INTERPRETING DRUG LABELS

The pharmaceutical companies label drugs with their brand name of the drug in large letters and the generic name in smaller letters. The form of the drug (tablet, capsule, liquid, or powder) and dosage are printed on the drug label.

Many of the calculation problems in this book use drug labels. By using drug labels, the student is able to practice solving drug problems that are applicable to clinical practice. The student should know what information is on a drug label and how this information is used in drug calculations. All drug labels provide seven basic items of data: (1) brand (trade) name, (2) generic name, (3) dosage, (4) form of the drug, (5) expiration date, (6) lot number, and (7) name of the manufacturer.

. . . .

example

DRUG LABEL

a. The brand (trade) name is the commercial name given by the pharmaceutical company (manufacturer of the drug). It is printed in large, bold letters.

b. The generic name is the chemical name given to the drug, regardless of the drug manufacturer. It is printed in smaller letters, usually under the brand name.

c. The dosage strength is the drug dose per drug form (tablet, capsule, liquid) as stated on the label.

d. The form of the drug (tablet, capsule, liquid) relates to the dosage strength.

e. The expiration date refers to the length of time the drug can be used before losing its potency. Drugs should not be administered after the expiration date. The nurse must check the expiration date of all drugs he or she administers.

f. The lot number identifies the drug batch in which the medication was produced. Occasionally, a drug is recalled according to the lot number.

g. The manufacturer is the pharmaceutical company that produces the brand name drug.

Examples of drug labels are given, and practice problems for reading drug labels follow the examples.

....

example 1

ORAL DRUG (SOLID FORM)

a. Brand (trade) name is Compazine

b. Generic name is prochlorperazine

c. Drug form is a sustained release capsule (SR capsule)

d. Dosage is 10 mg per capsule

e. Expiration date is 4/22/01 (after this date, the drug should be discarded)

f. Lot number is 764-RT-321

g. Manufacturer is SmithKline Beecham Pharmaceuticals

· ·

example 2

ORAL DRUG (LIQUID FORM)

a. Brand (trade) name is Duricef

b. Generic name is cefadroxil monohydrate

c. Drug form is oral suspension

d. Dosage is 500 mg per 5 mL

e. Manufacturer is Bristol-Myers Squibb Co.

f. Expiration date is 5/15/02

g. Lot number is 359-PR-246

· ·

example 3

INJECTABLE DRUG

a. Brand name is Mandol

b. Generic name is cefamandole nafate

c. Drug form is drug powder that must be reconstituted in a liquid form for use

d. Dosage is 500 mg drug powder

e. Drug container is vial

f. IV: reconstitute by using at least 5 mL of sterile water for injection which then must be diluted in 50 to 100 mL of IV fluids.
IM: 2 mL of a diluent should be added. The total amount of the drug would then equal 2.2 mL. The powder increases the liquid form by 0.2 mL.

I Practice Problems: Interpretation of Drug Labels

1.

a. Brand (trade) name _____

b. Generic name _____

c. Drug form _____

d. Dosage _____

e. Expiration date _____

f. Lot number _____

g. Manufacturer _____

2.

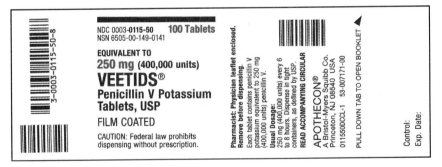

a. Brand (trade) name _____

b. Generic name _____

c. Drug form _____

d. Dosage _____ mg _____ units

e. Manufacturer _____

3.

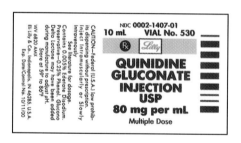

a. Brand (trade) name _____

b. Generic name _____

c. Drug form _____

d. Dosage _____

e. Expiration date _____

f. Manufacturer _____

4.

a. Brand (trade) name _____

b. Generic name _____

c. Drug form _____

d. Drug container _____

e. Dosage _____

f. Expiration date _____

5.

a. Brand (trade) name _____

b. Generic name _____

c. Drug form _____

d. Dosage _____

6.

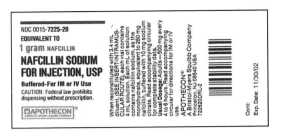

NDC 0015-7225-20
EQUIVALENT TO
1 gram NAFCILLIN
**NAFCILLIN SODIUM
FOR INJECTION, USP**
Buffered-For IM or IV Use
CAUTION: Federal law prohibits
dispensing without prescription.
▢APOTHECON®
A BRISTOL-MYERS SQUIBB COMPANY

Cont:
Exp. Date: 11/30/02

a. Brand name _____

b. Generic name _____

c. Drug form _____

d. Drug label suggests adding _____ diluent

e. Method of administration _____

f. Dosage 1 gram = _____ mL

g. Expiration date _____

h. Manufacturer _____

Military Time versus Traditional (Universal) Time

Many nursing settings currently are using military time, a 24-hour clock, when administering medications and treatments. For example, in military time, 3 AM is 0300 and 3 PM is 1500; 7:15 AM is 0715 and 7:30 PM is 1930. The AM hours are the same as on the traditional clock, and for hours after 12 noon, 12 is added to the PM hours; see Figure 3–1. The use of the 24-hour clock reduces drug administration errors.

Figure 3•1 _____
Military Clock

DRUG DIFFERENTIATION

Some drugs with similar names, such as quinine and quinidine, have different chemical drug structures. Extreme care must be exercised when administering drugs that "look alike" or that have similar spellings.

example 1

PERCOCET

PERCODAN

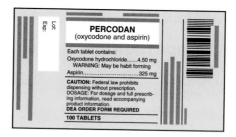

Percocet contains oxycodone and acetaminophen, whereas Percodan contains oxycodone and aspirin. A client may be allergic to aspirin or should not take aspirin; therefore, it is important that the client be given Percocet. *Read the drug labels carefully.*

example 2

HYDROXYZINE AND HYDRALAZINE

Hydroxyzine is an antianxiety drug and hydralazine is an antihypertensive drug.

example 3

QUINIDINE AND QUININE

Quinidine sulfate is an antidysrhythmic drug, and quinine sulfate is an antimalarial drug.

Drug Orders

Medication orders may be prescribed and written by a physician (MD), an osteopathic physician (DO), a dentist (DDS), a podiatrist (DPM), or a li-

PRESCRIPTION PAD MEDICATION ORDER

Roger J. Smith, Jr., M.D.
678 Apple Street
Wilmington, Delaware 19810

(123) 456-7891

NAME ———————————————————— Age ————

Address ——————————————————— Date ————

R$_{\text{X}}$

Generic permitted ——————
Label ——————
Safety Cap ——————
Refill —————— times

——————————————— M.D.

Figure 3•2

censed health care provider (HCP) who has been given authority by the state to write prescriptions. Drug prescriptions in private practice or in clinics are written on a small prescription pad and filled by a pharmacist at a drug store or hospital (see Fig. 3–2). For hospitalized patients, the drug orders are written on a doctor's order sheet and signed by the physician or licensed health provider (see Fig. 3–3). If the order is given by telephone (TO), the order must be cosigned by the physician within 24 hours. Most

PATIENT'S ORDERS

CITY HOSPITAL Dover, Delaware		PATIENT'S NAME Room #
Date	Time	Patient's Orders

Figure 3•3

health care institutions have policies concerning verbal or telephone drug orders. The nurse must know and must follow the institution's policy.

The basic components of a drug order are (1) date and time the order was written, (2) drug name, (3) drug dosage, (4) route of administration, (5) frequency of administration, and (6) physician or health care provider's signature. It is the nurse's responsibility to follow the physician's or HCP's order, but if any one of these components is missing, the drug order is incomplete and cannot be carried out. If the order is illegible, is missing a component, or calls for an inappropriate drug or dosage, clarification must be obtained before the order is carried out.

Examples of drug orders and their interpretation are:

6/3/01   9:10A   Digoxin 0.25 mg, po, qd
                    (give 0.25 mg of digoxin by mouth daily)
_____

                    Ibuprofen 400 mg, po, q4h, PRN
                    (give 400 mg of ibuprofen by mouth every 4 hours as needed)
_____

                    Cefadyl 500 mg, IM, q6h
                    (give 500 mg of Cefadyl intramuscularly every 6 hours)
_____

                    Prednisone 5 mg, po, q8h × 5 days
                    (give 5 mg of prednisone by mouth every 8 hours for 5 days)
_____

II Practice Problems: Interpretation of Drug Orders

Interpret these drug orders. For abbreviations that you do not know, see the section on abbreviations later in this chapter.

1. Tetracycline 250 mg, po, q6h

_____

2. HydroDIURIL 50 mg, po, qd

_____

3. Meperidine 50 mg, IM, q3−4h, PRN

_____

4. Ancef 1 g, IV, q8h

_____

5. Prednisone 10 mg, tid × 5 days

_____

List what is missing in these drug orders.

6. Codeine 30 mg, po, PRN for pain _____

7. Digoxin 0.25 mg, qd _____

8. Ceclor 125 mg, po _____

9. TheoDur 200 mg _____

10. Penicillin V K 200,000 U, for days _____

_____

There are four types of drug orders: (1) standing order, (2) one-time (single) order, (3) PRN (whenever necessary) order, and (4) STAT (immediately) order (Table 3–1). Many of the drugs ordered for nonhospitalized patients are normally standing orders that can be renewed (refilled) for 6 months. Narcotic orders are *not* automatically refilled; if the narcotic usage is extended, the physician writes another prescription or calls the pharmacy.

Charting Medications

Charting on medication records should be done immediately after the medications are given. Delay in charting could result in (1) forgetting to chart the drugs or (2) administration of the drugs by another nurse who thought the drugs were *not* given.

Medication records (charts) differ among health care facilities. Drug information that should be on the medication record includes (1) date drug was ordered, (2) drug name, (3) dosage, (4) route of administration, (5) frequency of administration, (6) date and time drug was given, and (7) nurse's signature and initials. An example of a medication record is illustrated in Figure 3–4.

table 3•1
TYPES OF DRUG ORDERS

TYPES/DESCRIPTION	EXAMPLES
Standing orders: A standing order may be typed or written on the doctor's order sheet. It may be an order that is given for a number of days, or it may be a routine order for all patients who had the same type of procedure. Standing orders may include PRN orders.	Erythromycin 250 mg, po, q6h, 5 days Demerol 50 mg, IM, q3–4h, PRN, pain Colace 100 mg, po, hs, PRN

One-time (single) orders:
   One-time orders are given once, usually at a specified time
	Preoperative orders:
	   Meperidine 75 mg, IM, 7:30 AM
	   Atropine SO$_4$ 0.4 mg, IM, 7:30 AM

PRN orders: PRN orders are given at the patient's request and at the nurse's judgment concerning safety and need	Pentobarbital 100 mg, hs, PRN Darvocet-N, tab 1, q4h, PRN
STAT orders: A STAT order is for a one-time drug given immediately	Regular insulin 10 U, SC, STAT

MEDICAL CENTER			PATIENT'S NAME *John Smith*
			ROOM # *6033*
Nurse's Signature/Title		Initial	
Sally Marshall, RN		SM	
Jack Kee, RN		JK	Allergies:
Thomas Jones, LPN		TJ	*Penicillin*

Continuing Medication Record

Date Order	Stop Date	Medication/ Dosage/Route/Frequency	Time	Date/ initials			
				5/14	5/15	5/16	5/17
5/14 JK		Digoxin 0.25 mg, po, qd	9	JK P.72	SM P.70	SM P.74	
5/14 JK	5/18 @ 24	Prednisone 5mg, po q8h x 5 days	8	JK	SM	SM	
			16	SM	TJ	TJ	
			24	TJ	JK	JK	

One-Time/PRN/STAT Medications

Date	Medication/Dose Route/Frequency	Time/ Initial	Reason	Result
5/15	Ibuprofen 400mg, po q4h, PRN	9:30A SM	Leg Pain	10:30A Relief from pain

Figure 3•4

Methods of Drug Distribution

Two methods of drug distribution frequently used for administering medications are the stock drug method and the unit dose method. Table 3–2 describes these methods and lists the advantages and disadvantages of each.

THE "5 RIGHTS" IN DRUG ADMINISTRATION

To provide safe drug administration, the nurse should practice the "5 rights": the right client, the right drug, the right dose, the right time, and

table 3•2
METHODS OF DRUG DISTRIBUTION

	STOCK DRUG METHOD	UNIT DOSE METHOD
Description	Drug is stored in a large container on the floor and is dispensed from the container for all patients	Drug is packaged in single doses by the pharmacy for 24-hour dosing
Advantages	Drug is always available, which eliminates time spent waiting for drug to arrive from the pharmacy Cost efficiency is enhanced by having large quantities of the drug	Packaging saves the nurse time otherwise spent in preparing the drug dose Correct dose is provided with *no* calculation needed Drug is billed for specific number of doses
Disadvantages	Drug error is more prevalent because the drug is "poured" by many persons More drugs to choose from, which may cause error Drug expiration date on the container may be missed	There is time delay in receiving the drug from the pharmacy If the doses are contaminated or damaged, they are not immediately replaceable

the right route (see "Checklist"). Three additional rights could be added: the right documentation, the right of the client to know the reason for administration of the drug, and the right of the client to refuse to take a medication.

RIGHT CLIENT: The client's identification band should always be checked before a medication is given. The nurse should:

- Verify client by checking his or her identification bracelet.
- Ask the client his or her name. Do not call the client by name. Some individuals answer to any name.
- Check the name on the client's medication label.

RIGHT DRUG: To avoid error, the nurse should:

- Check the drug label 3 times: (1) at first contact with the drug bottle, (2) before pouring the drug, and (3) after pouring the drug.
- Check that the drug order is complete and legible. If it is not, contact the physician or charge nurse.
- Know the drug action.
- Check the expiration date. Discard an outdated drug or return the drug to the pharmacy.
- If client questions the drug, recheck drug and drug dose. If in doubt, seek another health care personnel's advice, e.g., pharmacist, physician, licensed health care provider. Some generic drugs differ in shape or color.

RIGHT DOSE: Stock drugs and unit doses are the two methods frequently used for drug distribution. Not all health care institutions use the unit dose method (drugs prepared by dose in the pharmacy or by the pharmaceutical company). If the institution uses the unit dose method, drugs in bottles

CHECKLIST FOR THE "5 RIGHTS" IN DRUG ADMINISTRATION

Right Client

- Check client's identification bracelet. ☐
- Ask the client for his or her name. ☐
- Check the name on the client's medication label. ☐

Right Drug

- Check that the drug order is complete and legible. ☐
- Check the drug label 3 times. ☐
- Check the expiration date. ☐
- Know the drug action. ☐

Right Dose

- Calculate the drug dose. ☐
- Know the recommended dosage range for the drug. ☐
- Recalculate the drug dose with another nurse if in doubt. ☐

Right Time

- Administer drug at the specified time(s). ☐
- Document any delay or omitted drug dose. ☐
- Administer drugs that irritate gastric mucosa with food. ☐
- Administer antibiotics at even intervals (q6h, q8h). ☐

Right Route

- Know the route for administration of the drug. ☐
- Use aseptic techniques when administering a drug. ☐
- Document the injection site on the patient's chart. ☐

should *not* be administered without the consent of the physician or pharmacist. The nurse should:

- Be able to calculate drug dose using the ratio and proportion, basic formula, or dimensional analysis method.
- Know how to calculate drug dose by body weight (kg) or by body surface area (BSA; m^2). Drug doses for potent drugs (e.g., anticancer agents) and for children are frequently determined by body weight or BSA.
- Know the recommended dosage range for the drug. Check the *Physicians' Desk Reference*, the *American Hospital Formulary*, or another drug reference. If the nurse believes that the dose is incorrect or is not within the

therapeutic range, he or she should notify the charge nurse, physician, or pharmacist, and should document all communications.

- Recalculate drug dose if in doubt, or have a colleague recheck the dose.
- Question drug doses that appear to be incorrect.
- Have a colleague check the drug dose of potent or specified drugs such as insulin, digoxin, narcotics, and anticancer agents. This procedure is required by some facilities.

RIGHT TIME: The drug dose should be given at a specified time to maintain a therapeutic drug serum level. Too-frequent dosing can cause drug toxicity, and missed doses can nullify the drug action and its effect. The nurse should:

- Administer the drug at the specified time(s). Drugs can be given ½ hour before or after the time prescribed.
- Omit or delay a drug dose according to specific circumstance, e.g., laboratory and diagnostic tests. Notify the appropriate personnel of the reason.
- Administer drugs that are affected by foods, e.g., tetracycline, 1 hour before or 2 hours after meals.
- Administer drugs that can irritate the gastric mucosa, e.g., potassium or aspirin, with foods.
- Know that drugs with a long half-life ($t_{1/2}$), e.g., 20 to 36 hours, are usually given once per day. Drugs having a short half-life, e.g., 1 to 6 hours, are given several times a day.
- Administer antibiotics at even intervals [e.g., q8h (8-4-12) rather than tid (8-12-4); q6h (6-12-6-12) rather than qid (8-12-4-8)] to maintain a therapeutic drug serum level.

RIGHT ROUTE: The right route is necessary for appropriate absorption of the medication. The more common routes of absorption are (1) oral (by mouth, po) tablet, capsule, pill, liquid, or suspension; (2) sublingual (under the tongue for venous absorption, *not* to be swallowed); (3) buccal (between gum and check); (4) topical (applied to the skin); (5) inhalation (aerosol sprays); (6) instillation (in nose, eye, ear, rectum, or vagina); (7) and four parenteral routes: intradermal, subcutaneous, intramuscular, and intravenous. The nurse should:

- Know the drug route. If in doubt, check with the pharmacy. Ointment for the eye should have "ophthalmic" written on the tube. Drugs given sublingually (e.g., nitroglycerin tablet) should *not* be swallowed, because the effect of the drug would be lost.
- Administer injectables (subcutaneous and intramuscular) at appropriate sites (see Chapter 7).
- Use aseptic technique when administering drugs. Sterile technique is required with the parenteral routes.
- Document the injection site used on the client's chart or on another designated sheet.

ABBREVIATIONS

Selected abbreviations are given here in four categories: drug form, drug measurements, route of drug administration, and times of drug administration. These abbreviations are frequently used in drug therapy and in this text; therefore, nurses must know the meanings of these abbreviations.

A. Drug Form

ABBREVIATION	MEANING	ABBREVIATION	MEANING
aq	Water	SR	Sustained release
cap	Capsule	supp	Suppository
CD	Controlled dose	susp	Suspension
elix	Elixir	syr	Syrup
emuls	Emulsion	tab	Tablet
ext	Extract	tr, tinct	Tincture
mixt	Mixture	ung	Ointment
		XR	Extended release

B. Drug Measurements

ABBREVIATION	MEANING	ABBREVIATION	MEANING
cc	Cubic centimeter	mL	Milliliter
dL	Deciliter (one-tenth of a liter)	ℳ, min	Minim
		ng	Nanogram
dr	Dram	oz	Ounce
fl dr	Fluid dram (fl ʒ)	pt	Pint
fl oz	Fluid ounce (fl ℥)	qt	Quart
g, gm, G, Gm	Gram	s̄s̄	One-half
gr	Grain	T.O.	Telephone order
gtt	Drops	T, tbsp	Tablespoon
kg	Kilogram	t, tsp	Teaspoon
l, L	Liter	U	Unit
m², M²	Square meter	V.O.	Verbal order
mcg, μg	Microgram	×	Times
mEq	Milliequivalent	>	Greater than
mg	Milligram	<	Less than

C. Routes of Drug Administration

ABBREVIATION	MEANING	ABBREVIATION	MEANING
A.D., ad	Right ear	NGT	Nasogastric tube
A.S., as	Left ear	O.D., od	Right eye
A.U., au	Both ears	O.S., os	Left eye
ID	Intradermal	O.U., ou	Both eyes
IM	Intramuscular	P.O., po, os	By mouth
IV	Intravenous	PR	Per rectum
IVPB	Intravenous piggyback	Ⓡ	Right
		Rect	Rectal
KVO	Keep vein open	SC, subc, sc	Subcutaneous
Ⓛ	Left	Sl, sl, subl	Sublingual
		Vag	Vaginal

D. Times of Drug Administration

ABBREVIATION	MEANING	ABBREVIATION	MEANING
A.C., ac	Before meals	qd, od	Every day
ad lib	As desired	qh	Every hour
B.i.d., Bid, bid	Twice a day	q2h	Every 2 hours
BIW	Two times a week	q4h	Every 4 hours
c̄	With	q6h	Every 6 hours
h	Hour	q8h	Every 8 hours
hs	Hour of sleep	Q.i.d., Qid, qid	Four times a day
noct	At night	Qod, qod	Every other day
NPO	Nothing by mouth	s̄	Without
P.C., pc	After meals	SOS	Once if necessary, if
per	By		there is a need
PRN	Whenever neces-	STAT	Give immediately
	sary, as needed	T.i.d., Tid, tid	Three times a day
q	Every	TIW	Three times a week
qAM	Every morning,		
	every AM		

III Practice Problems: Abbreviations

If you have more than two incorrect answers, review the abbreviations and meanings. Then quiz yourself again.

1. cap _capsule_
2. SR _sustained release_
3. fl oz _fluid ounces_
4. g, G _gram_
5. gr _grain_
6. L _Liters_
7. mL _milliliters_
8. mcg, μg _micrograms_
9. mg _milligrams_
10. s̄s̄ _one half_
11. T _tablespoon_
12. t _teaspoon_
13. > _greater than_
14. A.U., au _both ears_
15. IM _intramuscular_

16. IV _intravenous_
17. KVO _keep vein open_
18. O.S. _left eye_
19. O.U. _both eyes_
20. SC _subcutaneous_
21. c̄ _with_
22. A.C., ac _before meals_
23. hs _hour of sleep_
24. NPO _nothing by mouth_
25. P.C., pc _after meals_
26. q4h _every 4 hours_
27. Qid, qid, q.i.d. _four times a day_
28. Tid, tid, t.i.d. _three times a day_
29. Bid, bid, b.i.d. _twice a day_
30. STAT _give immediately_

ANSWERS

I. Interpretation of Drug Labels

1. **a.** Coumadin
    b. warfarin sodium (crystalline)
    c. tablet
    d. 1 mg per tablet
    e. 3/22/97 (date expired, do not use, return to pharmacy)
    f. BD471CX
    g. Dupont Pharmaceuticals

2. **a.** Veetids
    b. penicillin V potassium
    c. tablet
    d. 250 mg per tablet; 400,000 units per tablet
    e. Apothecon

3. **a.** Tegopen
    b. cloxacillin sodium
    c. liquid for oral administration
    d. 125 mg per 5 mL
    e. 6/15/02
    f. Apothecon

4. **a.** quinidine gluconate
    b. quinidine gluconate (same as brand name)
    c. liquid for injection
    d. vial (multiple dose vial), total amount is 10 mL per vial
    e. 80 mg per mL
    f. 10/11/00

5. **a.** Decadron phosphate
    b. dexamethasone sodium phosphate
    c. liquid for injection
    d. 24 mg per mL

6. **a.** nafcillin sodium
    b. nafcillin sodium (same as brand name)
    c. drug powder to be reconstituted
    d. 3.4 mL diluent
    e. IM or IV
    f. 1 gram = 4 mL
    g. 11/30/02
    h. Apothecon

II. Interpretation of Drug Orders

1. Give 250 mg of tetracycline by mouth every 6 hours

2. Give 50 mg of HydroDIURIL by mouth every day

3. Give 50 mg of meperidine intramuscularly every 3 to 4 hours whenever necessary

4. Give 1 g of Ancef intravenously every 8 hours

5. Give 10 mg of prednisone three times a day for 5 days

6. frequency of administration

7. route of administration

8. frequency of administration

9. route and frequency of administration

10. route and frequency of administration and stop date

III. Abbreviations

1. capsule
2. sustained release
3. fluid ounce
4. gram
5. grain
6. liter
7. milliliter
8. microgram
9. milligram
10. one-half
11. tablespoon
12. teaspoon
13. greater than
14. both ears
15. intramuscular
16. intravenous
17. keep vein open
18. left eye
19. both eyes
20. subcutaneous
21. with
22. before meals
23. hour of sleep
24. nothing by mouth
25. after meals
26. every 4 hours
27. four times a day
28. three times a day
29. two times a day
30. immediately

alternative methods for drug administration

Objectives

- Recognize the various methods for drug administration.
- Explain the steps (methods) in drug administration using the various methods.

Outline

There are numerous methods for administering medications in addition to oral (tablets, capsules, liquid) and parenteral (subcutaneous, intramuscular, intravenous) routes. Alternative methods for drug administration include transdermal patches; inhalation sprays; nasal sprays and drops; eye drops and ointments; ear drops; pharyngeal (throat) sprays, mouthwashes, and lozenges; topical lotions, creams, and ointments; rectal suppositories; and vaginal suppositories, creams, and ointments.

TRANSDERMAL PATCH

Purpose

The transdermal patch contains medication (Fig. 4–1); the patch is applied to the skin for slow, systemic absorption, usually over 24 hours. Use of the transdermal route avoids the gastrointestinal problems associated with some oral medications and provides a more consistent drug level in the client's blood.

METHOD   **Transdermal Patch**

1. Cleanse the skin area where the patch will be applied. The area can be the chest, abdomen, arms, or thighs. Avoid areas that have hair.
2. Remove the transparent cover (inside) of the patch. Do not touch the inside of the patch.
3. Apply the patch to the chosen area with the dull, plastic side up.

INHALATION

Purpose

The drug inhaler delivers the prescribed dose to be absorbed by the mucosal lining of the respiratory tract (Fig. 4–2). The drug categories for respira-

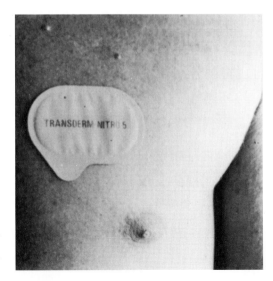

Figure 4•1 ————

Transdermal nitroglycerin patch. (Courtesy of Summit Pharmaceutical.)

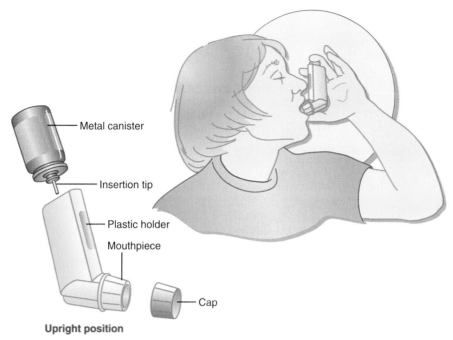

Metal canister

Insertion tip

Plastic holder

Mouthpiece

Cap

Upright position

Figure 4•2

Distribution of medication with and without a spacer. From American Lung Association (1993). *Understanding Lung Medications: How They Work—How to Use Them.* American Lung Association, p. 5.

tory inhalation are bronchodilators, which dilate bronchial tubes; glucocorticoids, which are anti-inflammatory agents; and mucolytics, which liquefy bronchial secretions.

Types

Two types of inhalers are the metered-dose inhaler (MDI) or nebulizer and the nasal inhaler.

The MDI can also be used with a spacer device, which enhances delivery of the medication. Figure 4–3 illustrates the advantage of a spacer device.

METHOD **Metered-Dose Inhaler**

1. Insert the medication canister into the plastic holder. If the inhaler has not been used recently or if it is being used for the first time, test spray before administering the metered dose.
2. Shake the inhaler well before using. Remove the cap from the mouthpiece.
3. Instruct the client to breathe out through the mouth, expelling air. Place the mouthpiece into the client's mouth, holding the inhaler upright (Fig. 4–2).
4. Instruct the client to keep his or her lips securely around the mouthpiece and inhale. While the client is inhaling, push the top of the medication canister once.

Without Spacer | With Spacer
10% Inhaler Device 57%
81% Mouth/Throat 22%
9% Lungs 21%

Figure 4•3

Technique for using the aerosol inhaler. From Kee, J., and Hayes, E. (2000). *Pharmacology: A Nursing Process Approach* (3rd ed.). Philadelphia: W. B. Saunders.

5. Instruct the client to hold his or her breath for a few seconds. Remove the mouthpiece and take your finger off the canister. Tell the client to exhale slowly.

6. If a second dose is required, wait 1 to 2 minutes and repeat steps 3 to 5.

7. Cleanse the mouthpiece.

METHOD **Metered-Dose Inhaler with Spacer**

1. Method is the same as the method used for the metered-dose inhaler just described (Fig. 4–3).

METHOD **Nasal Inhaler**

1. Instruct the client to blow his or her nose to clear the nostrils.

2. Insert the drug cartridge into the adapter (Fig. 4–4).

Figure 4•4

Nasal inhaler.

3. Shake the inhaler well before using. Remove the cap.
4. Place your finger on top of the cartridge.
5. Instruct the client to tilt his or her head back slightly. Place the tip of the adapter in one nostril; occlude the other nostril; and have client inhale while you press the adapter. Inform the client to exhale through his or her mouth.
6. Repeat the procedure with the other nostril if ordered.
7. Cleanse the tip of the adapter and dry thoroughly.

NASAL SPRAY AND DROPS

Purpose

Most drugs in nasal spray and drop containers are intended to relieve nasal congestion due to upper respiratory infection and polyps by shrinking swollen nasal membranes. Types of drugs given by this method are vasoconstrictors and glucocorticoids.

METHOD **Nasal Spray**

1. Instruct the client to sit with his or her head tilted slightly back or slightly forward, according to the directions on the spray container (Fig. 4–5).
2. Insert the tip of the container in one nostril and occlude the other nostril.
3. Instruct the client to inhale as you squeeze the drug spray container. Repeat with the same nostril if ordered.
4. Repeat the procedure with the other nostril if ordered.
5. Encourage the client to keep his or her head tilted for several minutes until the drug action is effective. The nose should not be blown until the head is upright.

Figure 4•5 ——————

Administering nasal spray. From Kee, J., & Hayes, E. (2000). *Pharmacology: A Nursing Process Approach* (3rd ed.). Philadelphia: W. B. Saunders.

Figure 4•6 ————————

Administering nose drops. From Kee, J., & Hayes, E. (2000). *Pharmacology: A Nursing Process Approach* (3rd ed.). Philadelphia: W. B. Saunders.

METHOD Nose Drops

1. Place the client in an upright position with his or her head tilted back.
2. Insert the dropper into the nostril without touching the nasal membranes.
3. Instill 2 drops of medications or the amount prescribed.
4. Instruct the client to keep his or her head back for 5 minutes and to breathe through the mouth.
5. Cleanse the dropper.
6. For the medication to reach the sinuses, the client should be in the supine position with head turned to one side and then the other so the medication can reach the frontal and maxillary sinuses. For the medication to reach the ethmoidal and sphenoidal sinuses, the client's head is lowered below his or her shoulders (Fig. 4–6).

EYE DROPS AND OINTMENT

Purpose

Eye medications are prescribed for various eye disorders, such as glaucoma, infection, and allergies, and for eye examination and eye surgery.

METHOD Eye Drops

1. Instruct the client to lie or sit with his or her head tilted back.
2. Instruct the client to look up toward the ceiling and away from the dropper. Pull down the lower lid of the affected eye (Fig. 4–7). Place one drop of medication into the lower conjunctival sac. This prevents the drug from dropping onto the cornea.

Figure 4•7

To administer eye drops, gently pull down the skin below the eye to expose the conjunctival sac. From Kee, J., & Hayes, E. (2000). *Pharmacology: A Nursing Process Approach* (3rd ed.). Philadelphia: W. B. Saunders.

3. Press gently on the medial nasolacrimal canthus (side closer to the nose) with a tissue to prevent systemic drug absorption.
4. If the other eye is affected, repeat the procedure in the other eye.
5. Inform the client to blink one or two times and then to keep the eyes closed for several minutes. Use a tissue to blot away excess drug fluid.

METHOD   Eye Ointment

1. Instruct the client to lie or sit with his or her head tilted back.
2. Pull down the lower lid to expose the conjunctival sac of the affected eye (Fig. 4–8).
3. Squeeze a strip of ointment about ¼ inch long (unless otherwise indicated) onto the conjunctival sac. Medication placed directly onto the cornea can cause discomfort or damage.
4. If the other eye is affected, repeat the procedure.
5. Instruct the client to close his or her eyes for 2 to 3 minutes. The client's vision may be blurred for a short time.

EAR DROPS

Purpose

Ear medication is frequently prescribed to soften and loosen the cerumen (wax) in the ear canal, for anesthetic effect, to immobilize insects in the ear canal, and to treat infection such as fungal infection.

Figure 4•8

To administer eye ointment, squeeze a ¼-inch-wide strip of ointment onto the conjunctival sac. From Kee, J., & Hayes, E. (2000). *Pharmacology: A Nursing Process Approach* (3rd ed.). Philadelphia: W. B. Saunders.

Ointment

METHOD   Ear Drops

1. Instruct the client to lie on the unaffected side or to sit upright with his or her head tilted toward the unaffected side.
2. Straighten the external ear canal (Fig. 4–9), as follows:
   Adult: Pull the auricle of the ear up and back.
   Child: Pull the auricle of the ear down and back.
3. Instill the prescribed number of drops. Avoid contaminating the dropper.
4. Instruct the client to remain in this position for 2 to 5 minutes to prevent the drop from leaking out of the ear.

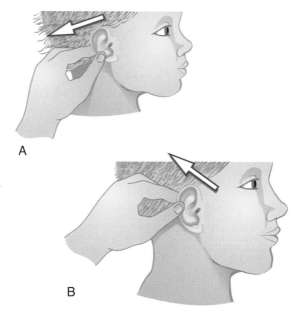

A

B

Figure 4•9

To administer ear drops, straighten the external ear canal by (*A*) pulling down on the auricle in children and (*B*) pulling up and back on the auricle in adults. From Kee, J., & Hayes, E. (2000). *Pharmacology: A Nursing Process Approach* (3rd ed.). Philadelphia: W. B. Saunders.

PHARYNGEAL SPRAY, MOUTHWASH, AND LOZENGE

Purpose

Sprays, mouthwashes, and lozenges can be prescribed to reduce throat irritation and for antiseptic and anesthetic effects. These methods are prescribed for a local effect on the throat and *not* for systemic use.

METHOD   Pharyngeal Spray

1. Instruct the client to sit upright.
2. Place a tongue blade over the client's tongue to prevent the tongue from becoming numb if an anesthetic is being administered.
3. Hold the spray pump nozzle outside the client's mouth, and direct the spray to the back of the throat.

METHOD   Pharyngeal Mouthwash

1. Instruct the client to sit upright.
2. Instruct the client to swish the solution around the mouth, but *not* to swallow the solution, and then to spit it into an emesis basin or sink.

METHOD   Pharyngeal Lozenge

1. Instruct the client to sit upright.
2. Instruct the client to place the lozenge in his or her mouth and suck until it is fully dissolved. The lozenge should *not* be chewed or swallowed whole.

TOPICAL PREPARATIONS: LOTION, CREAM, AND OINTMENT

Purpose

Topical lotions, creams, and ointments are useful to protect skin areas, prevent skin dryness, treat itching of skin areas, and relieve pain.

METHOD   Topical Lotion

1. Cleanse skin area with soap and water or other designated solution.
2. Shake the lotion container. Use clean or sterile gloves to apply the medicated lotion. Rub the lotion thoroughly into the skin unless otherwise indicated.

METHOD A   Topical Cream or Ointment

1. Cleanse the skin area.
2. Use clean or sterile glove(s) and a sterile tongue blade or gauze to apply the cream or ointment to the affected skin area. Use long, smooth strokes. A sterile gauze can be applied to the medicated area after application to prevent soiling of clothing.

METHOD B   Topical Cream or Ointment

1. Cleanse the skin area.
2. Squeeze a line of ointment from the tube onto your finger from the tip to the first skin crease; this is known as a fingertip unit (FTU). One FTU weighs about 0.5 g. Use the following guidelines for the number of FTUs to apply to various body areas:
   Face and neck: 2½ FTUs
   Arm: 3 FTUs
   Hand: 1 FTU
   Trunk (front and back): 14 FTUs
   Groin: 1 FTU
   Leg: 6 FTUs
   Foot: 2 FTUs
3. Apply the medication to the affected area.

RECTAL SUPPOSITORY

Purpose

Rectal medications are used to relieve vomiting when the client is unable to take oral medication, to relieve pain or anxiety, to promote defecation, and to administer drugs that could be destroyed by digestive enzymes.

METHOD   Rectal Suppository

1. Place the client on his or her left side in the Sims position (Fig. 4–10).
2. Use gloves or a finger cot on the index finger.
3. Expose the anus by lifting the upper portion of the buttock.
4. Lightly lubricate the suppository with water-soluble lubricant, and insert the narrow (pointed) end of the suppository through the anal sphincter muscle.
5. Instruct the client to remain in a supine position for 5 to 10 minutes.

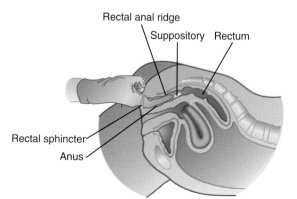

Figure 4•10

Inserting a rectal suppository. From Kee, J., & Hayes, E. (2000). *Pharmacology: A Nursing Process Approach* (3rd ed.). Philadelphia: W. B. Saunders.

Figure 4•11 ————————
Inserting a vaginal suppository. From Kee, J., & Hayes, E. (2000). *Pharmacology: A Nursing Process Approach* (3rd ed.). Philadelphia: W. B. Saunders.

VAGINAL SUPPOSITORY, CREAM, AND OINTMENT

Purpose

Vaginal medications are used to treat vaginal infection or inflammation.

METHOD   Vaginal Suppository, Cream, and Ointment

1. Wear clean gloves.
2. Place the client in lithotomy position (knees bent with feet on the table or bed).
3. Place the vaginal suppository at the tip of the applicator.

   or

   Connect the top of the vaginal cream or ointment tube with the tip of applicator. Squeeze the tube to fill the applicator.
4. Lubricate the applicator with water-soluble lubricant if necessary.
5. Insert applicator downward first and then upward and backward. (Fig. 4–11).
6. The client may use a light pad in the underwear to prevent soiling of clothing. Bedtime is the suggested time for vaginal drug administration.
7. Instruct the client to avoid using tampons after insertion of the vaginal medication.

methods of calculation

objectives

- Determine the amount of drug needed for a specified time.
- Select a dosage formula, such as basic formula, ratio and proportion, fraction equation, or dimensional analysis, for solving drug dosage problems.
- Convert units of measurement to the same system and unit of measurement prior to calculating drug dosage.
- Calculate the dosage amount of tablets, capsules, and liquid volume (oral or parenteral) needed to administer the prescribed drug.
- Calculate the drug dosage needed according to body weight and body surface area.

outline

Before drug dosage can be calculated, units of measurement must be converted to one system. If the drug is ordered in milligrams and comes in grains, then grains are converted to milligrams or milligrams are converted to grains.

Four methods for calculating drug dosages are: basic formula, ratio and proportion, fractional equation, and dimensional analysis. For drugs that require individualized dosing, body weight and body surface area are used. When body weight and body surface area calculations are used, one of the first three methods for calculation is necessary to determine the amount of drug needed from the container.

At some institutions, the nurse orders enough medication doses for a designated period. If the order requires 2 tablets, qid (4 times a day) for 5 days, then the number of tablets needed would be 2 tablets × 4 times a day × 5 days = 40 tablets.

DRUG CALCULATION

The four methods as mentioned for drug calculations are (1) basic formula, (2) ratio and proportion, (3) fractional equation, and (4) dimensional analysis (factor labeling).

METHOD 1: Basic Formula

The following formula is often used to calculate drug dosages. The basic formula is the most commonly used method, and it is easy to remember.

$$\frac{D}{H} \times V = \text{amount to give}$$

D or desired dose: Drug dose ordered by physician.

H or on-hand dose: Drug dose on label of container (bottle, vial, ampule).

V or vehicle: Form and amount in which the drug comes (tablet, capsule, liquid).

. . . .

examples

PROBLEM 1: Order: erythromycin (ERY-TAB) 0.5 g, po, q8h.
Drug available:

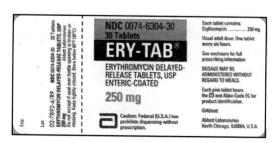

a. Both the dosage of the drug ordered and the dosage on the bottle are in the metric system; however, the units of measurement are different. Conversion is needed. To convert grams to milligrams move the decimal point three spaces to the right (see Chapter 1, Metric System):

$$0.5\ g = 0.500\ mg = 500\ mg$$

b. $\dfrac{D}{H} \times V = \dfrac{\overset{2}{\cancel{500}}}{\underset{1}{\cancel{250}}} \times 1\ tab = 2\ tablets$

Answer: erythromycin 0.5 g = 2 tablets

PROBLEM 2: Order: 0.5 g of ampicillin (Principen), po, bid.
Drug available:

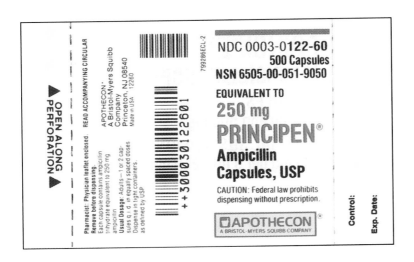

a. The unit of measurement that is ordered and the unit on the bottle are in the same system but in different units; therefore, conversion of units within the same system must be done first. To convert grams to milligrams, move the decimal point three spaces to the right (see Chapter 1, Metric System):

$$0.5\ g = 0.500\ mg = 500\ mg$$

b. $\dfrac{D}{H} \times V = \dfrac{500}{250} \times 1\ capsule = \dfrac{\overset{2}{\cancel{500}}}{\underset{1}{\cancel{250}}} = 2\ capsules$

Answer: ampicillin (Principen) 0.5 g = 2 capsules

PROBLEM 3: Order: phenobarbital gr ïi, STAT.
Drug available: phenobarbital 30 mg per tablet.

a. Before calculating drug dosage, convert to one unit of measurement. To convert grains to milligrams, *multiply* the number of grains by 60 (see Chapter 2, Grains and Milligrams):

$$2 \text{ gr} \times 60 = 120 \text{ mg}$$

b. $\dfrac{D}{H} \times V = \dfrac{120}{30} \times 1 = \dfrac{120}{30} = 4 \text{ tablets}$

Answer: phenobarbital gr ii = 4 tablets

PROBLEM 4: Order: meperidine (Demerol) 35 mg, IM, STAT. Drug available:

a. Conversion is not needed, because both are of the same unit of measurement.

b. $\dfrac{D}{H} \times V = \dfrac{35}{50} \times 1 \text{ mL} = \dfrac{35}{50} = 0.7 \text{ mL}$

Answer: meperidine (Demerol) 35 mg = 0.7 mL

METHOD 2: Ratio and Proportion

This is the oldest method used for calculating dosage problems:

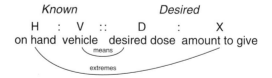

H and **V**: On the left side of the equation are the known quantities, which are dose on hand and vehicle.

D and **X**: On the right side of the equation are the desired dose and the unknown amount to give.

Multiply the means and the extremes. Solve for **X**.

examples

PROBLEM 1: Order: erythromycin (ERY-TAB) 0.5 g, po, q8h.
Drug available:

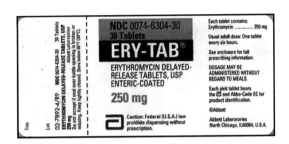

a. To convert grams to milligrams, move the decimal point three spaces to the right (see Chapter 1, Metric System):

$$0.5 \text{ g} = 0.500 \text{ mg} = 500 \text{ mg}$$

b. H : V :: D : X
  250 mg : 1 tab :: 500 mg : X tab

$$250 \text{ X} = 500$$
$$\text{X} = 2 \text{ tablets}$$

Answer: erythromycin 0.5 g = 2 tablets

Note: With ratio and proportion, the ratio on the left (milligrams to tablets) has the same relation as the ratio on the right (milligrams to tablets); the only difference is values.

PROBLEM 2: Order: aspirin (ASA) gr x, PRN.
Drug available: aspirin 325 mg per tablet.

a. To convert to one system and unit of measurement. To convert grains to milligrams, *multiply* the number of grains by 60 (65) (see Chapter 2, Grains and Milligrams).

$$10 \text{ gr} \times 60 \text{ (65)} = 600 \text{ or } 650 \text{ mg}$$

or

  gr : mg :: gr : mg
  1 : 60 (65) :: 10 : X
$$\text{X} = 600 \text{ or } 650 \text{ mg}$$

b. H : V :: D : X
  325 mg : 1 tablet :: 600 (650) mg : X tablet
$$325 \text{ X} = 600 \text{ (650)}$$
$$\text{X} = 1.8 \text{ tablets or } 2 \text{ tablets}$$
    (round off or use 650 instead of 600)

Answer: aspirin gr x = 2 tablets

PROBLEM 3: Order: amoxicillin 75 mg, po, qid.
Drug available:

a. Conversion is not needed because both use the same unit of measurement.

b.   H   :   V   : :   D   :   X
125 mg : 5 mL : : 75 mg : X mL

125 X = 375
X = 3 mL

Answer: amoxicillin 75 mg = 3 mL

PROBLEM 4: Order: meperidine (Demerol) 60 mg, IM, STAT.
Drug available: Meperidine in a prefilled syringe.

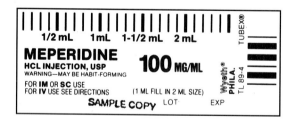

a. Conversion is not needed: the same unit of measurement is used.

b.   H   :   V   : :   D   :   X
100 mg : 1 mL : : 60 mg : X mL

100 X = 60
X = 0.6 mL

Answer: meperidine (Demerol) 60 mg = 0.6 mL

METHOD 3: Fractional Equation

This method *is similar* to ratio and proportion, except it is written as a fraction.

$$\frac{H}{V} = \frac{D}{X}$$

H: The dosage on hand or on the container.

V: The vehicle or the form in which the drug comes (tablet, capsule, liquid).

D: The desired dosage.

X: The unknown amount to give.

Cross-multiply and solve for **X**.

. . . .

examples

PROBLEM 1: Order: kanamycin sulfate (Kantrex) 1 g, po, q6h × 3d.
Drug available:

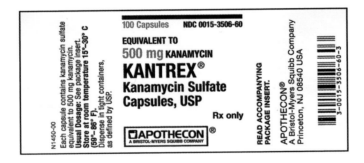

a. Convert grams to milligrams. Move the decimal point three spaces to the right.

$$1.0 \text{ g} = 1.000 \text{ mg} = 1000 \text{ mg}$$

b. $\dfrac{H}{V} = \dfrac{D}{X}$ $\dfrac{500 \text{ mg}}{1 \text{ capsule}} = \dfrac{1000}{X}$

$$500\ X = 1000$$
$$X = 2$$

Answer: *kanamycin 1 g = 2 capsules*

PROBLEM 2: Order: valproic acid (Depakene) 100 mg, po, tid.
Drug available: valproic acid (Depakene) 250 mg/5 mL suspension.

a. No unit conversion is needed.

b. $\dfrac{H}{V} = \dfrac{D}{X}$ $\dfrac{250}{5} = \dfrac{100}{X}$

250 X = 500

X = 2 mL

Answer: valproic acid (Depakene) 100 mg = 2 mL

PROBLEM 3: Order: atropine gr $\frac{1}{100}$, IM, STAT.
Drug available:

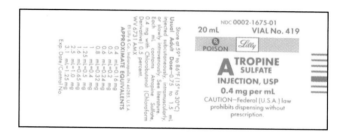

a. Two systems are involved: apothecary (grains) and metric (milligrams). Because the drug preparation is in milligrams, convert grains to milligrams (see Table 2–1 or Table 5–1; 0.6 mg = gr $\frac{1}{100}$).

table 5•1
METRIC AND APOTHECARY CONVERSIONS*

METRIC		APOTHECARY
Grams (g)	Milligrams (mg)	Grains (gr)
1	1000	15
0.5	500	1½
0.3	300 (325)	5
0.1	100	1½
0.06	60 (64)	1
0.03	30 (32)	½
0.015	15 (16)	¼
0.010	10	⅙
0.0006	0.6	$\frac{1}{100}$
0.0004	0.4	$\frac{1}{150}$
0.0003	0.3	$\frac{1}{200}$

LIQUID (APPROXIMATE)

30 mL (cc) = 1 oz (fl ʒ) = 2 tbsp (T) = 6 tsp (t)
15 mL (cc) = ½ oz = 1 T = 3 t
1000 mL (cc) = 1 quart (qt) = 1 liter (L)
500 mL (cc) = 1 pint (pt)
5 mL (cc) = 1 tsp (t)
4 mL (cc) = 1 fl dr (fl ʒ)
1 mL (cc) = 15 minims = 15 drops (gtt)

....
* Metric and apothecary equivalents frequently used in drug dosage conversions.

Also, you could use the ratio method:

$$gr:mg::gr:mg$$
$$1:60::\tfrac{1}{100}:X$$
$$X = \tfrac{60}{100}$$
$$X = 0.6 \text{ mg}$$

b. $\dfrac{H}{V} = \dfrac{D}{X}$ $\qquad \dfrac{0.4}{1} = \dfrac{0.6}{X}$

$$0.4\,X = 0.6$$
$$X = 1.5 \text{ mL}$$

Answer: atropine gr $\tfrac{1}{100}$ = 1.5 mL

METHOD 4: Dimensional Analysis

The dimensional analysis method (also called factor labeling or the label factor method) calculates dosages using three factors:

1. **Drug label factor:** The form of the drug dose (V) with its equivalence in units (H), e.g., 1 capsule = 500 mg.

2. **Conversion factor (C):** It will help if you memorize the following common conversions:

$$1 \text{ g} = 1000 \text{ mg}$$
$$1 \text{ g} = 15 \text{ gr}$$
$$1000 \text{ mg} = 15 \text{ gr}$$
$$1 \text{ gr} = 60 \text{ mg}$$

3. **Drug order factor:** The dosage desired (D).

These three factors are set up in an equation that allows you to cancel the units giving you the correct answer in the correct units for delivery.

$$V = \frac{V \text{ (vehicle)} \times \quad C \text{ (H)} \quad \times D \text{ (desired)}}{H \text{ (on hand)} \times \quad C \text{ (D)} \quad \times \quad 1}$$
$$\text{(drug label)} \quad \text{(conversion factor)} \quad \text{(drug order)}$$

As with other methods for calculation, the three components, **D, H,** and **V,** are necessary to solve the drug problem. With dimensional analysis, the conversion factor is built into the equation and is included when the units of measurements of the drug order and drug container differ. If the two are of the same units of measurement, the conversion factor is eliminated from the equation.

examples

PROBLEM 1: Order: kanamycin (Kantrex) 1 g, po, g6h × 3d.
Drug available:

Factors: 500 mg = 1 capsule (from drug label)
1 g/l (from drug order)
Conversion factor: 1 g = 1000 mg

$$cap = \frac{1 \text{ cap}}{\cancel{500} \text{ mg}} \times \frac{\overset{2}{\cancel{1000}} \text{ mg}}{1 \text{ g}} \times \frac{1 \text{ g}}{1}$$

(drug label) × (conversion factor) × (drug order)
(cancel units and numbers from numerator and
denominator)

$$1 \text{ cap} \times 2 = 2 \text{ caps}$$

Answer: *kanamycin 1 g = 2 capsules*

PROBLEM 2: Order: acetaminophen (Tylenol) gr XV, po, PRN.
Drug available:

Factors: 325 mg = 1 tablet (from drug label)
15 gr/1 (from drug order)
Conversion factor: 1000 mg = 15 gr
How many tablet(s) would you give?

$$tab = \frac{1 \text{ tab} \times 1000 \text{ mg} \times \cancel{15} \text{ gr}}{325 \text{ mg} \times \cancel{15} \text{ gr} \times 1} = \frac{1000}{325} = 3.07 \text{ tab or 3 tab}$$

Answer: acetaminophen gr XV = 3 tablets

Tylenol also is available in 500 mg tablets (extra-strength tablets).

CALCULATION FOR INDIVIDUALIZED DRUG DOSING

The two methods for individualizing drug dosing are body weight and body surface area (BSA).

Body Weight

Body weight allows the drug dose to be individualized and is often used for children and clients receiving chemotherapy. The first step is to convert pounds to kilograms (if necessary). The second step is to determine the drug dose per body weight by multiplying drug dose × body weight × frequency (day or per day in divided doses). The third step is to choose one of the three methods of drug calculation for the amount of drug to be given.

. . . .

examples

PROBLEM 1: Order: fluorouracil (5-FU), 12 mg/kg/day IV, not to exceed 800 mg/day. The adult weighs 140 pounds.

    a. Convert pounds to kilograms. Divide number of pounds by 2.2.
       Remember: 1 kg = 2.2 lb

$$140 \div 2.2 = 64 \text{ kg}$$

    b. mg × kg × 1 day =
       12 × 64 × 1   = 768 mg IV per day

Answer: fluorouracil (5-FU), 12 mg/kg/day = 768 mg or 750 to 800 mg

PROBLEM 2: Give cefaclor (Ceclor), 20 mg/kg/day in three divided doses. The child weighs 20 pounds.
Drug available:

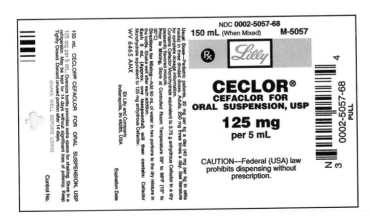

a. Convert pounds to kilograms.

$$20 \div 2.2 = 9 \text{ kg}$$

b. 20 mg $\times$ 9 kg $\times$ 1 day = 180 mg per day.

$$180 \text{ mg} \div 3 \text{ divided doses} = 60 \text{ mg}$$

$$\frac{D}{H} \times V = \frac{60}{125} \times 5 \qquad \textbf{or} \qquad \begin{array}{c} H : V :: D : X \\ 125 : 5 :: 60 : X \end{array} \qquad \textbf{or} \qquad \frac{125}{5} = \frac{60}{X}$$

$$= \frac{300}{125} = 2.4 \text{ mL} \qquad\qquad \begin{array}{c} 125\,X = 300 \\ X = 2.4 \text{ mL} \end{array} \qquad\qquad \begin{array}{c} 125\,X = 300 \\ X = 2.4 \text{ mL} \end{array}$$

Answer: cefacelor (Ceclor) 20 mg/kg/day = 2.4 mL per dose three times per day

Body Surface Area

Body surface area is an estimated mathematical function of height and weight. BSA is considered to be the most accurate way to calculate drug dosages for clients receiving chemotherapy and some drug dosages for infants and children. BSA can be determined by using nomograms, slide rules based on nomograms, or square roots.

BSA USING A NOMOGRAM

The BSA in square meters (m^2) is determined by the person's height and weight and where these points intersect on the nomogram scale (Figs. 5–1 and 5–2). The nomogram charts were developed from the square root formulas and correlated with heights and weights to simplify drug dosing before calculators were readily available. When a nomogram is used, points on the scale must be carefully plotted. An error in plotting points or drawing intersecting lines can lead to reading the incorrect BSA, resulting in dosing errors.

To calculate the dosage by BSA, multiply the drug dose $\times$ m^2, e.g., 100 mg $\times$ 1.6 m^2 = 160 mg/m^2. The advantage of using the nomogram is that no conversions from pounds to kilograms or inches to centimeters are needed.

examples

PROBLEM 1: Order: cyclophosphamide (Cytoxan) 100 mg/m^2/day, po. Client weighs 150 pounds and is 5'8" (68 inches) tall. Round off to the nearest tenth.

a. 68 inches and 150 pounds intersect the nomogram scale at 1.88 m^2 (BSA), 1.9 m^2 rounded off to the nearest tenth.

b. 100 mg $\times$ 1.9 m^2 = 190 mg/m^2/day of Cytoxan.

PROBLEM 2: Order: cytarabine (Cytosine) 200 mg/m^2/day IV $\times$ 5 days. For a client with myelocytic leukemia. The client is 64 inches tall and weighs 130 pounds. Round off to the nearest tenth.

BODY SURFACE AREA FOR ADULTS — NOMOGRAM

HEIGHT	BODY SURFACE AREA (BSA)	WEIGHT

Figure 5•1

Nomogram of body surface area (BSA) for adults. *Directions:* (1) find height; (2) find weight; (3) draw a straight line connecting the height and weight. Where the line intersects on the BSA column is the body surface area (m²). Sources: Deglin, J. H., Vallerand, A. H., and Russin, M. M. (1991). *Davis's Drug Guide for Nurses,* 2nd ed. Philadelphia: F. A. Davis, p. 1218. Used with permission from Lentner, C. (ed.) (1991). *Geigy Scientific Tables,* 8th ed., Vol. 1. Basel, Switzerland: Ciba-Geigy, pp. 226–227.

Figure 5•2

West nomogram for infants and children. *Directions:* (1) find height; (2) find weight; (3) draw a straight line connecting the height and weight. Where the line intersects on the SA column is the body surface area (m²). Modified from data of E. Boyd and C. D. West, in Behrman, R. E., Kliegman, R. M., and Arvin, A. M. (1996). *Nelson Textbook of Pediatrics,* 15th ed. Philadelphia: W. B. Saunders.

a. 64 inches and 130 pounds intersect the nomogram scale at 1.69 m² (BSA), or 1.7 m² (BSA) rounded off to nearest tenth.

b. 200 mg × 1.7 m² = 340 mg/m² IV daily for 5 days.

BSA USING SLIDE RULE

BSA slide rules based on nomograms are another tool used by practitioners to easily determine drug dosages.

Use a BSA slide rule as follows; Figure 5–3 shows an example of a BSA slide rule:

1. Slide the scale for wieght so that the client's weight is aligned with the mark, using the "lb" mark for client's weight in pounds or the "kg" mark for client's weight in kilograms.

2. On the scale for height, find the client's height, in either centimeters or inches.

3. Now look on the point on the "BSA" or "Surface Area" scale that corresponds directly with the client's height. The number at that point is the client's BSA.

BSA nomogram slide rules often have the adult values on one side and the children's values on the other.

BSA USING THE SQUARE ROOT

BSA can be calculated using the square root and a fractional formula of height and weight divided by a constant, one for the metric system and another for inches and pounds. Now that calculators are readily available, research has shown that this method results in fewer errors than drawing intersecting lines on a nomogram. Conversion of weight and height to the same system of measure is necessary first.

Figure 5•3

Using a body surface area calculator. Client, an adult, weighs 175 lb (1) and is 5′2″ or 62 in. (2). BSA, as shown on the calculator, is 1.8 m² (3).

The BSA metric formula is:

$$BSA = \sqrt{\frac{ht(cm) \times wt\ (kg)}{3600}}$$

The BSA Inches and Pounds Formula is:

$$BSA = \sqrt{\frac{ht(in) \times wt\ (lb)}{3131}}$$

....

examples

PROBLEM 1: Order: cisplatin (Platinol) 50 mg/m²/cycle IV. Client weighs 84.5 kg and is 168 cm tall. Use the BSA metric formula.

a. $BSA = \sqrt{\dfrac{168\ cm \times 84.5\ kg}{3600}}$

$BSA = \sqrt{\dfrac{14196}{3600}}$

$BSA = \sqrt{3.94}$

$BSA = 1.98\ m^2$

b. 50 mg × 1.98 m² = 99 mg/m², or 100 mg/m².

PROBLEM 2: Order: melphalon (Alkeran) 16 mg/m² q 2 weeks. Client is 68 inches tall and weighs 172 pounds. Use the BSA inches and pounds formula.

a. $BSA = \sqrt{\dfrac{68\ in \times 172\ lbs.}{3131}}$

$BSA = \sqrt{\dfrac{11696}{3131}}$

$BSA = \sqrt{3.73}$

$BSA = 1.9\ m^2$

b. 16 mg × 1.9 m² = 30.4 mg/m² or 30 mg/m².

NOTE The future of individualizing drug dosages may be based on calculating Lean Body Mass, which involves height, weight and age values, or dosage that is based on renal and hepatic plasma clearance of a drug.

SUMMARY PRACTICE PROBLEMS

Solve the following calculation problems using Method 1, 2, or 3. To convert units within the metric system (grams to milligrams), refer to Chapter 1. To convert apothecary to metric systems and vice versa, refer to Chapter 2 or Table 5–1. For reading drug labels, refer to Chapter 3. Several of the calculation problems have drug labels. Drug dosage and drug form are printed on the drug label.

Extra practice problems are available in the chapters on oral drugs, injectable drugs, and pediatric drug administration.

1. Order: lorazepam (Ativan) 1 mg, po, tid.
   Drug available:

How many tablet(s) would you give? _____

2. Order: sulfisoxazole (Gantrisin) 1 g.
   Drug available: sulfisoxazole (Gantrisin) 250 mg per tablet.
   How many tablet(s) would you give? _____

3. The physician ordered erythromycin 500 mg, po, q8h, for 7 days. Drug available:

   a. How many tablets would you order for 7 days? _____

   b. How many tablets would you give every 8 hours? _____

4. Order: clarithromycin (Biaxin) 100 mg, po, q6h.
   Drug available:

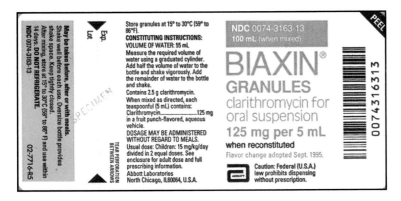

How many milliliters (mL) should the client receive per dose?

5. Order: phenytoin (Dilantin) 50 mg, po, bid.
Drug available:

a. Which Dilantin container would you select? _____

b. How many Dilantin capsules would you give per dose? _____

6. Order: methyldopa (Aldomet) 150 mg, po, tid.
Drug available:

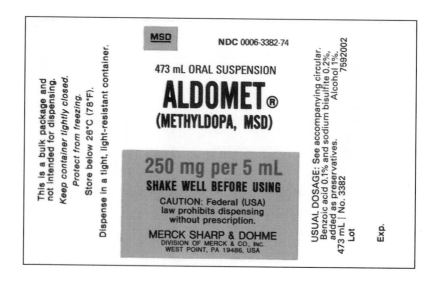

How many mL would you give per dose? _____

7. Order: dexamethasone (Decadron) 0.5 mg, po, qid.
Drug available:

a. How many tablets would you give per dose? _____

b. How many milligrams would the client receive per day? _____

8. Order: diltiazem (Cardizem) SR 120 mg, po, bid for hypertension.
Drugs available:

a. Which drug bottle should be selected? _____

b. How many tablet(s) should the client receive per dose? _____

9. Order: cimetidine (Tagamet) 0.2 g, po, qid.
   Drug available:

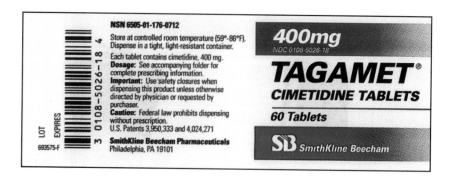

How many tablet(s) would you give per dose? _____

10. Order: codeine gr 1, po, STAT.
    Drug available:

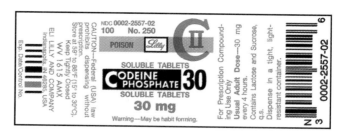

How many tablet(s) should the client receive? _____

11. Order: methylprednisolone (Medrol) 75 mg, IM.
    Drug available: Medrol 125 mg per 2 mL per ampule.

    How many mL would you give? _____

12. Order: sulfisoxazole (Gantrisin) 50 mg/kg daily in 4 divided doses (q6h).
    The client weighs 44 pounds.

    How many milligrams should the client receive per dose? _____

13. Order: ticarcillin disodium (Ticar), 200 mg/kg/d in 4 divided doses, IV.
    Client weighs 176 pounds.
    Max dose: 40 q/d.
    Drug available:

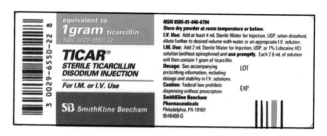

a. How many kilograms does the client weigh? _____

b. How many milligrams per day _____ mg/d; and how many milligrams per dose? _____ mg, q6h; or how many grams per dose? _____ g, q6h.

14. Order: kanamycin (Kantrex) 15 mg/kg/day in 3 divided doses (q8h), IV. Drug is to be diluted in 100 mg of D_5W. The client weighs 180 pounds. Drug available:

a. How many mg should the client receive per day? _____

b. How many mg should the client receive per dose? _____

c. How many mL should the client receive per dose? _____

15. Order: sulfisoxazole (Gantrisin) 2 g/m^2 daily in 4 divided doses (q6h). The client weighs 110 pounds and is 60 inches tall.

How many milligrams should the client receive per dose? _____

16. Order: doxorubicin (Adriamycin) 60 mg/m^2 IV per month. Client weighs 120 pounds and is 5'2" (62 inches) tall.

How many milligrams should the client receive? _____

17. Order: etoposide (VePesid) 100 $mg/m^2/d \times 5d$. Client weighs 180 pounds and is 70 inches tall. Drug available:

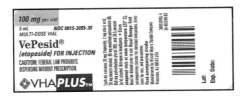

a. What is the BSA? _____

b. How many milligrams (mg) should the client receive? _____

c. How many milliliters are needed? _____

Dimensional Analysis (Factor Labeling)

18. Order: aminocaproic acid 1.5 g, po, STAT.
    Drug available: aminocaproic acid 500 mg tablet.
    Factors: 500 mg = tablet (drug label)
    Conversion factor: 1 g = 1000 mg

    How many tablet(s) would you give? _____

19. Order: ampicillin (Principen) 50 mg/kg/day, po, in 4 divided doses (q6h).
    Client weighs 88 pounds, or 40 kg (88 ÷ 2.2 = 40 kg).
    Drug available:

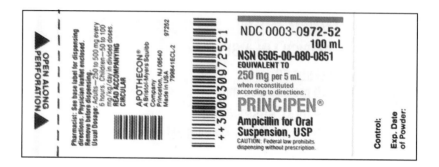

    Factors: 250 mg = 5 mL (drug label)
    Conversion factor: none (both are in milligrams)

    a. How many milligrams per day should the client receive? _____

    b. How many milligrams per dose should the client receive?

    _____

    c. How many milliliters should the client receive per dose (q6h)?

    _____

20. Order: cimetidine (Tagamet) 0.8 g, po, hs.
    Drug available:

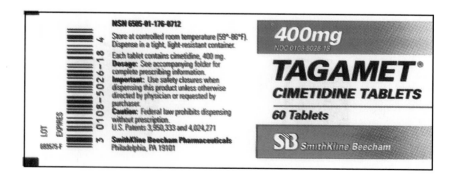

    Factors: 400 mg = 1 tablet (drug label)
           0.8 g/l (drug order)

Conversion factor: 1 g = 1000 mg (units of measurements are not the same; conversion factor is needed)

How many tablet(s) would you give? _____

21. Order: codeine gr i (1), po, STAT.
Drug available:

Factors: 30 mg = 1 tablet (drug label)
　　　　 gr 1/1 (drug order)
Conversion factor: 1 gr = 60 mg

How many tablet(s) would you give? _____

22. Order: amikacin (Amikin) 250 mg, IM, q6h.
Drug available:

Factors: 1 g = 4 mL (drug label)
　　　　 250 mg/1 (drug order)
Conversion factor: 1 g = 1000 mg

How many milliliters would you give? _____

BSA by Square Root

23. Order: Vinblastine sulfate (Velban) 7.4 mg/m² IV × 1. Client's height is 115 cm and weight is 52 kg. Use BSA metric formula to determine dosage.

Drug available:

How many milligrams should the client receive?

24. Order: Etoposide (VePesid) 50 mg/m² day IV. Client's height is 72 inches and weight is 190 pounds.
How many milligrams should the client receive?

ANSWERS

1. $\dfrac{D}{H} \times V = \dfrac{1}{0.5} \times 1$ **or**   H : V :: D : X   **or** $\dfrac{0.5}{1} = \dfrac{1}{X}$
                          0.5 mg : 1 tab :: 1 mg : X tab

          $= \dfrac{1}{0.5} = 2$ tablets   0.5 X = 1   0.5 X = 1
                             X = 2 tablets   X = 2 tablets

2. 4 tablets

3. a. 2 tablets × 3 doses per day × 7 days = 42 tablets

   b. 2 tablets every 8 hrs

4. $\dfrac{D}{H} \times V = \dfrac{100}{\underset{25}{\cancel{125}}} \times \dfrac{\overset{1}{\cancel{5}}}{1} =$ H : V :: D : X
                               125 : 5 :: 100 : X

                               125 X = 500

    $\dfrac{100}{25} = 4$ mL   X $= \dfrac{500}{125} = 4$ mL

5. a. The nurse could *not* use either of the Dilantins.

   b. A capsule *cannot* be cut in half. The physician should be notified. Dilantin dose should be changed.

6. $\dfrac{D}{H} \times V = \dfrac{150}{50} \times \cancel{5}^{1}$ **or**   H : V :: D : X
                           250 : 5 :: 150 : X

    $\dfrac{150}{50} = 3$ mL   250 X = 750
                        X = 3 mL

7. a. $\dfrac{D}{H} \times V = \dfrac{0.5}{0.25}$ **or**   H : V :: D : X
                         0.25 : 1 tablet :: 0.5 : X tablets

      $0.25\overline{)0.50}^{\,2.} = 2$ tablets   0.25 X = 0.5
                          X = 2 tablets

   b. 2 mg

8. a. Cardizem SR 60 mg

   b. 2 SR capsules per dose

9. Change grams to milligrams by moving the decimal three spaces to the right (see Chapter 1, Metric System).

$$0.2 \text{ g} = 0.200 \text{ mg (200 mg)}$$

$\dfrac{D}{H} \times V = \dfrac{200}{400} \times 1 \text{ tablet}$ **or**

$\qquad = \dfrac{200}{400} = \text{½ tablet}$

H : V :: D : X
400 mg : 1 tablet : : 200 mg : X tablet
$\qquad 400 \text{ X} = 200$
$\qquad \text{X} = \dfrac{200}{400} = 0.5 \text{ or ½ tablet}$

10. Change grains to milligrams (see Chapter 2 or Table 5–1): 1 gr = 60 mg.

$\dfrac{D}{H} \times V = \dfrac{60}{30} \times 1$ **or**

$\qquad = \dfrac{60}{30} = 2 \text{ tablets}$

H : V :: D : X
30 mg : 1 tablet : : 60 mg : X tablet
$\qquad 30 \text{ X} = 60$
$\qquad \text{X} = 2 \text{ tablets}$

11. $\dfrac{D}{H} \times V = \dfrac{75}{125} \times 2$ **or**

$\qquad = \dfrac{150}{125} = 1.2 \text{ mL}$

H : V : : D : X
125 : 2 : : 75 : X
$\qquad 125 \text{ X} = 150$
$\qquad \text{X} = 1.2 \text{ mL}$

or

$\dfrac{125}{2} = \dfrac{75}{\text{X}}$
$\qquad 125 \text{ X} = 150$
$\qquad \text{X} = 1.2 \text{ mL}$

12. Change 44 pounds to kilograms: 44 ÷ 2.2 = 20 kg.

$$50 \text{ mg} \times 20 \text{ kg} \times 1 \text{ day} = 1000 \text{ mg of Gantrisin per day}$$

$$1000 \text{ mg} \div 4 \text{ times per day (q6h)} = 250 \text{ mg q6h}$$

13. **a.** Client weighs 80 kg

b. 200 mg × 80 = 16,000 mg per day; 4,000 mg per dose or 4 g per dose (q6h)

14. Change 180 pounds to kilograms: 180 ÷ 2.2 = 81.8 kg
a. 15 mg × 82 kg = 1230 mg per day
b. 1230 ÷ 3 times a day (q8h) = 410 mg (400 mg, q8h)

c. $\dfrac{D}{H} \times V = \dfrac{400}{500} \times 2$ **or**

$\qquad = \dfrac{800}{500} = 1.6 \text{ mL}$

H : V :: D : X
500 mg : 2 mL : : 400 mg : X mL
$\qquad 500 \text{ X} = 800$
$\qquad \text{X} = 1.6 \text{ mL}$

Give kanamycin 1.6 mL

15. 60 inches and 110 pounds intersect the nomogram scale at 1.5 m².

$$2 \text{ g} \times 1.5 \text{ m}^2 = 3 \text{ g or 3000 mg per day}$$

$$3000 \text{ mg} \div 4 \text{ times per day} = 750 \text{ mg}$$

16. 62 inches and 120 pounds intersect the nomogram scale at 1.6 m².

$$60 \text{ mg} \times 1.6 \text{ m}^2 = 96 \text{ mg of Adriamycin}$$

17. **a.** With the use of the nomogram, the BSA is 2.06
b. 100 mg × 2.06 = 206 mg or 200 mg.

c. The amount of VePesid use should be 10 mL

$$\frac{D}{H} \times V = \frac{200}{100} \times 5 = 10 \text{ mL}$$

Dimensional Analysis (Factor Labeling)

18. $\text{Tablets} = \dfrac{1 \text{ tablet} \times \overset{2}{\cancel{1000 \text{ mg}}} \times 1.5 \cancel{g}}{\underset{1}{\cancel{500 \text{ mg}}} \times 1 \cancel{g} \times 1} = \dfrac{3.0}{1} = 3 \text{ tablets}$

19. a. 50 mg/kg/day
$50 \times 40 = 2000 \text{ mg}$
   b. $2000 \text{ mg} \div 4 = 500 \text{ mg per dose.}$

   c. $\text{mL} = \dfrac{5 \text{ mL} \times \overset{2}{\cancel{500 \text{ mg}}}}{\underset{1}{\cancel{250 \text{ mg}}} \times 1} = \dfrac{10}{1} = 10 \text{ mL}$

20. $\text{Tablets} = \dfrac{1 \text{ tablet} \times \overset{10}{\cancel{1000 \text{ mg}}} \times 0.8 \cancel{g}}{\underset{4}{\cancel{400 \text{ mg}}} \times 1 \cancel{g} \times 1} = \dfrac{10 \times 0.8}{4} = \dfrac{8}{4} = 2 \text{ tablets}$

21. $\text{Tablets} = \dfrac{1 \text{ tablet} \times \overset{2}{\cancel{60 \text{ mg}}} \times 1 \cancel{gr}}{\underset{1}{\cancel{30 \text{ mg}}} \times 1 \cancel{gr} \times 1} = 2 \text{ tablets}$

22. $\text{Milliliters} = \dfrac{4 \text{ mL} \times 1 \cancel{g} \times \overset{1}{\cancel{250 \text{ mg}}}}{1 \cancel{g} \times \underset{4}{\cancel{1000 \text{ mg}}} \times 1} = \dfrac{4}{4} = 1 \text{ mL}$

BSA by Square Root

23. a. $\text{BSA} = \sqrt{\dfrac{115 \text{ cm} \times 52 \text{ kg}}{3600}}$

   $\text{BSA} = \sqrt{\dfrac{5980}{3600}}$

   $\text{BSA} = \sqrt{1.66}$

   $\text{BSA} = 1.28 \text{ m}^2$

   b. $7.4 \text{ mg} \times 1.28 \text{ m}^2 = 9.4 \text{ mg/m}^2$

24. a. $\text{BSA} = \sqrt{\dfrac{72 \text{ in} \times 190 \text{ lbs}}{3131}}$

   $\text{BSA} = \sqrt{\dfrac{13680}{3131}}$

   $\text{BSA} = \sqrt{4.36}$

   $\text{BSA} = 2.0 \text{ m}^2$

   b. $50 \text{ mg} \times 2.0 \text{ m}^2 = 100 \text{ mg/m}^2$

part

three

calculations for oral, injectable, and intravenous drugs

oral and enteral preparations with clinical applications

Objectives

- State the advantages and disadvantages of administering oral medications.
- Calculate oral dosages from tablets, capsules, and liquids using given formulas.
- Give the rationale for diluting and not diluting oral liquid medications.
- Explain the method for administering sublingual medication.
- Calculate the amount of drug to be given per day in divided doses.
- Determine the amount of tube feeding solution needed for dilution according to the percent ordered.
- Determine the amount of water needed to dilute liquid medication.

Outline

Oral administration of drugs is considered a convenient and economical method of giving medications. Oral drugs are available as tablets, capsules, powders, and liquids. Oral medications are referred to as po (per os, or by mouth) drugs and are absorbed by the gastrointestinal tract, mainly from the small intestine.

There are some disadvantages in administering oral medications, such as: (1) variation in absorption rate due to gastric and intestinal pH and food consumption within the gastrointestinal tract; (2) irritation of the gastric mucosa causing nausea, vomiting, or ulceration, e.g., with oral potassium chloride; (3) retention or inactivation of the drug in the body because of reduced liver function; (4) destruction of drugs by digestive enzymes; (5) aspiration of drugs into the lungs by seriously ill or confused patients; and (6) discoloration of tooth enamel, e.g., with a saturated solution of potassium iodide (SSKI). Oral administration is an effective way to give medications in many instances, and at times it is the route of choice.

Body weight and body surface area were discussed in Chapter 5. When solving drug problems that require body weight or body surface area, refer to Chapter 5.

Enteral nutrition and enteral medication are discussed toward the end of the chapter. Calculations of percent for enteral feeding solutions and enteral medication are discussed.

TABLETS AND CAPSULES

Most tablets are scored and can be broken in halves and sometimes in quarter (Fig. 6–1). Half of a tablet may be indicated when the drug does not come in a lesser strength. Half-tablets may not be broken equally; therefore, the patient may receive less than or more than the required dose. Also, crushing a drug tablet does not ensure that the patient will receive the entire drug dose. Some of the crushed tablet could be lost. Instead of halving or crushing a drug tablet, use the liquid form of the drug, if available, to ensure proper drug dosage.

Capsules are gelatin shells containing powder or time pellets. Time-release capsules should remain intact and not be divided in any way. Many drugs that come in capsules also come in liquid form. When a smaller dose is indicated and is not available in tablet or capsule, the liquid form of the drug is used (Fig. 6–2).

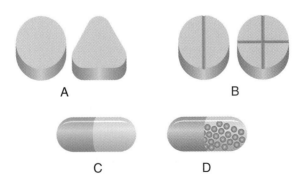

A   B

C   D

Figure 6•1
Shapes of tablets (*A* and *B*) and capsules (*C* and *D*). From Kee, J., & Hayes, E. (2000). *Pharmacology: A Nursing Process Approach* (3rd ed.). Philadelphia: W.B. Saunders.

Figure 6•2
Medicine cup for liquid measurement. From Kee, J.,
& Hayes, E. (2000). *Pharmacology: A Nursing Process
Approach* (3rd ed.). Philadelphia: W.B. Saunders.

CAUTION

- A tablet that is NOT scored should not be broken.
- Instead of breaking or crushing a tablet, use the liquid form if available.
- Time-release capsules should not be crushed and diluted, because the entire medication could be absorbed rapidly.
- Enteric-coated tablets must NOT be crushed, because the medication could irritate the stomach. Enteric-coated tablets are absorbed by the small intestine.
- Tablets or capsules that are irritating to the gastric mucosa should be taken with 6 to 8 ounces of fluid, with meals, or immediately after meals.

Calculation of Tablets and Capsules

To determine the drug dose, the following steps should be taken:

1. Check the drug order.
2. Determine the drug available (generic name, brand name, and dosage per drug form).
3. Set up the method for drug calculation (basic formula, ratio and proportion, fraction equation, or dimensional analysis).
4. Convert to the like units of measurement within the same system before solving the problem. Use the unit of measure on the drug container to calculate the drug dose.
5. Solve for the unknown (**X**).

Decide which of the methods of calculation you wish to use and then use that same method for calculating all dosages. In the following examples, the basic formula and the ratio and proportion methods are used.

Basic Formula

$$\frac{D \text{ (desired dose)}}{H \text{ (on-hand dose)}} \times V = \text{(vehicle)}$$

Ratio and proportion

$$H : V :: D : X$$
on hand vehicle desired dose X

PROBLEM 1: Order: pravastatin sodium (Pravachol) 20 mg, q.d.
Drug available:

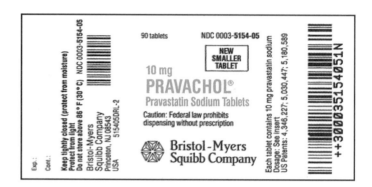

Methods: $\dfrac{D}{H} \times V$

$$H \quad : \quad V \quad :: \quad D \quad : \quad X$$
$$10\ mg : 1\ tab :: 20\ mg : X\ tab$$

$$\frac{20}{10} \times 1 = 2\ tablets$$

$$10\,X = 20$$
$$X = 2\ tablets$$

Answer: Pravachol 20 mg = 2 tablets, daily.

PROBLEM 2: Order: erythromycin (ERY-TAB) 0.5 g, qid.
Drug available:

Note: Gram (g) and milligram (mg) are both units in the metric system. *Remember:* when changing grams (larger unit) to milligrams (smaller unit), move the decimal point three spaces to the right. Refer to Chapter 1, Table 2–1, or Table 5–1. Because the drug dose on the drug label is in milligrams, conversion should be from grams to milligrams.

Methods: 0.5 g = 0.500 mg (Method A)

$$\frac{D}{H} \times V = \frac{500}{250} \times 1 \quad \textbf{or} \quad H \quad : \quad V \quad :: \quad D \quad : \quad X$$
$$250\ mg : 1\ tab :: 500\ mg : X\ tab$$

$$= \frac{500}{250} = 2\ tablets$$

$$250\,X = 500$$
$$X = 2\ tablets$$

Answer: ERY-TAB 0.5 g = 2 tablets

PROBLEM 3: Order: aspirin gr x, po, STAT.

Drug available: aspirin 325 mg per tablet.

Note: *The dose is ordered in the apothecary system, gr x, and the label on the drug bottle is in the metric system (325 mg). Use Table 2−1 or Table 5−1 to convert units.*

Methods: 325 mg = gr v (5) and 650 mg = gr X (10)

$$\frac{D}{H} \times V = \frac{10 \text{ gr}}{5 \text{ gr}} \times 1 = \frac{10}{5} = 2 \text{ tablets} \quad \textbf{or} \quad \begin{array}{c} H \;:\; V \;::\; D \;:\; X \\ 5 \text{ gr} : 1 \text{ tab} :: 10 \text{ gr} : X \text{ tab} \end{array}$$

$$5 X = 10$$
$$X = 2 \text{ tablets}$$

or

$$\frac{D}{H} \times V = \frac{650 \text{ mg}}{325 \text{ mg}} \times 1 = \frac{650}{325} = 2 \text{ tablets}$$

Answer: *Aspirin gr x = 2 tablets.*

LIQUIDS

Liquid medications come as tinctures, elixirs, suspensions, and syrups. Some liquid medications are irritating to the gastric mucosa and must be well diluted before being given, e.g., KCl (potassium chloride). Usually, liquid cough medicines are not diluted. Medications in tincture form are always diluted.

- Concentrated liquid medication that can irritate the gastric mucosa should be diluted in *at least* 4 ounces of fluid.

- Liquid medication that can discolor the teeth *should be well diluted* and taken through a drinking straw.

CAUTION

Calculation of Liquid Medications

examples

PROBLEM 1: Order: potassium chloride (KCl) 20 mEq, bid.

Drug available: liquid potassium chloride 10 mEq per 5 mL.

Methods: $\dfrac{D}{H} \times V = \dfrac{20}{10} \times 5$ **or** $\begin{array}{c} H \;:\; V \;::\; D \;:\; X \\ 10 \text{ mEq} : 5 \text{ mL} :: 20 \text{ mEq} : X \text{ mL} \end{array}$

$$= \frac{100}{10} = 10 \text{ mL} \qquad \qquad 10 X = 100$$
$$X = 10 \text{ mL}$$

Answer: Potassium chloride 20 mEq = 10 mL

PROBLEM 2: Order: amoxicillin (Amoxil) 0.25 g, po, tid.
Drug available:

Change grams to milligrams: 0.25 g = 0.250 mg.

Methods: $\dfrac{D}{H} \times V = \dfrac{250}{125} \times 5$ **or**

$$H \quad : \quad V \quad :: \quad D \quad : \quad X$$
$$125 \text{ mg} : 5 \text{ mL} :: 250 \text{ mg} : X \text{ mL}$$

$$= \dfrac{1250}{125} = 10 \text{ mL}$$

$$125 \, X = 1250$$
$$X = 10 \text{ mL}$$

Answer: Amoxil 0.25 g = 10 mL

PROBLEM 3: Give SSKI 300 mg, q6h, diluted in water.
Drug available: saturated solution of potassium iodide, 50 mg per drop (gt), drops (gtt).

Methods: $\dfrac{D}{H} \times V = \dfrac{300}{50} \times 1$ **or**

$$H \quad : \quad V \quad :: \quad D \quad : \quad X$$
$$50 \text{ mg} : 1 \text{ gt} :: 300 \text{ mg} : X \text{ gtt}$$

$$= \dfrac{300}{50} = 6 \text{ gtt}$$

$$50 \, X = 300$$
$$X = 6 \text{ gtt}$$

Answer: SSKI 300 mg = 6 gtt (drops)

SUBLINGUAL TABLETS

Few drugs are administered sublingually (tablet placed under the tongue). Sublingual tablets are small and soluble and are quickly absorbed by the numerous capillaries on the underside of the tongue.

> - *Do not* swallow a sublingual tablet, e.g., nitroglycerin (NTG). If the drug is swallowed, the desired immediate action of the drug is decreased or lost.
> - Fluids *should not* be taken until the drug has dissolved.

CAUTION

Calculation of Sublingual Medications

examples

PROBLEM 1: Order: nitroglycerin (Nitrostat) 0.6 mg, sublingually (SL).
Drug available:

Note: The systems and weights must be the same. See Table 2–1 or Table 5–1. The label has both systems of measurement.

$$0.6 \text{ mg} = \text{gr } \tfrac{1}{100}$$

Methods:

$$\frac{D}{H} \times V = \frac{0.6}{0.6} \times 1 \quad \textbf{or}$$

$$
\begin{array}{ccccc}
H & : & V & :: & D & : \\
\dfrac{1}{100} \text{ gr} & : 1 \text{ tab} & :: & \dfrac{1}{100} \text{ gr} & : X \text{ tab}
\end{array}
$$

$$\frac{1}{100} X = \frac{1}{100}$$

$$= \frac{0.6}{0.6} = 1 \text{ SL tablet} \qquad X = \frac{1}{100} \times \frac{100}{1} = 1 \text{ SL tablet}$$

Answer: nitroglycerin (Nitrostat) 0.6 mg = 1 SL tablet

PROBLEM 2: Order: isosorbide dinitrate (Isordil) 5 mg sublingually.
Drug available: Isordil 2.5 mg per tablet.

Method: $\dfrac{D}{H} \times V = \dfrac{5}{2.5} \times 1 \quad \textbf{or}$

$$
\begin{array}{ccccccc}
H & : & V & :: & D & : & X \\
2.5 \text{ mg} & : 1 \text{ tab} & :: & 5 \text{ mg} & : X \text{ tab}
\end{array}
$$

$$2.5 X = 5$$

$$= 2 \text{ SL tablets} \qquad X = 2 \text{ SL tablets}$$

Answer: Isordil 5 mg = 2 SL tablets

I Practice Problems: Oral Medications

For each question, calculate the correct dosage that should be administered.

1. Order: Coumadin 5 mg, po, qd.
Drug available:

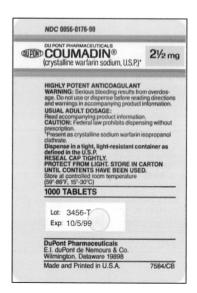

a. How many tablet(s) would you give? _____

b. Check the expiration date. Would you give the drug from this bottle? Explain.

2. Order: sulfisoxazole (Gantrisin) 0.5 g.
Drug available: Gantrisin 250 mg per tablet.

3. Order: digoxin (Lanoxin) 0.5 mg.
Drug available:

4. Order: codeine gr 1, PRN, q4h.
Drug available:

5. Order: potassium chloride 40 mEq, po.
Drug available: potassium chloride 20 mEq/15 mL.

6. Order: Cefaclor (Ceclor) 250 mg, q8h.
Drug available:

a. Which Ceclor bottle would you select? Why? _____

b. How many mL per dose should the patient receive? _____

7. Order: ProSom (estazolam) 2 mg, po, hs.
Drug available: 1 mg tablet

a. How many tablet(s) should be given? _____

b. What time of day would you administer ProSom? _____

8. Order: cefuroxime axetil (Ceftin) 400 mg, q12h.
Drug available:

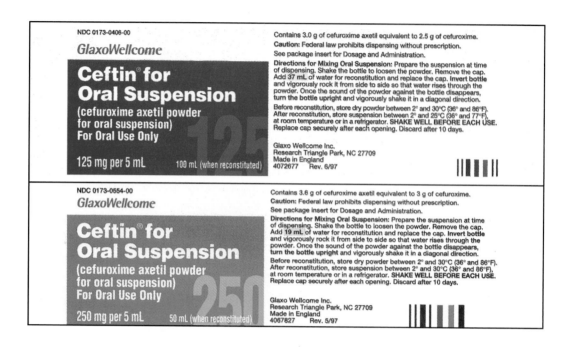

a. How many mL should the client receive? _____

b. Which drug bottle would you use? _____

Why? _____

9. Order: Dicloxacillin (Dynapen) 100 mg, q6h.
Drug available:

How many mL should the client receive? _____

10. Order: HydroDiuril 50 mg, po, qd.
    Drug available:

    a. Which drug bottle would you use? _____

    b. How many tablet(s) would you give, if the tablet(s) are not

       scored? _____

       Explain. _____

11. Order: simvastatin (Zocor) 30 mg, qd.
    Drug available:

a. Which bottle(s) of Zocor would you select? Why?

_____

b. How many tablet(s) should the client receive? _____

12. Order: cefadroxil (Duricef) 0.4 g, po, q6h.
    Drug available:

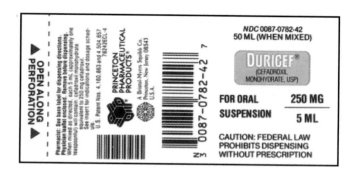

How many mL should the client receive per dose? _____

13. Order: phenobarbital gr $\overline{ss}$.
    Drug available: phenobarbital 15 mg per tablet.

14. Order: cefprozil (Cefzil) 100 mg, po, q12h.
    Drug available:

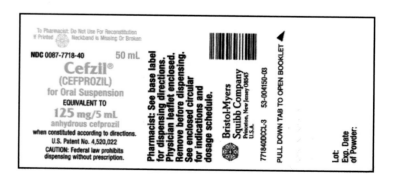

How many mL should the client receive per dose? _____

15. Order: meperidine (Demerol) 100 mg, po, q4h, PRN for pain.
Drug available: (unit [individualized] packaged doses)

How many tablet(s) of meperidine would you give? _____

16. Order: nitroglycerin gr $\frac{1}{150}$, SL, STAT.
Drug available:

Which Nitrostat SL tablet would you give? (Refer to Table 2–1 or Table 5–1 if needed.) _____

17. Order: Mycostatin 250,000 U oral swish and swallow, qid.
Drug available:

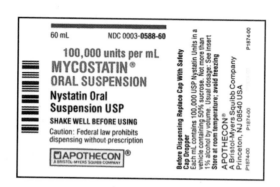

Calculate the correct dosage.

18. Order: diazepam (Valium) 2½ mg.
Drug available: Valium 5 mg scored tablet.
Calculate the correct dosage.

19. Order: ondansetron HCl (Zofran) 6 mg, 30 min before chemotherapy, then q8h × 2 more doses.
Drug available:

How many milliliters (mL) would you give per dose?

_____

20. Order: allopurinol 450 mg, po, qd.
Drug available: allopurinol 300 mg scored tablet.
Calculate the correct dosage.

21. Order: cefadroxil (Duricef) 1 g, po, as a loading dose; then cefadroxil 0.5 g, po, q12h.

Drug available:

a. Which drug bottle would you select? _____

b. How many milliliters would you give as the loading dose?

_____

c. How many milliliters per 0.5 g? _____

22. Order: lorazepam (Ativan) 0.5 mg, po, q6h.
Drug available: scored tablet.

Calculate the correct dosage.

Questions 23–27 relate to body weight and body surface area. Refer to Chapter 5 as necessary.

23. Order: valproic acid (Depakene) 10 mg/kg/day in three divided doses (tid), po. Client weighs 165 pounds. How much Depakene should be administered tid? _____

24. Order: cyclophosphamide (Cytoxan) 4 mg/kg/day, po. Client weighs 154 pounds. How much Cytoxan would you give per day?

_____

25. Order: mercaptopurine 2.5 mg/kg/day po or 100 mg/m² body surface area po. The client weighs 132 pounds and is 64 inches tall. The estimated body surface area according to the nomogram is 1.7 m². The amount of drug the client should receive according to body weight is

_____ and according to body surface area is _____.

26. Order: ethosuximide (Zarontin) 20 mg/kg/day in 2 divided doses (q12h). Client weighs 110 pounds (110 ÷ 2.2 = 50 kg). Drug available:

a. How many milligrams should the client receive per day? _____

b. How many tablet(s) should the client receive per dose? _____

27. Order: minocycline HCl (Minocin) 4 mg/kg/day in 2 divided doses (q12h). Client weighs 132 pounds (132 ÷ 2.2 = 60 kg). Drug available: Minocin 50 mg/5 mL.

a. How many milligrams should the client receive per day? _____

b. How many milliliters (mL) should the client receive per dose?

_____

Questions 28–32 relate to dimensional analysis (factor labeling). Refer to Chapter 5 as necessary.

28. Order: methyldopa (Aldomet) 0.5 g, po, qd.

Drug available: drug label: _____ mg = _____ tablet.

Factors: 250 mg = 1 tablet (drug label)
        0.5 g/l (drug order)
Conversion factors: 1 g = 1000 mg

How many tablet(s) of methyldopa 250 mg would you give? _____

29. Order: Vasotec 5 mg, po, bid.
Drug available:

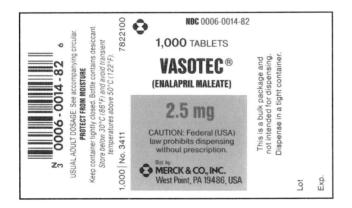

Factors: 2.5 mg = 1 tablet (drug label); 5 mg/l (drug order)
Conversion factor: none

How many tablet(s) should the client receive? _____

30. Order: amoxicillin (Amoxil) 0.4 g, po, q6h.
Drug available:

Factors: 250 mg/5 mL (drug label); 0.4 g/l (drug order)
Conversion factor: 1 g = 1000 mg

How many mL would you give? _____

31. Order: acetaminophen (Tylenol) gr x, po.
Drug available:

Factors: _____

Conversion factor: _____

How many acetaminophen tablets would you give? _____

32. Order: oxacillin sodium 125 mg, po, q6h.
Drug available:

Factors: _____

Conversion factor: _____

How many mL of oxacillin would you give? _____

ENTERAL NUTRITION AND DRUG ADMINISTRATION

When the client is unable to take nourishment by mouth, enteral feeding (tube feeding) is usually preferred over intravenous therapy. Candidates for enteral feedings are clients with neurologic deficits who have difficulty swallowing; debilitated clients; clients with burns and malnutrition disorders; clients with upper gastric obstructions; and clients who have undergone radical head and neck surgery. The cost of enteral feedings is much less than that of intravenous therapy and there is less risk for infection.

Drugs that can be administered orally can be given via enteral tube. The drug must be in liquid form or dissolved into a liquid. The only exceptions are medications in time-release form, enteric-coated form or sublingual form, and bulk-forming laxatives.

Enteral Feedings

Enteral feeding can be administered through a tube inserted into the nose (nasogastric), mouth (orogastic), stomach (gastrostomy), or jejunum (jejunostomy) (Fig. 6–3). The nasogastric and orogastric routes are primarily for short-term use and cause nasal and pharyngeal irritation if usage is prolonged. The gastrostomy and jejunostomy routes are for long-term feeding and require a surgical procedure for insertion.

Enteral feedings may be given as a bolus (intermittent) or as a continuous drip feeding over a specified period. With bolus feedings, the amount of solution administered is approximately 200 mL or less, and feeding times per day are more frequent. Continuous feedings can be given by gravity flow from a bag or by infusion pump (Fig. 6–4).

There are many types of enteral feeding solutions designed to meet the nutritional needs of clients. Names of common feeding solutions are listed in Table 6–1.

Although enteral feeding solutions are formulated to be given full strength, this strength may not be tolerated. Solutions that are highly concentrated (hyperosmolar or hypertonic) when given in full strength can

table 6•1 COMMON ENTERAL FORMULATIONS		
Ensure	Isocal	Nepho
Ensure Plus	Sustacal	Ultracal
Ensure HN	Sustacal HC	Jevity
Osmolite	Vital	Criticare
Osmolite HN	Pulmocare	Promote

Nasogastric   Nasoduodenal/nasojejunal

Gastrostomy   Jejunostomy

Figure 6•3

Types of gastrointestinal tubes for enteral feedings. A *nasogastric* tube is passed from the nose into the stomach. A weighted *nasoduodenal/nasojejunal* tube is passed through the nose into the duodenum/jejunum. A *gastrostomy* tube is introduced through a temporary or permanent opening on the abdominal wall (stoma) into the stomach. A *jejunostomy* tube is passed through a stoma directly into the jejunum. From Kee, J., & Hayes, E. (2000). *Pharmacology: A Nursing Process Approach* (3rd ed.). Philadelphia: W.B. Saunders. With adaptation from Davis, J. R., and Sherer, K.: Applied Nutrition and Diet Therapy for Nurses, 2nd ed. Philadelphia: W.B. Saunders, p. 354, 1994.

cause vomiting, cramping, or excessive diarrhea. When gastrointestinal symptoms occur, the enteral solution can be diluted with water. In many situations, clients develop better gastrointestinal tolerance when the strength of the solution is gradually increased. It may take 3 to 5 days for gastrointestinal tolerance to appear. When enteral feedings are less than full strength, they are ordered in percent (%). The nurse must calculate the amount of solution and the amount of water that should be given.

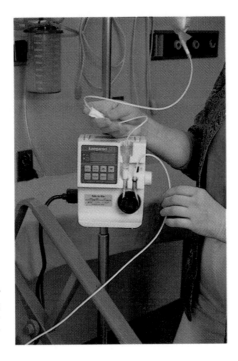

Figure 6•4
Enteral infusion pump. From Lindeman, C., &
McAthie, M. (1999). *Fundamentals of Contemporary Nursing Practice.* Philadelphia: W.B. Saunders.

CALCULATION OF PERCENT FOR ENTERAL FEEDING SOLUTIONS

Percent (%) of a solution indicates its strength. Percent is a portion of 100, e.g., 20% is 20 of 100 parts (20/100). To find percent, the basic formula, ratio and proportion, or a percentage problem can be used.

D: desired percent

H: on-hand volume (100)

V: desired total volume

X: unknown amount of solution

METHODS A & B   Basic Formula *and* Ratio and Proportion

$$\frac{D}{H}\left(\frac{\text{desired \%}}{\text{on-hand volume}}\right) \times V \text{ (desired total volume)}$$

or

H   :   V   ::   D   :   X
on-hand : desired :: desired : unknown
volume total volume % amount of
solution

or

METHOD C   Percentage Problem

Desired total volume × desired % (in hundredths) = amount of tube feeding (TF) solution

Following the tube feeding, 30 mL (cc) of water should be given to clear the tubing. The tube is clamped after a bolus feeding.

· ·

examples

PROBLEM 1: A client has been receiving intravenous fluids for 5 days. A nasogastric tube was inserted, and 250 mL (cc) of 50% Ensure solution was ordered q4h for 1 day. Calculate how much Ensure and water are needed to make 250 mL (50% solution).

Methods: 50% solution is 50 in 100 parts.

$$\frac{D}{H}\left(\frac{\text{desired \%}}{\text{on-hand volume}}\right) \times V\,(\text{desired total volume}) \quad \textbf{or} \quad H : V :: D : X$$
$$100 : 250\,\text{mL} :: 50 : X\,\text{mL}$$

$$\frac{50}{100} \times 250 = \frac{12,500}{100} \qquad\qquad 100\,X = 12,500$$
$$X = 125\,\text{mL of Ensure}$$
$$= 125\,\text{mL of Ensure}$$

or

$$250\,\text{mL} \times 0.50\,(50\%) = 125\,\text{mL of TF solution}$$

How much water should be added?

$$\text{Total amount} - \text{amount of TF} = \text{amount of water}$$
$$250\,\text{mL} \quad - \quad 125\,\text{mL} \quad = \quad 125\,\text{mL}$$

Answer: 125 mL of Ensure + 125 mL of water

PROBLEM 2: Three days later, the client's tube feeding order is changed. The client is to receive 250 mL (cc) of 70% Osmolite solution q6h.

How much Osmolite solution and water should be mixed to equal 250 mL?

Methods: 70% solution is 70 in 100 parts.

$$\frac{D}{H} \times V = \frac{70}{100} \times 250 \quad \textbf{or} \quad H : V :: D : X$$
$$100 : 250\,\text{mL} :: 70 : X\,\text{mL}$$

$$= \frac{17,500}{100} = \begin{array}{l}175\,\text{mL of}\\ \text{Osmolite}\end{array} \qquad \begin{array}{l}100\,X = 17,500\\ X = 175\,\text{mL of}\\ \qquad\text{Osmolite}\end{array}$$

or

$$250\,\text{mL} \times 0.70\,(70\%) = 175\,\text{mL of TF solution}$$

How much water should be added?

$$\text{Total amount} - \text{amount of TF} = \text{amount of water}$$
$$250\,\text{mL} \quad - \quad 175\,\text{mL} \quad = \quad 75\,\text{mL}$$

Answer: 175 mL of Osmolite + 75 mL of water.

PROBLEM 3: One week later, the client's tube feeding order is changed to 250 mL (cc) of 40% Ensure Plus. How much Ensure Plus and water should be mixed to equal 250 mL?

Methods: 40% solution is 40 in 100 parts.

$$\frac{D}{H} \times V = \frac{40}{100} \times 250 \quad \textbf{or} \quad \begin{array}{l} H: \quad V \quad :: D: \quad X \\ 100: 250 \text{ mL}:: 40: X \text{ mL} \end{array}$$

$$= \frac{10,000}{100} = \begin{array}{l} 100 \text{ mL of} \\ \text{Ensure Plus} \end{array} \quad \begin{array}{l} 100 \, X = 10,000 \\ X = 100 \text{ mL of} \\ \quad \text{Ensure Plus} \end{array}$$

or

250 mL $\times$ 0.40 (40%) = 100 mL of TF solution

How much water should be added?

$$\begin{array}{ccccc} \text{Total amount} & - & \text{amount of TF} & = & \text{amount of water} \\ 250 \text{ mL} & - & 100 \text{ mL} & = & 150 \text{ mL} \end{array}$$

Answer: 100 mL of Ensure Plus + 150 mL of water.

II Practice Problems: Percent of Enteral Solutions

1. Order: 200 mL of 25% Sustacal solution q4h through a nasogastric tube. How much Sustacal solution and water should be mixed to equal 200

   mL? _____

2. Order: 300 mL of 75% Pulmocare solution q6h through a nasogastric tube. How much Pulmocare solution and water should be mixed to equal

   300 mL? _____

3. Order: 500 mL of 60% Ensure Plus solution q8h through a nasogastric tube. How much Ensure Plus solution and water should be mixed to

   equal 500 mL? _____

4. Order: 400 mL of 30% Osmolite solution q6h through a nasogastric tube. How much Osmolite solution and water should be mixed to equal 400

   mL? _____

Enteral Medications

Oral medications in liquid, tablet, or capsule form can be administered when properly diluted through the feeding tube as a bolus and then flushed from the enteral tube with water. All liquid medication is hyperosmolar (>1000 mOsm/kg) when compared with the osmolality of the secretions of the gastrointestinal tract (130 to 350 mOsm/kg). Although the hyperosmolality of liquid medication was once thought to be well tolerated by the gastrointestinal tract, research indicates that cramping, distention, vomiting, and diarrhea can be caused by the administration of undiluted hypertonic liquid medications and electrolyte solutions. Liquid medication should be diluted with water to reduce osmolality to 500 mOsm/kg to decrease gastrointestinal intolerance.

Table 6–2 lists the osmolalities of various commercial drug solutions and suspensions.

table 6·2

OSMOLALITIES OF VARIOUS COMMERCIAL DRUG SOLUTIONS AND SUSPENSIONS

PRODUCT	MANUFACTURER	AVERAGE OSMOLALITY (m/Osm/kg)
Acetaminophen elixir, 65 mg/mL	Roxane	5400
Acetaminophen with codeine elixir	Wyeth-Ayerst	4700
Amoxicillin suspension, 50 mg/mL	Squibb	2250
Ampicillin suspension, 50 mg/mL	Squibb	2250
Cascara aromatic fluid extract	Roxane	1000
Cephalexin suspension, 50 mg/mL	Dista	1950
Cimetidine solution, 60 mg/mL	SmithKline Beecham	5500
Co-trimoxazole suspension	GlaxoWellcome	2200
Dexamethasone solution, 1 mg/mL	Roxane	3100
Dextromethorphan HBr syrup, 2 mg/mL	Parke-Davis	5950
Digoxin elixir, 50 μg/mL	GlaxoWellcome	1350
Diphenhydramine HCl elixir, 2.5 mg/mL	Roxane	850
Diphenoxylate/atropine suspension	Roxane	8800
Docusate sodium syrup, 3.3 mg/mL	Roxane	3900
Erythromycin E.S. suspension, 40 mg/mL	Abbott	1750
Ferrous sulfate liquid, 60 mg/mL	Roxane	4700
Furosemide solution, 10 mg/mL	Hoechst Marion Roussel	2050
Haloperidol concentrate, 2 mg/mL	McNeil	500
Hydroxyzine HCl syrup, 2 mg/mL	Roerig	4450
Kaolin-pectin suspension	Roxane	900
Lactulose syrup, 0.67 g/mL	Roerig	3600
Lithium citrate syrup, 1.6 mEq/mL	Roxane	6850
Magnesium citrate solution	Medalist	1000
Metoclopramide HCl syrup, 1 mg/mL	A. H. Robins	8350
Milk of magnesia suspension	Pharmac. Assoc.	1250
Multivitamin liquid	Upjohn	5700
Nystatin suspension, 100,000 U/mL	Squibb	3300
Paregoric tincture	Roxane	1350
Phenytoin sodium susp., 25 mg/mL	Parke-Davis	1500
Potassium chloride liquid, 10%	Roxane	3550
Potassium iodide sat sol (SSKI), 1 g/mL	Upsher-Smith	10950
Prochlorperazine syrup, 1 mg/mL	SmithKline Beecham	3250
Promethazine HCl syrup, 1.25 mg/mL	Wyeth-Ayerst	3500
Sodium phosphate liquid, 0.5 g/mL	C. B. Fleet	7250
Theophyline solution, 5.33 mg/mL	Berlex	800
Thioridazine suspension, 20 mg/mL	Sandoz	2050

From: Estoup, M. (1994). Approaches and limitations of medication delivery in patients with enteral feeding tubes. *Critical Care Nurse*, Vol 14(1), Table 2, p. 70. Reprinted with permission of *Critical Care Nurse*, February, 1994.

CALCULATION OF DILUTION FOR ENTERAL MEDICATIONS

To determine the amount of water needed to dilute a liquid medication, the following information must be obtained:

1. Calculate the drug order to find the volume of the drug.
2. Find the osmolality of the drug (check drug literature or pharmacist).
3. Use 500 mOsm as a constant for the desired osmolality.

METHOD

Step 1 Calculate the volume of drug:

$$\frac{D}{H} \times V \quad \textbf{or} \quad H:V::D:X$$

Step 2 Find osmolality of drug:

$$\frac{\text{known mOsm}}{\text{desired mOsm}} \times \text{volume of drug} = \text{total volume of liquid}$$

Step 3 Water for dilution:

$$\text{total volume of liquid} - \text{volume of drug} = \text{volume of water for dilution}$$

examples

PROBLEM 1: Order: acetaminophen 650 mg, q6h, PRN for pain.
Drug available: acetaminophen elixir 65 mg/mL.
Average mOsm/kg = 5400.

Step 1: Calculate the volume of drug:

$$\frac{D}{H} \times V = \frac{650}{65} \times 1 \quad \textbf{or} \quad \begin{array}{c} H \ : \ V \ :: \ D \ : \ X \\ 65\ mg : 1\ mL :: 650\ mg : X\ mL \\ 65\ X = 650 \\ X = 10\ mL \end{array}$$
$$= 10\ mL$$

Step 2: Find osmolality of drug:

$$\frac{\text{known mOsm (5400)}}{\text{desired mOsm (500)}} \times \text{volume of drug (10)}$$
$$= \frac{5400}{500} \times 10 = 108\ mL$$

Step 3: Water for dilution:

$$\text{total volume of drug (108 mL)} - \text{volume of drug (10 mL)}$$
$$= 98\ mL\ \text{volume of water for dilution}$$

PROBLEM 2: Order: Colace 50 mg bid.
Drug available: docusate sodium 3.3 mg/mL.
Average mOsm/kg = 3900.

Step 1: Calculate the volume of drug:

$$\frac{D}{H} \times V = \frac{50}{3.3} \times 1 \quad \textbf{or} \quad \begin{array}{c} H \ : \ V \ :: \ D \ : X \\ 3.3\ mg : 1\ mL :: 50\ mg : X \\ 3.3\ X = 50 \\ X = 15.1\ or\ 15\ mL \end{array}$$
$$= 15.1\ mL$$

Step 2: Find osmolality of drug:

$$\frac{\text{known mOsm (3900)}}{\text{desired mOsm (500)}} \times \text{volume of drug (15 mL)}$$
$$= \frac{3900}{500} \times 15 = 117\ mL$$

Step 3: Water for dilution:

$$\text{total volume of drug (117 mL)} - \text{volume of drug (15 mL)}$$
$$= 102 \text{ mL volume of water for dilution}$$

III Practice Problems: Enteral Medications

Calculate the amount of water needed to reduce the osmolality to 500 mOsm for the following medications:

1. Order: amoxicillin suspension 250 mg by tube, qid.
Drug available: amoxicillin suspension 50 mg/mL.

2. Order: metoclopramide HCl syrup 10 mg, q ac and hs per tube.
Drug available: metoclopramide 1 mg/mL.

3. Order: KCl oral solution 40 mEq, qd by tube.
Drug available: KCl 10% oral solution, 20 mEq/15 mL.

4. Order: thioridazine suspension 50 mg, tid by tube.
Drug available: thioridazine suspension 20 mg/mL.

ANSWERS

I. Practice Problems: Oral Medications

1. a. $\dfrac{D}{H} \times V = \dfrac{5}{2.5} \times 1$ **or**   H : V :: D : X
2.5 mg : 1 tab :: 5 mg : X tab

$= 2.5\overline{)5.0}$ (=2.)

$= 2$ tablets

2.5 X = 5
X = 2 tablets

b. No. Expiration date has expired.

2. 0.5 g = 500 mg (Method A) or see Table 2−1 or Table 5−1.

$$\dfrac{D}{H} \times V = \dfrac{500}{250} \times 1 \quad \textbf{or} \quad$$

H : V :: D : X
250 mg : 1 tab :: 500 mg : X tab

$= \dfrac{500}{250} = 2$ tablets

250 X = 500
X = 2 tablets

3. 2 tablets

4. Change grains to milligrams (milligram value is on the drug label).
Refer to Chapter 2, Table 2−1, or Table 5−1: 1 gr = 60 mg.

$$\dfrac{D}{H} \times V = \dfrac{60}{30} \times 1 \quad \textbf{or} \quad$$

H : V :: D : X
30 mg : 1 tab :: 60 mg : X tab

$= 2$ tablets

30 X = 60
X = 2 tablets

5. 30 mL

6. a. Select the 125 mg/5 mL bottle. It is a fractional dosage with the 375 mg/5 mL bottle (3.3 mL).

b. $\dfrac{D}{H} \times V = \dfrac{250}{125} \times 5 \text{ mL}$ **or**

$$= \dfrac{1250}{125} =$$

$$= 10 \text{ mL of Ceclor}$$

$$H : V :: D : X$$
$$125 : 5 :: 250 : X$$
$$125 \text{ X} = 1250$$
$$X = 10 \text{ mL of Ceclor}$$

7. a. 2 tablets of ProSom

   b. hs : hour of sleep or at bedtime

8. a. $\dfrac{D}{H} \times V = \dfrac{400}{125} \times 5 = \dfrac{2000}{125} = 16 \text{ mL of Ceftin}$

or

$$\dfrac{D}{H} \times V = \dfrac{400}{250} \times 5 = \dfrac{2000}{250} = 8 \text{ mL of Ceftin}$$

   b. Either Ceftin bottle could be used. For fewer mLs, select the 250 mg/5 mL bottle.

9. $\dfrac{D}{H} \times V = \dfrac{100}{62.5} \times 5 \text{ mL} = \dfrac{500}{62.5}$ **or**

$$= 8 \text{ mL of Dynapen}$$

$$H : V :: D : X$$
$$62.5 : 5 :: 100 : X$$
$$62.5 \text{ X} = 500$$
$$X = 8 \text{ mL}$$

10. a. The HydroDiuril 25 mg tablet bottle is preferred. A half-tablet from the HydroDiuril 100 mg tablet bottle can be used; however, breaking or cutting the 100 mg tablet can result in an inaccurate dose.

   b. From the HydroDiuril 25 mg bottle, give 2 tablets. From the HydroDiuril 100 mg bottle, give ½ tablet (if the tablet is scored).

11. a. Select a 10 mg and 20 mg Zocor bottle.

   b. Give 1 tablet from each bottle.

12. Change grams to milligrams by moving the decimal point three spaces to the right: 0.400 g = 400 mg. Also see Table 2−1 or Table 5−1.

$$\dfrac{D}{H} \times V = \dfrac{400}{250} \times 5 \text{ mL} \quad \textbf{or}$$

$$= \dfrac{2000}{250} = 8 \text{ mL}$$

$$H : V :: D : X$$
$$250 \text{ mg} : 5 \text{ mL} :: 400 \text{ mg} : X \text{ mL}$$
$$250 \text{ X} = 2000$$
$$X = 8 \text{ mL}$$

13. Use the metric system. According to Table 2−1 or Table 5−1, gr $\overline{ss}$ = 30 mg. Give 2 tablets.

14. $\dfrac{D}{H} \times V = \dfrac{100}{125} \times 5 \text{ mL}$ **or**

$$= \dfrac{500}{125} = 4 \text{ mL}$$

$$H : V :: D : X$$
$$125 \text{ mg} : 5 \text{ mL} :: 100 \text{ mg} : X$$
$$125 \text{ X} = 500$$
$$X = 4 \text{ mL}$$

15. Give 2 tablets of meperidine

16. Nitrostat 0.4 mg

17. 2½ mL

18. ½ tablet

19. $\dfrac{D}{H} \times V = \dfrac{6}{4} \times 5 = \dfrac{30}{4} = 7.5$ mL of Zofran

20. 1½ tablets

21. **a.** For loading dose and maintenance doses, the 500 mg/5 mL is preferred, but either bottle could be used.

    b. Loading dose: change grams to milligrams:

    $$1.000\,g = 1000 \text{ mg}$$

    Using the 250 mg/5 mL bottle:

    $\dfrac{D}{H} \times V = \dfrac{1000}{\cancel{250}_{50}} \times \cancel{5}^{1}$ mL   **or**

    $= \dfrac{1000}{50} = 20$ mL

    H : V :: D : X
    250 mg : 5 mL : : 1000 mg : X mL
    250 X = 5000
    X = 20 mL

    Using the 500 mg/5 mL bottle: give 10 mL per dose of Duricef.

    c. Maintenance doses per dose, change grams to milligrams

    $$0.500\,g = 500 \text{ mg}$$

    Using the 250 mg/5 mL bottle:

    $\dfrac{D}{H} \times V = \dfrac{500}{250} \times 5$ mL   **or**

    $= 10$ mL

    H : V :: D : X
    250 mg : 5 mL : : 500 mg : X
    250 X = 2500
    X = 10 mL

    Using the 500 mg/5 mL: give 5 mL per dose of Duricef.

22. ½ tablet

23. 165 lb = 75 kg (change pounds to kilograms by dividing by 2.2 into 165 pounds, or 165 ÷ 2.2)

    $$10 \text{ mg} \times 75 = 750 \text{ mg}$$

    $$750 \div 3 = 250 \text{ mg, tid}$$

24. 154 lb = 70 kg
    4 mg × 70 = 280 mg/day

25. 132 lb = 60 kg
    2.5 mg × 60 = 150 mg **or** 100 × 1.7 = 170 mg

26. **a.** 20 mg/50 kg/day = 20 × 50 = 1000 mg per day

    b. 2 tablets of Zarontin per dose (500 mg per dose)

27. **a.** 4 mg/60 kg/day = 4 × 60 = 240 mg per day **or** 120 mg, q12h

    b. $\dfrac{D}{H} \times V = \dfrac{120}{\cancel{50}_{10}} \times \cancel{5}^{1}$ mL   **or**

    $= \dfrac{120}{10} = 12$ mL

    H : V : : D : X
    50 : 5 : : 120 : X
    50 X = 600
    $X = \dfrac{600}{50} = 12$ mL

Give 12 mL per dose of minocycline.

28. Drug label: 250 mg = 1 tablet

$$\text{tablets} = \frac{1\text{ tab} \times \overset{4}{\cancel{1000}\text{ }\cancel{mg}} \times 0.5\text{ }\cancel{g}}{\underset{1}{\cancel{250}\text{ }\cancel{mg}} \times 1\text{ }\cancel{g} \times 1} = 0.5 \times 4 = 2\text{ tablets}$$

29. $$\text{tablets} = \frac{1 \times \overset{2}{\cancel{5.0}\text{ }\cancel{mg}}}{\underset{1}{\cancel{2.5}\text{ }\cancel{mg}} \times 1} = 2\text{ tablets of Vasotec}$$

30. $$\text{mL} = \frac{5\text{ mL} \times \overset{4}{\cancel{1000}\text{ }\cancel{mg}} \times 0.4\text{ }\cancel{g}}{\underset{1}{\cancel{250}\text{ }\cancel{mg}} \times 1\text{ }\cancel{g} \times 1} = 8\text{ mL}$$

Give 8 mL per dose of amoxicillin.

31. Factors: 325 mg = 1 tablet; gr × (10)/1
Conversion factor: 1 gr = 60 mg

$$\text{tablets} = \frac{1\text{ tab} \times \overset{12}{\cancel{60}\text{ }\cancel{mg}} \times \overset{2}{\cancel{10}\text{ }\cancel{gr}}}{\underset{\underset{13}{65}}{\cancel{325}\text{ }\cancel{mg}} \times 1\text{ }\cancel{gr} \times 1} = \frac{24}{13} = 1.84\text{ or 2 tablets}$$

60 (64) mg = 1 gr (approximate weights). Round off to the nearest whole number.

32. Factors: 250 mg = 5 mL; 125 mg/1
Conversion factor: *none*

$$\text{mL} = \frac{5\text{ mL} \times \overset{1}{\cancel{125}\text{ }\cancel{mg}}}{\underset{2}{\cancel{250}\text{ }\cancel{mg}} \times 1} = \frac{5}{2} = 2\tfrac{1}{2}\text{ or 2.5 mL}$$

II. Percent of Enteral Solutions

1. $\dfrac{D}{H} \times V = \dfrac{25}{100} \times 200$ **or** $100:200::25:X$

$$= \frac{200}{4} = 50\text{ mL of Sustacal} \qquad \begin{array}{l}100\,X = 5000 \\ X = 50\text{ mL of Sustacal}\end{array}$$

or

200 mL × 0.25 (25%) = 50 mL of Sustacal

Total amount − amount of TF = amount of water
200 mL − 50 mL = 150 mL

50 mL of Sustacal + 150 mL of water

2. 225 mL of Pulmocare + 75 mL of water

3. $\dfrac{D}{H} \times V = \dfrac{60}{100} \times 500$ **or** $100:500::60:X$

$$= \frac{30,000}{100} = 300\text{ mL of Ensure Plus} \qquad \begin{array}{l}100\,X = 30,000 \\ X = 300\text{ mL of Ensure Plus}\end{array}$$

or

500 mL $\times$ 0.60 (60%) = 300 mL of Ensure Plus

Total amount $-$ amount of TF = amount of water

500 mL $-$ 300 mL   =   200 mL

300 mL of Ensure Plus + 200 mL of water

4. 120 mL of Osmolite + 280 mL of water

III. Enteral Medications

1. *Step 1* $\dfrac{D}{H} \times V = \dfrac{\overset{5}{\cancel{250}}}{\underset{1}{\cancel{50}}} \times 1$ **or** $\begin{array}{c} H : V : : \ D \ : X \\ 50 : 1 : : 250 : X \end{array}$

= 5 mL   50 X = 250

X = 5 mL

Step 2 $\dfrac{\text{known mOsm (2250)}}{\text{desired mOsm (500)}} \times$ volume of drug (5)

$= \dfrac{2250}{500} \times 5 \text{ mL} = 22.5 \text{ mL}$

Step 3 total volume of liquid (22.5) $-$ volume of drug (5) = 17.5 mL

Total: 22.5 mL to be administered

2. *Step 1* $\dfrac{D}{H} \times V = \dfrac{10}{1} \times 1 = 10$ **or** $\begin{array}{c} H \ : \ V \ : : \ \ D \ : X \\ 1 \text{ mg} : 1 \text{ mL} : : 10 \text{ mg} : X \end{array}$

X = 10 mL

Step 2 $\dfrac{\text{known mOsm (8350)}}{\text{desired mOsm (500)}} \times$ volume of drug (10)

$= \dfrac{8350}{500} \times 10 = 167 \text{ mL}$

Step 3 total volume of liquid (167 mL) $-$ volume of drug (10 mL) = 157 mL

3. *Step 1* $\dfrac{D}{H} \times V = \dfrac{\overset{2}{\cancel{40}}}{\underset{1}{\cancel{20}}} \times 15 = 30 \text{ mL}$ **or** $\begin{array}{c} H \ : \ V \ : : \ \ D \ \ : X \\ 20 \text{ mEq} : 15 \text{ mL} : : 40 \text{ mEq} : X \end{array}$

20 X = 600

X = 30 mL

Step 2 $\dfrac{\text{known mOsm (3550)}}{\text{desired mOsm (500)}} \times$ volume of drug (30)

$= \dfrac{3550}{500} \times 30 = 213 \text{ mL}$

Step 3 total volume of liquid (213) $-$ volume of drug (30) = 183 mL

4. *Step 1* $\dfrac{D}{H} \times V = \dfrac{\overset{}{\cancel{50}}}{\underset{2}{\cancel{20}}} \times 1 = 2.5 \text{ mL}$ **or** $\begin{array}{c} H \ : \ V \ : : \ \ D \ \ : X \\ 20 \text{ mg} : 1 \text{ mL} : : 50 \text{ mEq} : X \end{array}$

20 X = 50

X = 2.5 mL

Step 2 $\dfrac{\text{known mOsm (2050)}}{\text{desired mOsm (500)}} \times \text{volume of drug (2.5)} = 10.25 \text{ mL}$

Step 3 total volume of liquid (10.25 mL) − volume of drug (2.5 mL) =
7.75 mL

injectable preparations with clinical applications

Objectives

- Select the correct syringe and needle for a prescribed injectable drug.
- Calculate dosage of drugs for subcutaneous and intramuscular routes from solutions in vials and ampules.
- Explain the procedure for preparing and calculating medications in powder form for injectable use.
- Determine prescribed insulin dosage in units using an insulin syringe.
- Explain the methods for mixing two insulin solutions in one insulin syringe and for mixing two injectable drugs in one syringe.
- State the various sites for intramuscular injections.
- Explain how to administer intradermal, subcutaneous, and intramuscular injections.

Outline

Medications administered by injection can be given intradermally (under the skin), subcutaneously (SC, into fatty tissue), intramuscularly (IM, into the muscle), and intravenously (IV, into the vein). Intravenous injectables are discussed in Chapter 8. Injectable drugs are ordered in grams, milligrams, micrograms, grains, or units. The preparations of injectable drugs may be packaged in a solvent (diluent or solution) or in a powdered form.

This chapter is divided into five sections: (1) injectable preparations, such as vials, ampules, syringes, needles, and pre-filled cartridges; (2) intradermal injections; (3) subcutaneous injections, including heparin; (4) insulin injections; and (5) intramuscular injections from prepared liquid and reconstituted powder in vials and ampules, and the mixing of drugs in a syringe. Examples and practice problems follow each section, and the answers to the practice problems are located at the end of the chapter.

INJECTABLE PREPARATIONS

Vials and Ampules

Drugs are packaged in vials (sealed rubber-top containers) for single and multiple doses and in ampules (sealed glass containers) for a single dose. Multiple-dose vials can be used more than once because of their self-sealing rubber top; however, ampules are used only once after the glass-necked container is opened. The drug is in either liquid or powder form in vials and ampules. When drugs in solution deteriorate rapidly, they are packaged in dry form and solvent (diluent) is added prior to administration. If the drug is in powdered form, mixing instructions and dose equivalents such as milligrams (mg) per milliliter (mL) are usually given; if not, check the drug information insert. After the dry form of the drug is reconstituted with sterile water, bacteriostatic water, or saline, the drug is used immediately or must be refrigerated. Usually, the reconstituted drug in the vial is used within 48 hours to 1 week; check the drug information insert. A vial and an ampule are shown in Figure 7–1.

The route by which the injectable drug can be given, such as SC, IM, or IV, is printed on the drug label.

Vial   Ampule

Figure 7•1 ——————————

(A) vial. *(B)* ampule. From Kee, J., & Hayes, E. (2000). *Pharmacology: A Nursing Process Approach* (3rd ed.). Philadelphia: W.B. Saunders.

A   B

Tip   Barrel   Plunger

Figure 7•2 ——————————————————

Parts of a syringe. From Kee, J., & Hayes, E. (2000). *Pharmacology: A Nursing Process Approach* (3rd ed.). Philadelphia: W.B. Saunders.

Syringes

Types of syringes used for injections include 3-mL and 5-mL calibrated syringes, metal and plastic syringes for pre-filled cartridges, tuberculin syringes, and insulin syringes. There are 10-mL, 20-mL, and 50-mL syringes that are used mostly for drug preparations. A syringe is composed of a barrel (outer shell), plunger (inner part), and the tip, where the needle joins the syringe (Fig. 7–2).

THREE-MILLILITER SYRINGE

The 3-mL syringe is calibrated in tenths (0.1 mL) and minims (♏). The amount of fluid in the syringe is determined by the rubber end of the plunger that is closer to the tip of the syringe (Fig. 7–3). Remember, millili-

THREE MILLILITER SYRINGE

½   1   1½   2   2½   3

A

B

C

Figure 7•3 ——————————————————

Three-milliliter syringes: *(A)* 3-mL syringe with 0.1-mL markings; *(B)* 3-mL syringe with a needle cover; *(C)* 3-mL syringe with a protective cover over the needle after injection. From Kee, J., & Hayes, E. (2000). *Pharmacology: A Nursing Process Approach* (3rd ed.). Philadelphia: W.B. Saunders.

Figure 7•4

SafetyGlide needle. Courtesy of Bectin Dickson Division, Franklin Lakes, NJ.

ter (mL) and cubic centimeter (cc) are used interchangeably. An advance in safety needle technology is the SafetyGlide shielding hypodermic needle (Fig. 7–4). The purpose for this type of needle is to reduce needlestick injuries.

FIVE-MILLILITER SYRINGE

The 5-mL syringe is calibrated in 0.2 mL. A 5-mL syringe is usually used when the fluid needed is more than 2½ mL. This syringe is frequently used to reconstitute a dry drug form with sterile water, bacteriostatic water, or saline. Figure 7–5 shows the 5-mL syringe and its markings and the 5-mL needleless syringe.

FIVE MILLILITER SYRINGE

A

B

Figure 7•5

Five-milliliter syringes: *(A)* 5-mL syringe with 0.2-mL markings; *(B)* needleless 5-mL syringe that can penetrate a rubber-top vial. From Kee, J., & Hayes, E. (2000). *Pharmacology: A Nursing Process Approach* (3rd ed.). Philadelphia: W.B. Saunders.

TUBERCULIN SYRINGE

Figure 7•6

Tuberculin syringe. From Kee, J., & Hayes, E. (2000). *Pharmacology: A Nursing Process Approach* (3rd ed.). Philadelphia: W.B. Saunders.

TUBERCULIN SYRINGE

The tuberculin syringe is a 1-mL, slender syringe that is calibrated in tenths (0.1 mL), hundredths (0.01 mL), and minims (Fig. 7–6). This syringe is used when the amount of drug solution to be administered is less than 1 mL and for pediatric and heparin dosages. The tuberculin syringe is also available in a one-half milliliter (mL) syringe. Figure 7–7 illustrates the ½-mL and the 1-mL tuberculin syringes.

INSULIN SYRINGE

The insulin syringe has a capacity of 1 mL. Insulin is measured in units, and insulin dosage *must NOT* be calculated in milliliters. Insulin syringes are calibrated as 2 units per mark, and 100 units equal 1 mL (Fig. 7–8). *Insulin syringes, NOT tuberculin syringes, must be used for administering insulin.* Insulin syringes are available in lo-dose, ½-mL, and 1-mL sizes. The 1-mL insulin syringe may be purchased with a permanently attached needle or detachable needle (Fig. 7–9).

PRE-FILLED DRUG CARTRIDGE AND SYRINGE

Many injectable drugs are packaged in pre-filled disposable cartridges. The disposable cartridge is placed into a reusable metal or plastic holder. A pre-

Figure 7•7

Two types of tuberculin syringes: *(A)* ½-cc tuberculin syringe with a permanently attached needle; *(B)* 1-cc tuberculin syringe with a detachable needle. (Courtesy of Bectin Dickson Division, Franklin Lakes, NJ.)

INSULIN SYRINGE

Figure 7•8

Insulin syringe. From Kee, J., & Hayes, E. (2000). *Pharmacology: A Nursing Process Approach* (3rd ed.). Philadelphia: W.B. Saunders.

filled cartridge usually contains 0.1 to 0.2 mL of excess drug solution. On the basis of the amount of drug to be administered, the excess solution must be expelled prior to administration. Figure 7–10A illustrates the Tubex syringe with cartridge. Injectables are also supplied by pharmaceutical companies in ready-to-use pre-filled syringes that do not require a holder. Figure 7–10B illustrates a BD Hypak pre-filled syringe.

Needles

A needle consists of (1) a hub (large metal or plastic part attached to the tip of the syringe), (2) a shaft (thin needle length), and (3) a bevel (end of the needle). Figure 7–11 illustrates the parts of a needle.

Needle size is determined by gauge (diameter of the lumen) and by

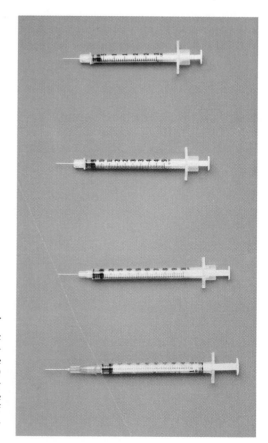

Figure 7•9

Four types of insulin syringes: *(A)* ³⁄₁₀-cc insulin syringe with a permanently attached needle; *(B)* ½-cc insulin syringe with a permanently attached needle; *(C)* 1-cc insulin syringe with a permanently attached needle; *(D)* 1-cc insulin syringe with a detachable needle. (Courtesy of Bectin Dickson Division, Franklin Lakes, NJ.)

Figure 7•10

(A) Tubex syringe with cartridge. (B) BD Hypak pre-filled syringe. (B) (A, courtesy of Wyeth-Ayerst Laboratories, Philadelphia, PA; B, courtesy of Bectin Dickson Division, Franklin Lakes, NJ.)

length. The larger the gauge number, the smaller the diameter of the lumen. The smaller the gauge number, the larger the diameter of the lumen. The usual range of needle gauges is from 18 to 26. Needle length varies from ⅜ inch to 2 inches. Table 7–1 lists the needle sizes and lengths for use in intradermal, subcutaneous, and intramuscular injections.

When choosing the needle length for an intramuscular injection, the nurse must consider the size of the client and the amount of fatty tissue. A client with minimal fatty (subcutaneous) tissue may need a needle length of 1 inch. For an obese client, the length of the needle for an intramuscular injection may be 1½ to 2 inches.

Insulin syringes and pre-filled cartridges have permanently attached needles. With other syringes, needle sizes can be changed. Needle gauge and length are indicated on the syringe package or on the top cover of the syringe. These values appear as gauge / length, such as 21g / 1½ inch. Figure 7–12 illustrates two types of needle gauge and length.

PARTS OF A NEEDLE

Figure 7•11

Parts of a needle. From Kee, J., & Hayes, E. (2000). *Pharmacology: A Nursing Process Approach* (3rd ed.). Philadelphia: W.B. Saunders.

table 7•1
NEEDLE SIZE AND LENGTH

TYPE OF INJECTION	NEEDLE GAUGE	NEEDLE LENGTHS (inch)
Intradermal	25, 26	⅜, ½, ⅝
Subcutaneous	23, 25, 26	⅜, ½, ⅝
Intramuscular	19, 20, 21, 22	1, 1½, 2

Research has shown that after an injection, medication remains in the hub of the syringe, where the needle joins the syringe. This volume can be as much as 0.2 mL. There is controversy as to whether air should be added to the syringe prior to administration to ensure that the total volume is given. The best practice is to follow the institution's policy.

ANGLES FOR INJECTION

For injections, the needle enters the skin at different angles. Intradermal injections are given at a 10- to 15-degree angle, subcutaneous injections at a 45- to 90-degree angle, and intramuscular injections at a 90-degree angle. Figure 7–13 illustrates the angles for intradermal, subcutaneous, and intramuscular injections.

I Practice Problems: Needles

1. Which would have the larger needle lumen: a 21-gauge needle or a 25-gauge needle? _____

2. Which would have the smaller needle lumen: an 18-gauge needle or a 26-gauge needle? _____

3. Which needle would have a length of 1½ inches: a 20-gauge needle or a 25-gauge needle? _____

4. Which needle would have a length of ⅝ inch: a 21-gauge needle or a 25-gauge needle? _____

5. Which needle would be used for an intramuscular injection: a 21-gauge needle with a 1½-inch length or 25-gauge needle with a ⅝-inch length? _____

A 25 g/½   B 21 g/1½

Figure 7•12 ————————————————————

Two combinations of needle gauge and length.

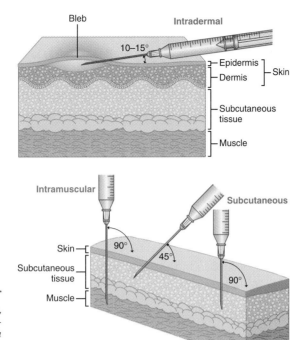

Figure 7•13

Angles for injection. From Kee, J., & Hayes, E. (2000). *Pharmacology: A Nursing Process Approach* (3rd ed.). Philadelphia: W.B. Saunders.

INTRADERMAL INJECTIONS

Usually, an intradermal injection is used for skin testing for diagnostic purposes. Primary uses are for tuberculin and allergy testing. The tuberculin syringe (25 g / ½ inch) holds 1 mL (16 minims) and is calibrated in 0.1 to 0.01 mL.

The inner aspect of the forearm is often used for diagnostic testing because there is less hair in the area and the test results are easily seen. The upper back can also be used as a testing site. The needle is inserted with the bevel upward at a 10- to 15-degree angle. Do not aspirate. Test results are read 48 to 72 hours after the intradermal injection. A reddened or raised area indicates a positive reaction.

SUBCUTANEOUS INJECTIONS

Drugs injected into the subcutaneous (fatty) tissue are absorbed slowly because there are fewer blood vessels in the fatty tissue. The amount of drug solution administered subcutaneously is generally 0.5 to 1 mL at a 45-, 60-, or 90-degree angle. Irritating drug solutions are given intramuscularly because they could cause sloughing of the subcutaneous tissue.

The two types of syringes used for subcutaneous injections are the tuberculin syringe (1 mL), which is calibrated in 0.1 and 0.01 mL, and the 3-mL syringe which is calibrated in 0.1 mL (Fig. 7–14). The needle gauge commonly used is 25- or 26-gauge, and the length is usually ⅜ to ⅝ inch.

Figure 7•14

Syringes used for subcutaneous injections.

Insulin is also administered subcutaneously and is discussed later in this chapter.

Calculation for Subcutaneous Injections

Formulas for solving problems of subcutaneous injections are the basic formula, ratio and proportion, and fractional equation (see Chapter 5). The following problems are examples of injections that can be given subcutaneously.

. . . .

examples

PROBLEM 1: Order: heparin 5000 U, SC.
Drug available:

Methods:

Basic formula

$$\frac{D}{H} \times V = \frac{5000}{10,000} \times 1 \quad \textbf{or}$$

$$= \frac{5}{10} = 0.5 \text{ mL}$$

Ratio and proportion

$$H \quad : \quad V \quad :: \quad D \quad : \quad X$$

$$10,000 \text{ U} : 1 \text{ mL} :: 5000 \text{ U} : X \text{ mL}$$

$$10,000 \text{ X} = 5000$$

$$X = \frac{5000}{10,000} = \frac{5}{10} =$$

$$0.5 \text{ mL}$$

Answer: Heparin 5000 U = 0.5 mL

PROBLEM 2: Order: morphine 10 mg, SC.
Drug available:

See label with approximate equivalents.

Methods: $\dfrac{D}{H} \times V = \dfrac{10}{15} \times 1$ **or**

$$H : V :: D : X$$
$$15 \text{ mg} : 1 \text{ mL} :: 10 \text{ mg} : X \text{ mL}$$

$= \dfrac{2}{3} = 0.67 \text{ mL}$
or 0.7 mL

$15 X = 10$

$X = \dfrac{\overset{2}{\cancel{10}}}{\underset{3}{\cancel{15}}} = \dfrac{2}{3} = 0.67 \text{ mL}$
or 0.7 mL

Answer: Morphine 10 mg = 0.67 or 0.7 mL (use a tuberculin syringe or a 3-mL syringe)

II Practice Problems: Subcutaneous Injections

Use the formula you chose for calculating oral drug dosages in Chapter 6.

1. Which needle gauge and length should be used for a subcutaneous injection:

   a 25 g/⅝ inch or 26 g/⅜ inch? _____

2. Order: heparin 4000 U, SC.
   Drug available:

   a. How many milliliters of heparin would you give? _____

   b. At what angle would you administer the drug? _____

3. Order: heparin 7500 U, SC.
Drug available:

a. How many milliliters of heparin would you give? _____

b. This drug is supplied in a cartridge. What type of syringe should be used? _____

4. Order: atropine SO$_4$ gr $\frac{1}{100}$, SC.
Drug available:

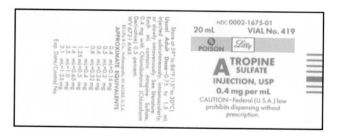

How many milliliters of atropine would you give? _____

5. Order: erythropoietin (Epogen) 50 units/kg SC.
Drug available: Epogen 10,000 units/mL.
Client weighs 65 kg.

a. What is the correct dosage? _____

b. How many milliliters would you give? _____

6. Order: filgrastim (Neupogen) 6 mcg/kg SC BID.
Drug available: Neupogen 300 mcg/ml.
Client weighs 198 pounds.

a. How many kg does the client weigh? _____

b. How many milliliters would you give? _____

c. Explain how the drug should be drawn up. _____

INSULIN INJECTIONS

Insulin is prescribed and measured in USP units. Most insulins are manufactured in concentrations of 100 units per mL. Insulin should be administered with an insulin syringe, which is calculated to correspond with the U 100 insulin. Insulin bottles and syringes are color-coded. The U 100 insulin bottle and the U 100 syringe are color-coded orange.

The insulin syringe may be marked on one side in even units (10, 20, 30) and on the other side in odd units (5, 15, 25).

Insulin is easy to prepare and administer as long as the nurse uses the *same insulin concentration with the same calibrated insulin syringe*, e.g., a U 100 insulin bottle and a U 100 insulin syringe. For example, if the prescribed insulin dosage is 30 units, withdraw 30 units from a bottle of U 100 insulin using a U 100–calibrated insulin syringe.

Administering insulin with a tuberculin syringe is *not* suggested and *should be avoided.*

Types of Insulin

Insulin is categorized as fast-acting, intermediate-acting, or long-acting. The following drug labels are arranged according to insulin action.

A: Fast-Acting Insulin

B: Intermediate-Acting Insulin

C: Long-Acting Insulin

Insulins are clear (regular or crystalline insulin) or cloudy (NPH, Lente) because of the substances (protamine and zinc) used to prolong the action of insulin in the body. Only clear (regular) insulin can be given intravenously as well as subcutaneously. Insulin that contains protamine and zinc can be administered only subcutaneously.

A new fast-acting insulin that was approved for use in 1996 is lispro insulin (Humalog). Lispro insulin acts faster than regular insulin and thus can be administered 5 minutes before mealtime, whereas regular insulin is given 30 minutes before meals. Lispro insulin is formed by reversing two amino acids in human regular insulin (Humulin).

The use of commercially premixed combination insulins has become popular for the diabetic client who mixes fast-acting and intermediate-acting insulins. Examples of combination insulins are Humulin 70/30, Novolin 70/30, and Humulin 50/50. The 70/30 vial contains 70% NPH insulin and 30% regular insulin, and the 50/50 vial contains 50% NPH insulin and 50% regular insulin. The client does not have to mix regular and NPH insulins as long as this combination is effective. Some people, however, need less than 30% regular insulin and more NPH; they will need to mix the two insulins together in the prescribed proportions.

The sources of insulins are beef, pork, beef-pork, and human (Humulin). Some individuals are allergic to beef insulin, so pork insulin is used because it has biologic properties similar to those of human insulin.

Insulin is administered subcutaneously at a 45-, 60-, or 90-degree angle into the subcutaneous tissue. The angle for administering insulin depends on the amount of fatty tissue in the client. For a very thin person, a 45-degree angle is suggested. A 90-degree angle should be used on obese or average-sized persons. When using a 90-degree angle, pinch the skin upward so the insulin is deposited into the fatty tissue.

Mixing Insulins

Regular insulin is frequently mixed with insulins containing protamine, such as NPH, and zinc, such as Lente.

. . . .

example

Problem and method for mixing insulin.

PROBLEM 1: Order: Regular insulin U 10 and Lente insulin U 40, SC.
Drug available: Regular insulin U 100 and Lente insulin U 100, both in multidose vials. The insulin syringe is marked U 100.

Methods: 1. Cleanse the rubber tops or diaphragms of the insulin bottles.

2. Draw up 40 U of air* and inject into the Lente insulin bottle. Do not allow the needle to come into contact with the Lente insulin solution. Withdraw the needle.

3. Draw up 10 U of air and inject into the regular insulin bottle.

4. Withdraw 10 U of regular insulin. Regular insulin is withdrawn before Lente and NPH.

5. Withdraw 40 U of Lente insulin.

6. Administer the two insulins immediately after mixing. Do not allow the insulin mixture to stand, because unpredicted physical changes might occur. Unpredicted changes are more common with protamine insulins such as NPH than with Lente insulin.

III Practice Problems: Insulin

1. Order: NPH insulin 35 U, SC.
Drug available: NPH insulin U 100 and U 100 insulin syringe.

---

*You may draw up 50 units of air; inject 40 units into the NPH bottle and 10 units into the regular insulin bottle.

Indicate on the insulin syringe the amount of insulin that should be withdrawn.

2. Order: Lente insulin 50 U, SC.
Drug available: Lente U 100 and U 100 insulin syringe.
Indicate on the insulin syringe the amount of insulin that should be withdrawn.

3. Order: regular insulin U 8 and NPH insulin U 52.
Drug available: regular insulin U 100 and NPH insulin U 100.
The insulin syringe is U 100.
Explain the method for mixing the two insulins.

_____

Indicate on the U 100 insulin syringe how much regular insulin should be withdrawn and how much NPH insulin should be withdrawn.

4. Order: regular insulin U 15 and Lente insulin U 45.
Drug available: regular insulin U 100 and Lente insulin U 100.
The insulin syringe is U 100.

Explain the method for mixing the two insulins.

_____

Indicate on the U 100 insulin syringe how much regular insulin and how much Lente insulin should be withdrawn.

Continuous Subcutaneous Insulin Infusion (CSII) Pumps

CSII pumps are small (pager-sized), battery-powered, programmable devices that constantly infuse a rapid-acting 100 U insulin at a set rate of units per hour. The pump holds a small syringe, which is attached to an infusion set with a soft catheter or needle. The catheter or needle is inserted into the subcutaneous tissue, most often the abdomen, and secured with a transparent film. The pump can be programmed to: (1) infuse at a set basal rate of units per hour; (2) deliver bolus infusions to cover meals ranging from over a few minutes to a few hours; (3) change delivery rates at specific times of the day, i.e., 3 AM to 9 AM, to avoid the phenomenon of early morning hyperglycemia; and (4) override set basal rate to allow for unexpected changes in activity, such as early morning exercise.

The pump can deliver smaller amounts of insulin, 0.1 or 0.2 units, more accurately than a syringe. Because the pump can provide many variations in insulin regimens and improve glycemic control, a CSII pump can be used as an integral part of insulin therapy for the diabetic client. Figure 7–15 shows an example of an insulin pump.

INTRAMUSCULAR INJECTIONS

The IM injection is a common method of administering injectable drugs. The muscle has many blood vessels (more than fatty tissue), so medications given by intramuscular injections are absorbed more rapidly than those given by SC injections. The volume of solution for an IM injection is 0.5 to 3.0 mL, with the average being 1 to 2 mL. A volume of drug solution greater than 3 mL causes increased muscle tissue displacement and possible tissue damage. Occasionally, 5 mL of certain drugs, such as magnesium sulfate, may be injected in a large muscle, such as the dorsogluteal. Dosages greater than 3 mL are usually divided and given at two different sites.

Needle gauges for IM injections containing thick solutions are 19 and 20, and for thin solutions, 20 to 21. IM injections are administered at a 90-

Figure 7•15

Portable insulin pump. (Courtesy of Disetronic Medical Systems, Inc., Minneapolis, MN.)

degree angle. The needle length depends on the amount of adipose (fat) and muscle tissue; the average needle length is 1½ inches.

The common sites for IM injections are the deltoid, dorsogluteal, ventrogluteal, and vastus lateralis muscles. Figure 7–16 displays the sites for each muscle used with IM injection. Table 7–2 gives the volume for drug administration, common needle size, client's position, and angle of injection for the four IM injection sites.

The discussion on intramuscular injection is divided into three subsections: (1) drug solutions for injection, (2) reconstitution of powdered drugs, and (3) mixing of injectable drugs. An example is given for each type, and practice problems follow.

Drug Solutions for Injection

Commercially premixed drug solutions are stored in vials and ampules for immediate use. At times, there may be enough drug solution left in a vial for another dose, and the vial may be saved. The balance of a drug solution

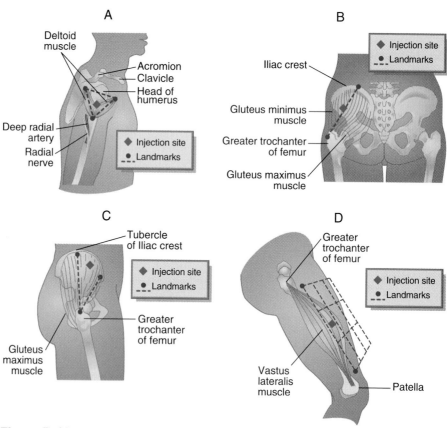

Figure 7•16

Intramuscular injection sites. *(A)* deltoid; *(B)* dorsogluteal; *(C)* ventrogluteal; *(D)* vastus lateralis. From Kee, J., & Hayes, E. (2000). *Pharmacology: A Nursing Process Approach* (3rd ed.). Philadelphia: W.B. Saunders.)

table 7•2
INTRAMUSCULAR INJECTION SITES IN THE ADULT

	DELTOID	DORSOGLUTEAL	VENTROGLUTEAL	VASTUS LATERALIS
Volume for drug administration	*Usual:* 0.5–1 mL *Maximum:* 2.0 mL	*Usual:* 1.0–3 mL *Maximum:* 3 mL; 5 mL gamma-globulin	*Usual:* 1–3 mL *Maximum:* 3–4 mL	*Usual:* 1–3 mL *Maximum:* 3–4 mL
Common needle size	23–25 gauge; ⅝–1½ inches	18–23 gauge; 1¼–3 inches	20–23 gauge; 1¼–2½ inches	20–23 gauge; 1¼–1½ inches
Client's position	Sitting; supine; prone	Prone	Supine; lateral	Sitting (dorsal flex foot); supine
Angle of injection	90° angle, angled slightly toward the acromion	90° angle to flat surface; upper outer quadrant of the buttock *or* outer aspect of line from the posterior iliac crest to the greater trochanter of the femur	80°–90° angle; angle the needle slightly toward the iliac crest	80°–90° angle For thin person: 60°–75° angle

in an ampule is *always* discarded after the ampule has been opened and used.

examples

Two problems are given as examples for calculating IM dosage. Choose one of the four methods for calculating drug dosage.

PROBLEM 1: Order: gentamycin 60 mg, IM.
Drug available: gentamycin 80 mg/2 mL in a vial.

Methods: $\dfrac{D}{H} \times V = \dfrac{60}{80} \times 2$ **or**

$$= \dfrac{120}{80} = 1.5 \text{ mL}$$

$$H \ : \ V \ :: \ D \ : \ X$$
$$80 \text{ mg} : 2 \text{ mL} :: 60 \text{ mg} : X \text{ mL}$$
$$80 X = 120$$
$$X = \dfrac{120}{80} = 1.5 \text{ mL}$$

Answer: *gentamycin 60 mg = 1.5 mL*

PROBLEM 2: Order: Naloxone 0.5 mg, IM, STAT.
Drug available:

Methods: $\dfrac{D}{H} \times V = \dfrac{0.5}{0.4} \times 1$

$$= \quad \textbf{or} \quad \begin{array}{l} H \; :V: \; : \; D \; :X \\ 0.4 : 1 : : 0.5 :X \end{array}$$

$$\begin{array}{r} 1.25 \text{ mL} \\ 0.4\overline{)0.500} \end{array}$$

$(0.4) X = 0.5$

$X = 1.25 \text{ mL}$

Answer: Naloxone 0.5 mg = 1.25 mL

Reconstitution of Powdered Drugs

Certain drugs lose their potency in liquid form. Therefore, manufacturers package these drugs in powdered form, and they are reconstituted prior to administration. To reconstitute a drug, look on the drug label or in the drug information insert (circular or pamphlet) for the type and amount of diluent to use. Sterile water, bacteriostatic water, and normal saline are the primary diluents. If the type and amount of diluent are not specified on the drug label or in the drug information insert, call the pharmacy.

The powdered drug occupies space and therefore increases the volume of drug solution. Usually, manufacturers determine the amount of diluent to mix with the drug powder to yield 1 to 2 mL per desired dose. After the powdered drug has been reconstituted, the unused drug solution should be dated, initialed, and refrigerated. Most drugs retain their potency for 48 hours to 1 week when refrigerated. Check the drug information insert or drug label for how long the reconstituted drug may be used.

· ·

e x a m p l e s

PROBLEM 1: Order: oxacillin sodium 500 mg, IM, q6h.
Drug available:

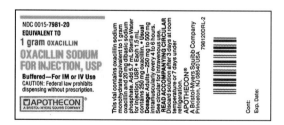

According to the label on the bottle, the amount of powdered drug in the vial is 1 g. The drug label states:
Add 5.7 mL of sterile water (diluent) to the vial. Each 250 mg = 1.5 mL or 1 g = 6 mL.

Methods: Change grams to milligrams or change milligrams to grams (see Table 5–1). 1 gram = 1000 mg or 500 mg = 0.500 g (0.5 g).

Move the decimal point three spaces to the left.

Milligrams   *Grams*

$$\frac{D}{H} \times V = \frac{500}{1000} \times 6 \text{ mL} \quad \textbf{or}$$

$$H : V :: D : V$$
$$1\,g : 6\,mL :: 0.5\,g : X$$

$$= \frac{3000}{1000} = 3 \text{ mL}$$

$$X = 3.0$$
$$X = 3.0 \text{ mL}$$

or

$$\frac{D}{H} \times V = \frac{\overset{2}{\cancel{500}}}{\underset{1}{\cancel{250}}} \times 1.5 \text{ mL} = 3 \text{ mL}$$

Answer: oxacillin sodium 500 mg = 3 mL

PROBLEM 2: Order: nafcillin sodium 250 mg, IM, q6h.
Drug available:

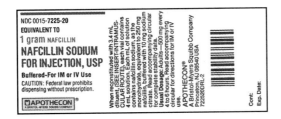

The drug label reads to add 3.4 mL of sterile or bacteriostatic water. Each 4 mL contains 1 gram (1000 mg) of nafcillin.

Methods: $\frac{D}{H} \times V = \frac{250}{1000} \times 4 \text{ mL}$ **or**

$$H : V :: D : X$$
$$1000\,mg : 4\,mL :: 250\,mg : X$$

$$= \frac{1000}{1000}$$

$$1000\,X = 1000$$

$$= 1 \text{ mL nafcillin}$$

$$X = \frac{1000}{1000}$$

$$= 1 \text{ mL of nafcillin}$$

Answer: nafcillin 250 mg = 1 mL

Mixing of Injectable Drugs

Drugs mixed together in the same syringe must be compatible to prevent precipitation. To determine drug compatibility, check drug references or check with a pharmacist. When in doubt about compatibility, do *not* mix drugs.

The three methods associated in drug mixing are (1) mixing two drugs in the same syringe from two vials, (2) mixing two drugs in the same syringe from one vial and one ampule, and (3) mixing two drugs in a prefilled cartridge and from a vial.

METHOD 1   Mixing Two Drugs in the Same Syringe from *Two Vials*

1. Draw air into the syringe to equal the amount of solution to be withdrawn from the first vial, and inject the air into the first vial. Do *not* allow the needle to come into contact with the solution. Remove the needle.
2. Draw air into the syringe to equal the amount of solution to be withdrawn from the second vial. Invert the second vial and inject the air.
3. Withdraw the desired amount of solution from the second vial.
4. Change the needle unless you will use the entire volume in the first vial.
5. Invert the first vial and withdraw the desired amount of solution.

or

1. Draw air into the syringe to equal the amount of solution to be withdrawn and inject the air into the first vial. Withdraw the desired drug dose.
2. Insert a 25-g needle into the rubber top (not in the center) of the second vial. This acts as an air vent. Injecting air into the second vial is *not* necessary.
3. Insert the needle in the center of the rubber-top vial (beside the 25-g needle–air vent), invert the second vial, and withdraw the desired drug dose.

METHOD 2   Mixing Two Drugs in the Same Syringe from *One Vial and One Ampule*

1. Remove the amount of desired solution from the vial.
2. Aspirate the amount of desired solution from the ampule.

METHOD 3   Mixing Two Drugs in a *Pre-filled Cartridge from a Vial*

1. Check the drug dose and the amount of solution in the pre-filled cartridge. If a smaller dose is needed, expel the excess solution.
2. Draw air into the cartridge to equal the amount of solution to be withdrawn from the vial. Invert the vial and inject the air.
3. Withdraw the desired amount of solution from the vial. Make sure the needle remains in the fluid, and do *not* take more solution than needed.

examples

Mixing drugs in the same syringe.

PROBLEM 1: Order: meperidine (Demerol) 60 mg and atropine SO_4 gr $1/150$, IM.
The two drugs are compatible.
Drugs available:

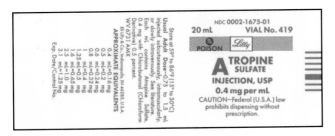

Note: Meperidine is in a pre-filled Tubex cartridge, and atropine sulfate is in a vial.

> How many milliliters of each drug would you give?
> Explain how to mix the two drugs.

Methods: meperidine

$$\frac{D}{H} \times V = \frac{60}{100} \times 1 \quad \textbf{or} \quad \begin{array}{c} H \quad : \quad V \quad :: \quad D \quad : \quad X \\ 100 \text{ mg} : 1 \text{ mL} :: 60 \text{ mg} : X \text{ mL} \end{array}$$

$$= 0.6 \text{ mL} \qquad\qquad \begin{array}{c} 100 \, X = 60 \\ X = 0.6 \text{ mL} \end{array}$$

atropine SO_4

gr $\frac{1}{150}$ = 0.4 mg (see Tables 2–1 and 5–1).

Answer: meperidine (Demerol) 60 mg = 0.6 mL
atropine gr $\frac{1}{150}$ = 1 mL

Procedure: Mix two drugs in a cartridge with one drug from a vial:

1. Check drug dose and volume on pre-filled cartridge.
2. Expel 0.4 mL and any excess of drug solution from cartridge; 0.6 mL remains in the cartridge.
3. Draw 1 mL of air in the cartridge and inject into the vial.
4. Withdraw 1 mL of atropine from vial into the pre-filled cartridge.

PROBLEM 2: Order: meperidine 25 mg, Vistaril 25 mg, and Robinul 0.1 mg, IM. All three drugs are compatible.
Drugs available: meperidine (Demerol) is in a 2-mL Tubex cartridge labeled 50 mg/mL. Hydroxyzine (Vistaril) is in a 50 mg/mL ampule. Glycopyrrolate (Robinul) is in a 0.2 mg/mL vial.

> How many milliliters of each drug would you give?
> Explain how the drugs could be mixed together.

Methods: a. meperidine 25 mg. Label: 50 mg/mL

$$\frac{D}{H} \times V = \frac{25}{50} \times 1 \quad \textbf{or} \quad H : V :: D : X$$
$$50 \text{ mg} : 1 \text{ mL} :: 25 \text{ mg} : X \text{ mL}$$

$$= 0.5 \text{ mL} \qquad 50 \text{ X} = 25$$
$$X = \frac{1}{2} \text{ mL or } 0.5 \text{ mL}$$

b. Vistaril 25 mg. Label: 50 mg/mL ampule.

$$\frac{D}{H} \times V = \frac{25}{50} \times 1 \quad \textbf{or} \quad H : V :: D : X$$
$$50 \text{ mg} : 1 \text{ mL} :: 25 \text{ mg} : X \text{ mL}$$
$$= 0.5 \text{ mL} \qquad 50 \text{ X} = 25$$
$$X = \frac{1}{2} \text{ mL or } 0.5 \text{ mL}$$

c. Robinul 0.1 mg. Label: 0.2 mg/mL.

$$\frac{D}{H} \times V = \frac{0.1}{0.2} \times 1 \quad \textbf{or} \quad H : V :: D : X$$
$$0.2 \text{ mg} : 1 \text{ mL} :: 0.1 \text{ mg} : X \text{ mL}$$
$$= 0.5 \text{ mL} \qquad 0.2 \text{ X} = 0.1$$
$$X = 0.5 \text{ mL}$$

Answer: meperidine (Demerol) 25 mg = 0.5 mL; Vistaril 25 mg = 0.5 mL; Robinul 0.1 mg = 0.5 mL

Procedure: Mix three drugs in the cartridge:

1. Check drug dose and volume on pre-filled cartridge. Expel 0.5 mL of meperidine and any excess of drug solution from cartridge.

2. Draw 0.5 mL of air into the cartridge and inject into the vial containing the Robinul.

3. Withdraw 0.5 mL of Robinul from the vial into the pre-filled cartridge containing meperidine.

4. Withdraw 0.5 mL of Vistaril from the ampule into the cartridge.

IV Practice Problems: Intramuscular Injections

1. Order: tobramycin (Nebcin) 50 mg, IM, q8h.
   Drug available:

How many mL of tobramycin would you give? _____

2. Order: methylprednisolone (Solu-Medrol) 75 mg, IM, qd.
   Drug available: 125 mg/2 mL in vial.

   How many mL would you give? _____

3. Order: vitamin B$_{12}$ (cyanocobalamin) 30 mcg (μg), IM, qd.
   Drug available:

How many mL of cyanocobalamin would you give? _____

4. Order: Naloxone 0.2 mg, IM, STAT.
   Drug available:

How many mL would you give? _____

5. Order: cefepime HCl (Maxipime) 500 mg, IM, q12h.
   Drug available:

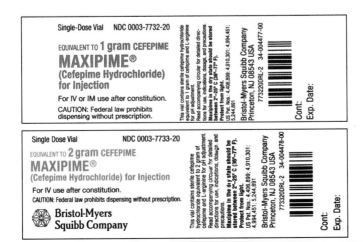

   a. Which single dose vial of Maxipime would you select? _____

   Explain. _____

   b. How many milliliters (mL) of diluent should you use for reconstitution

   of the drug? _____

> **Note:** The drug label does not indicate the amount of diluent to use. This may be found in the drug information insert. Usually, if you inject 2.6 mL of diluent, the amount of drug solution may be 3.0 mL. If you inject 3.4 or 3.5 mL of diluent, the amount of drug solution should be 4.0 mL.

   c. How many mL of drug solution should the client receive? _____

6. Order: prochlorperazine (Compazine) 4 mg, IM, q8h, as needed.
Drug available:

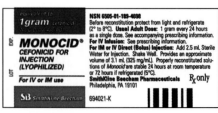

How many mL should the client receive? _____

7. Order: secobarbital (Seconal) 125 mg, IM, 1 hour prior to surgery.
Drug available: Seconal 50 mg/mL.

How many mL would you give? _____

8. Order: Thiamine HCl 75 mg, IM, qd.
Drug available: 100 and 200 mg/mL vials.

   a. Which vial would you use? _____

   b. How many mL would you give? _____

9. Order: hydroxyzine (Vistaril) 25 mg, deep IM, STAT.
Drug available: Vistaril 100 mg/2 mL in a vial.

How many mL would you give? _____

10. Order: cefonicid (Monocid) 750 mg, IM, qd.
Drug available:

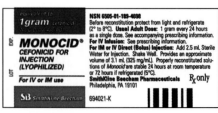

Change grams to milligrams (3 spaces to the right) or milligrams to gram (3 spaces to the left).

1.000 g = 1000 mg (the label is in milligrams)

a. How many gram(s) is 750 mg, IM, qd.?

b. How many milliliters (mL) of diluent should be injected into the vial

(see drug label)? _____

c. How many milliliters of cefonicid (Monocid) should the client receive

per day? _____

11. Order: meperidine (Demerol) 35 mg and promethazine (Phenergan) 10 mg, IM.
Drugs available: meperidine 50 mg/mL in a pre-filled cartridge that holds 2 mL of solution (2-mL cartridge); promethazine 25 mg/mL in an ampule.

a. How many mL of meperidine would you give? _____

b. How many mL of promethazine would you give? _____

c. Explain how the two drugs would be mixed in the cartridge.

_____

12. Order: meperidine (Demerol) 50 mg and atropine SO_4 0.3 mg, IM.
Drugs available:

a. How many mL of meperidine would you give? _____

b. How many mL of atropine would you give? _____

c. Explain how the two drugs are mixed in the cartridge.

_____

13. Order: procaine penicillin G (Wycillin) 400,000 U, IM, q12h.
Drug available:

600,000 U = 1 mL.

How many mL of procaine penicillin would you withdraw? _____

14. Order: heparin 2500 U, SC, q6h.
Drug available:

a. Which drug cartridge would you use? _____

b. How many mL of heparin would you give? _____

15. Order: chlordiazepoxide HCl (Librium) 50 mg, IM, STAT.
Drug available: 5 mL of dry Librium (100 mg) powder in ampule.
Add 2 mL of special intramuscular diluent to the ampule. When diluted,
the powder content may increase the volume.

How many mL would be equivalent to 50 mg? _____

Explain. _____

16. Order: cefamandole (Mandol) 500 mg, IM, q6h.
Drug available:

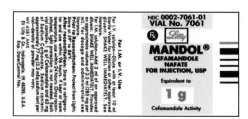

a. Change milligrams to grams (see Chapter 1).

_____

b. How many mL of diluent would you add (see drug label)?

_____

c. What size syringe would you use? _____

d. How many mL = 1 g; how many mL = 500 mg? _____

17. Order: ticarcillin (Ticar), 400 mg, IM, q6h.
Drug available:

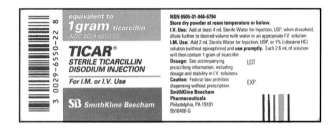

Drug label reads to add 2 mL of diluent. Total volume of solution is

_____ .

How many mL of ticarcillin should be withdrawn? _____

18. Order: morphine gr ⅙, IM, STAT.
Drug available:

Change grains to milligrams (see Chapter 1 or Tables 2–1 and 5–1).

_____

How many mL of morphine would you give? _____

19. Order: ceftazidime (Fortaz) 500 mg, IM, q8h.
Add 2.0 mL of diluent = 2.6 mL drug solution. Check the drug information insert.

Drug available:

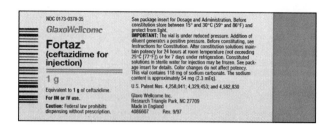

a. How many gram(s) of ceftazidime (Fortaz) should the client receive per day? _____

b. How many milliliters (mL) of ceftazidime would you give per dose?

_____

20. Order: ampicillin 0.25 g, IM, q6h.
Drug available:

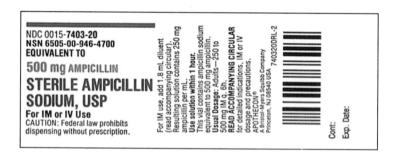

a. To change grams to milligrams, move the decimal point 3 spaces to the _____.

b. How many mL of diluent would you add to the vial? _____

c. How many mL should the client receive? _____

21. Order: diazepam 8 mg, IM, STAT and repeat in 4 hours if necessary.
Drug available:

a. Which ampule or vial of diazepam would you select? _____

b. How many milliliters (mL) of diazepam should the client receive?

_____

22. Order: benztropine mesylate (Cogentin) 1.5 mg, IM, qd.
Drug available:

How many milliliters (mL) of Cogentin should the client receive?

_____

23. Order: interferon alfa-2b (Intron A) 10 million IU IM TIW (3 × week).
Drug available: interferon alfa-2b (Intron A) 25 million IU/5 mL vials.

a. How many milliliters would you give per dose? _____

b. Explain how the drug should be drawn up. _____

24. Order: vitamin K (AquaMEPHYTON) 2.5 mg IM × 1.
Drug available: AquaMEPHYTON 10 mg/mL ampule.

How many milliliters would you give? _____

Questions 25 through 27 relate to drug dosage per body weight.

25. Order: amikacin (Amikin) 15 mg/kg/day, q8h, IM.
Drug available:

Client weighs 140 pounds.

   a. How many kilograms does the client weigh? _____

   b. How many milligrams should the client receive daily? _____

   c. How many milligrams should the client receive q8h (three divided doses)? _____

   d. How many mL should the client receive q8h? _____

26. Order: netilmicin SO_4 (Netromycin) 2.0 mg/kg, q8h, IM.
Patient weighs 174 pounds.
Drug available: netilmicin 100 mg/mL.

   a. How many kilograms does the client weigh? _____

   b. How many milligrams should the client receive daily? _____

   c. How many milligrams should the client receive q8h? _____

   d. How many mL should the client receive q8h? _____

27. Order: kanamycin (Kantrex) 15 mg/kg/day, q12h.
Drug available: (drug is also available in 1 g = 3 mL vial).

NDC 0015-3502-20
EQUIVALENT TO
500 mg KANAMYCIN per 2 mL
KANTREX®
Kanamycin Sulfate
Injection, USP
FOR I.M. OR I.V. USE
CAUTION: Federal law prohibits
dispensing without prescription.

0.66% sodium bisulfite added as
an antioxidant, buffered with 2.2%
sodium citrate. • Adjusted to pH
4.5 with H_2SO_4. • Kantrex
injection should not be physically
mixed with other antibacterial
agents.
READ ACCOMPANYING CIRCULAR
Distributed by APOTHECON®
A Bristol-Myers Squibb Co.
Princeton, NJ 08540
Made in USA   3502200RL-1

MAXIMUM DAILY DOSE: 1.5 gram

Cont:
Exp. Date:

Client weighs 67 kg.

   a. How many milligrams should the client receive per day? _____

   b. How many milligrams should the client receive every 12 hours?

   _____

   c. How many mL should the client receive per dose? _____

   d. How many mL from the 1 g = 3 mL vial should the client receive per dose? _____

Questions 28 through 32 relate to dimensional analysis. Refer to Chapter 5.

28. Order: droperidol 2 mg, IM, STAT.
Drug available: droperidol 5 mg/2 mL.
Factors: 5 mg/2 mL; 2 mg/1
Conversion factor: *none;* order and drug available are both in milligrams.

How many mL of droperidol should be given? _____

29. Order: codeine gr ½, IM, PRN.
Drug available:

Factors: 60 mg = 1 mL
        gr ½/1
Conversion factor: 1 gr = 60 mg

How many milliliters of codeine would you give? _____

30. Order: cephapirin (Cefadyl) 500 mg, IM, q6h.
Drug available:

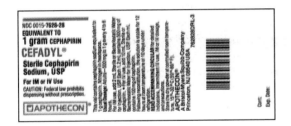

How many mL of diluent would you add? _____

Cefadyl 1 g = _____ mL; 500 mg = _____ mL

Factors: 1 g/ _____ mL; 500 mg/1

Conversion factor: 1 g = 1000 mg

How many milliliters of Cefadyl would you give? _____

31. Order: oxacillin 300 mg, IM, q8h.
Drug available:

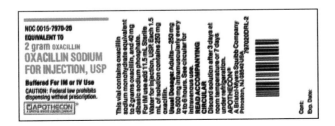

    a. Factors (drug label and drug order): _____

    b. Conversion factor: _____

    c. How many mL of oxacillin would you give? _____

32. Order: cefazolin (Ancef) 0.25 g, IM, q12h.
Drug available:

Note: *Change grams to milligrams; drug label is in milligrams.*

    a. Label states to add _____ mL or _____
diluent.

    b. How many mL of Ancef would you give? _____

ANSWERS

I. Needles

1. The 21-gauge needle, because it is the smaller gauge number.

2. The 26-gauge needle, because it is the larger gauge number.

3. The 20-gauge needle, because it has the larger lumen (small gauge). A needle with a 20 gauge and 1½-inch length is used for IM injection.

4. The 25-gauge needle, because it has the smaller lumen (larger gauge). It is used for SC injections. The needle is not long enough for an IM injection.

5. The 21-gauge needle with 1½-inch length (21 g/1½ inch). Muscle is under subcutaneous or fatty tissue, so a longer needle size is needed.

II. Subcutaneous Injections

1. *Both* needle gauge and length combinations could be used.

2. a. 0.4 mL

    b. 45- to 60-degree angle. The angle depends on the amount of fatty tissue in the client.

3. a. ¾ mL or 0.75 mL

    b. Tubex syringe, a reusable plastic or metal syringe.

4. Change grains (apothecary system) to milligrams (metric system). See Table 2–1. gr ⅟₁₀₀ = 0.6 mg.

$$\frac{D}{H} \times V = \frac{0.6}{0.4} \times 1 \quad \textbf{or}$$

$$\text{H} \quad : \text{V} \; :: \quad \text{D} \quad : \text{X}$$
$$0.4 \text{ mg} : 1 \text{ mL} : : 0.6 \text{ mg} : \text{X mL}$$

$$= \frac{0.6}{0.4} = 1.5 \text{ mL}$$

$$0.4 = 0.6$$

$$\text{X} = \frac{0.6}{0.4} = 1.5 \text{ mL}$$

5. a. 50 units/kg × 65 kg = 3250 units

b. $\frac{D}{H} \times V = \frac{3250}{10,000} \times 1 \quad \textbf{or}$

$$\text{H} \quad : \text{V} \; :: \quad \text{D} \quad : \text{X}$$
$$10,000 \text{ U} : 1 \text{ mL} : : 3250 \text{ U} : \text{X}$$

$$= 0.325 \text{ mL}$$

$$10,000 \text{ X} = 3250$$
$$\text{X} = 0.325 \text{ mL}$$

Answer: Epogen 3250 units = 0.325 mL

6. a. 198 lb ÷ 2.2 kg = 90 kg

b. 90 kg × 6 mcg/kg = 540 mcg

c. $\frac{D}{H} \times V = \frac{540 \text{ mcg}}{300 \text{ mcg}} \times 1 \text{ mL}$

$$= 1.8 \text{ mL}$$

Answer: Neupogen 540 mcg (μg) = 1.8 mL

d. Drug can be prepared in two syringes, one with 1 mL, and the other with 0.8 mL.

III. Insulin

1. Withdraw 35 U of NPH insulin to the 35 mark on the insulin syringe. Both the insulin and the syringe have the same concentration: U 100.

2. Withdraw 50 U of Lente insulin to the 50 mark on the insulin syringe. Both the insulin and the syringe have the same concentration: U 100.

3. Inject 52 U of air into the NPH insulin bottle. Do not allow the needle to touch the insulin solution. Inject 8 U of air into the regular insulin bottle, and withdraw 8 U of regular insulin. Withdraw 52 U of NPH insulin. Total amount of insulin should be 60 U. Do *not* allow the insulin mixture to stand. Administer immediately, because NPH contains protamine, and unpredicted physical changes could occur with a delay in administration.

4. Inject 45 U of air into the Lente insulin bottle. Inject 15 U of air into the regular insulin bottle, and withdraw 15 U of regular insulin. Withdraw 45 U of Lente insulin. Total amount of insulin should be 60 U. Insulin mixture can stand for a short period of time because it is Lente insulin.

IV. Intramuscular Injections

1. $\dfrac{D}{H} \times V = \dfrac{50}{80} \times 2\ \text{mL}$ **or**

$$= \dfrac{100}{80} = 1.25\ \text{mL}$$

H : V :: D : X
80 mg : 2 mL : : 50 mg : X mL
80 X = 100
$$X = \dfrac{100}{80} = 1.25\ \text{mL}$$

Answer: tobramycin 50 mg = 1.25 mL

2. $\dfrac{D}{H} \times V = \dfrac{\overset{3}{\cancel{75}}}{\underset{5}{\cancel{125}}} \times 2\ \text{mL}$ **or**

$$= \dfrac{6}{5} = 1.2\ \text{mL}$$

H : V :: D : X
125 mg : 2 mL : : 75 mg : X mL
125 X = 150
X = 1.2 mL

Answer: methylprednisolone 75 mg = 1.2 mL

3. 0.3 mL of vitamin B_{12} (cyanocobalamin)

4. 0.5 mL of Naloxone (Narcan)

5. **a.** Select the Maxipime 1-gram vial. Maxipime 2-gram vial is for intravenous use according to the drug label and cannot be used for intramuscular injection.

   b. The amount of diluent is 3.4 mL; 2.6 mL of diluent could also be used.

c. Change 500 mg to 0.5 g or 1 g to 1000 mg

$$\frac{D}{H} \times V = \frac{0.5 \text{ g}}{1 \text{ g}} \times 4 \text{ mL} = 2 \text{ mL of cefepime twice a day}$$

6. $\dfrac{D}{H} \times V = \dfrac{4}{5} \times 1 \text{ mL} = \dfrac{4}{5}$ **or**

$$\begin{array}{c} \text{H} : \text{V} :: \text{D} : \text{X} \\ 5 \text{ mg}:1 \text{ mL}::4 \text{ mg}:\text{X} \end{array}$$

0.8 mL of compazine

$$5 \text{ X} = 4$$
$$\text{X} = 0.8 \text{ mL}$$

7. 2.5 mL of secobarbital

8. a. 100 mg vial

   b. 0.75 mL of thiamine

9. ½ or 0.5 mL of hydroxyzine

10. a. 750 mg of cefonicid (Monocid) is equivalent to 0.75 g.

   b. Drug label indicates that 2.5 mL of diluent should be added to the drug powder, which yields 3.1 mL of drug solution.

   c. $\dfrac{D}{H} \times V = \dfrac{0.75 \text{ g}}{1 \text{ g}} \times 3.1 \text{ mL}$

   $= 2.33 \text{ mL or } 2.3 \text{ mL of cefonicid solution}$

11. a. meperidine 35 mg = 0.7 mL

   b. promethazine 10 mg = 0.4 mL

   c. Procedure: **1.** Check meperidine dose and volume in pre-filled cartridge.

   2. Expel 0.3 mL and any excess in pre-filled cartridge; 0.7 mL of solution should remain.

   3. Withdraw 0.4 mL of promethazine from ampule into cartridge.

12. a. meperidine 50 mg = ½ or 0.5 mL

   b. atropine 0.3 mg = 0.75 or 0.8 mL

   Atropine:

   $$\frac{D}{H} \times V = \frac{0.3}{0.4} \times 1 \text{ mL} \quad \textbf{or}$$

   $$\begin{array}{c} \text{H} : \text{V} :: \text{D} : \text{X} \\ 0.4 \text{ mg}:1 \text{ mL}::0.3 \text{ mg}:\text{X mL} \end{array}$$

   $$0.4 \text{ X} = 0.3$$

   $$\frac{0.75}{0.4)\overline{0.3\,00}} = 0.75 \text{ or } 0.8 \text{ mL}$$

   $$\text{X} = \frac{0.3}{0.4} = 0.75 \text{ or } 0.8 \text{ mL}$$

   c. 1. The two drugs are compatible.

   2. Pre-filled cartridge contains 100 mg = 1 mL. Expel 0.5 mL and any excess in the prefilled cartridge; 0.5 mL drug remains.

   3. Inject 0.75 (0.8) mL of air into the vial, and withdraw the same amount of atropine into the cartridge.

13. $\dfrac{D}{H} \times V = \dfrac{400,000}{600,000} \times 1 \text{ mL} \quad \textbf{or}$

$$\begin{array}{c} \text{H} : \text{V} :: \text{D} : \text{X} \\ 600,000 \text{ U}:1 \text{ mL}::400,000 \text{ U}:\text{X mL} \end{array}$$

$$= \frac{4}{6} = 0.66 \text{ or } 0.7 \text{ mL}$$

$$600,000 \text{ X} = 400,000$$
$$\text{X} = 0.66 \text{ or } 0.7 \text{ mL}$$

Answer: procaine penicillin U 400,000 = 0.7 mL

14. **a.** Use either heparin cartridge: 5000 U/0.5 mL or 10,000 U/1 mL

    b. 0.25 mL of heparin

15. Librium 50 mg = 1 mL (100 mg = 2 mL)

After adding 2 mL of diluent, withdraw the entire drug solution to determine the total volume of drug solution. Expel half of the solution; the remaining drug solution is equivalent to chlordiazepoxide (Librium) 50 mg.

16. **a.** Change milligrams to grams (smaller to larger number) by moving the decimal point three spaces to the *left*. 500. mg = 0.5 g.

Because the drug weight on the label is in grams, the conversion is to grams. However, the drug can be converted to milligrams by changing grams to milligrams (moving the decimal point three spaces to the *right*): 1 g = 1.000 mg = 1000 mg.

    b. Drug label states to add 3 mL of diluent and, after reconstituted, the drug solution will be 3.5 mL. Mandol 1 g = 3.5 mL.

    c. A 5-mL syringe is preferred: however, a 3-mL syringe can be used because less than 3 mL of the drug solution is needed.

    d. $\dfrac{D}{H} \times V = \dfrac{0.5}{1} \times 3.5$ mL **or**   H : V :: D : X

$$1000 \text{ mg} : 3.5 \text{ mL} :: 500 \text{ mg} : X \text{ mL}$$

           = 1.75 or 1.8 mL   1000 X = 1750

                                             X = 1.75 or 1.8 mL

Answer: cefamandole (Mandol) 500 mg = 1.8 mL

17. Change 400 milligrams to grams

$$400 \text{ mg} = 0.400 \text{ g or } 0.4 \text{ g}$$

$\dfrac{D}{H} \times V = \dfrac{0.4}{1} \times 2.6$ **or**   H : V :: D : X

                              1 g : 2.6 mL :: 0.4 mg : X mL

        = 1 mL   X = 2.6 × 0.4

                                    X = 1 mL

ticarcillin 400 mg or 0.4 g = 1.0 mL

18. 1 gr = 60 mg; gr ⅙ = 10 mg

$\dfrac{D}{H} \times V = \dfrac{\overset{2}{\cancel{10}}}{\underset{3}{\cancel{15}}} \times 1$ mL **or**   H : V :: D : X

                           15 mg : 1 mL :: 10 mg : X mL

          $= \dfrac{2}{3}$ = 0.66 or 0.7 mL   15 X = 10

                                      X = 0.66 or 0.7 mL

19. **a.** Change milligrams to grams; move the decimal point three spaces to the left: 500. mg = 0.5 g

$$0.5 \text{ g} \times 3 \text{ (q8h)} = 1.5 \text{ g per day}$$

    b. Add 2 mL of diluent to yield 2.6 mL (check drug information insert):

$$\frac{D}{H} \times V = \frac{0.5 \text{ g}}{1 \text{ g}} \times 2.6 \text{ mL} = 1.3 \text{ mL per dose}$$

20. **a.** right, 0.25 g = 250 mg

    b. 1.8 mL (after dilution, 2 mL)

    c. 1 mL = 250 mg of ampicillin

21. **a.** Either the ampule or the vial could be used. The diazepam 5 mg/mL is a multiple-dose vial that contains 10 mL of drug solution.

    b. Ampule: $\dfrac{8 \text{ mg}}{10 \text{ mg}} \times 2 \text{ mL} = 1.6 \text{ mL of diazepam}$

    Vial: $\dfrac{8 \text{ mg}}{5 \text{ mg}} \times 1 \text{ mL} = 1.6 \text{ mL of diazepam}$

22. $\dfrac{D}{H} \times V = \dfrac{\overset{}{\cancel{1.5 \text{ mg}}}}{\underset{1}{\cancel{2 \text{ mg}}}} \times \overset{1}{\cancel{2}} \text{ mL} = 1.5 \text{ mL of Cogentin}$

23. $\dfrac{D}{H} \times V = \dfrac{10}{25} \times 5$ **or**

    $$= 0.4 \times 5$$
    $$= 2 \text{ mL}$$

H	:	V	::	D	:	X

    25 million units : 5 mL : : 10 million units : X mL

    $$25 \text{ X} = 50$$
    $$\text{X} = 2 \text{ mL}$$

    Answer: Intron A 2 mL three times a week

24. $\dfrac{D}{H} \times V = \dfrac{2.5}{10} \times 1$ **or**

    $$= 0.25 \text{ mL}$$

    H : V :: D :X

    10 mg : 1 mL : : 2.5 mg : X

    $$10 \text{ X} = 2.5$$
    $$\text{X} = 0.25 \text{ mL}$$

    Answer: AquaMEPHYTON 2.5 mg = 0.25 mL

25. **a.** 140 ÷ 2.2 = 63.6 kg

    b. 15 mg × 63.6 × 1 = 954 mg daily

    c. 954 ÷ 3 = 318 mg of amikacin q8h

    d. $\dfrac{D}{H} \times V = \dfrac{318}{500} \times 2$ **or**

    $$= \frac{636}{500} = 1.27 \text{ or } 1.3 \text{ mL}$$

    H : V :: D : X

    500 mg : 2 mL : : 318 mg : X mL

    $$500 \text{ X} = 636$$
    $$\text{X} = 1.27 \text{ or } 1.3 \text{ mL}$$

    Answer: give 1.27 or 1.3 mL of amikacin q8h (three times a day)

26. **a.** 174 ÷ 2.2 = 79.1 kg

    b. 2 mg × 79.1 = 158 mg daily

    c. 158 ÷ 3 = 52 mg or 50 mg q8h

    d. $\dfrac{D}{H} \times V = \dfrac{\overset{5}{\cancel{50}}}{\underset{10}{\cancel{100}}} \times 1 \text{ mL}$ **or**

    $$= \frac{5}{10} = 0.5 \text{ mL}$$

    H : V :: D : X

    100 mg : 1 mL : : 50 mg : X mL

    $$100 \text{ X} = 50$$
    $$\text{X} = 0.5 \text{ mL}$$

    Answer: netilmicin 50 mg = 0.5 mL

27. a. 15 mg/67 kg/day = 15 × 67 = 1005 mg/day.

  b. 500 mg (1005 mg ÷ 2 = 500 mg)

  c. $\dfrac{\overset{1}{\cancel{500}}}{\underset{1}{\cancel{500}}} \times 2 = 2$ mL per dose of Kantrex

  d. 1 g = 1000 mg $\dfrac{D}{H} \times V = \dfrac{\overset{1}{\cancel{500}}}{\underset{2}{\cancel{1000}}} \times 3 = \dfrac{3}{2} = 1.5$ mL

28. milliliters $= \dfrac{2 \text{ mL} \times 2 \cancel{\text{mg}}}{5 \cancel{\text{mg}} \times 1} = \dfrac{4}{5} = 0.8$ mL

  0.8 mL of droperidol

29. milliliters $= \dfrac{1 \text{ mL} \times \cancel{60 \text{ mg}} \times 0.5 \cancel{\text{gr}}}{\cancel{60 \text{ mg}} \times 1 \cancel{\text{gr}} \times 1} = 0.5$ mL

30. a. 2 mL of diluent (sterile or bacteriostatic water)

  b. 1 g = 2.4; 500 mg = 1.2 mL (as stated on the label)

  c. Factors: 1 g/2.4 mL; 500 mg/1

  d. milliliters $= \dfrac{2.4 \times 1 \cancel{\text{g}} \times \overset{1}{\cancel{500 \text{ mg}}}}{1 \cancel{\text{g}} \times \underset{2}{\cancel{1000 \text{ mg}}} \times 1} = \dfrac{2.4}{2} = 1.2$ mL

  Give 1.2 mL of Cefadyl.

31. a. Factors: drug label: 2 g = 12 mL (add 11.5 mL) **or** 250 mg = 1.5 mL **or** 0.25 g = 1.5 mL

  drug order: 300 mg/1

  b. Conversion factor: 1 g = 1000 mg

  c. milliliters $= \dfrac{1.5 \text{ mL} \times 1 \cancel{\text{g}} \times \overset{3}{\cancel{300 \text{ mg}}}}{0.25 \cancel{\text{g}} \times \underset{10}{\cancel{1000 \text{ mg}}} \times 1} = \dfrac{4.5}{2.5} =$

  1.8 mL of oxacillin per dose

32. 0.25 g = 0.025 mg (250 mg)

  a. Drug label: add 2 mL diluent = 2.2 mL of drug solution.

  b. Give 1.1 mL of Ancef.

intravenous preparations with clinical applications

Objectives

- Name catheter sites for intravenous access.
- Examine the three methods for calculating intravenous (IV) flow rate and select one of the methods for IV calculation.
- Calculate drops per minute of prescribed IV solutions for IV therapy.
- Determine the drop factor according to the manufacturer's product specification.
- Calculate the drug dosage for IV medications.
- Calculate the flow rate for IV drugs being administered in a prescribed amount of solution.
- Explain the types and uses of electronic IV delivery devices.
- Calculate the rate of direct IV injection.

Outline

Intravenous (IV) therapy is used for administering fluids containing water, dextrose, fat emulsions, vitamins, electrolytes, and drugs. Approximately 90% of all hospitalized clients, some outpatients, and some home-care clients receive IV therapy. Drugs are administered intravenously for direct absorption and fast action. Many drugs cannot be absorbed through the gastrointestinal tract, and the IV route provides bioavailability. Certain drugs that need to be absorbed immediately are administered by direct intravenous injection—diluted, over several minutes. However, many drugs administered IV are irritating to the veins because of the drugs' pH or osmolality and must be diluted and administered slowly.

Advantages of IV drug therapy are (1) rapid drug distribution into the bloodstream, (2) rapid onset of action, and (3) no drug loss to tissues. There are many complications of IV therapy, some of which are sepsis, thrombosis, phlebitis, air emboli, infiltration, and extravasation. The nurse must monitor for signs of these complications during the course of IV therapy.

Three methods are used to administer IV fluid and drugs: (1) direct IV drug injection, (2) continuous IV infusion, and (3) intermittent IV infusion. Continuous IV administration replaces fluid loss, maintains fluid balance, and is a vehicle for drug administration. Intermittent IV administration is primarily used for giving IV drugs.

Nurses play an important role in preparing and administering IV solutions and drugs. Nursing functions and responsibilities include (1) knowledge of intravenous sets and their drop factors, (2) calculating IV flow rates, (3) verifying compatibility of the IV solution and the drug, (4) mixing drugs and diluting in IV solution, (5) regulating IV infusion devices, and (6) maintaining patency of IV accesses.

INTRAVENOUS ACCESS SITES

The successful administration of IV drugs and fluids depends on a patent IV access. The most common site for short-term therapy is the peripheral site, in which a short catheter or needle is inserted in a vein in the hand or arm. Feet and legs can be used, but the risk of a deep vein thrombus is always present. For individuals without adequate peripheral sites or those requiring long-term IV therapy, a central venous site is chosen. Central venous sites are the superior vena cava and the inferior vena cava. The superior vena cava is accessed from the internal jugular vein and the right or left subclavian vein, whereas the inferior vena cava is accessed from the femoral vein. The insertion requires a minor surgical procedure: percutaneous vein cannulation with the introduction of a catheter. The catheter may be single-lumen or multilumen. A long-line peripheral catheter can also be used to access the superior vena cava. The long-line catheter is inserted in a large vein (the basilic) and advanced through the subclavian vein to the superior vena cava. In some states, peripherally inserted central catheters (PICCs), are inserted by registered nurses.

Clients who need IV access for long-term use, such as chemotherapy, antibiotic therapy, or nutritional support, are given much longer catheters, which are tunneled under the skin after the vein is cannulated. The catheter and its drug infusion port exit from the subcutaneous tissue to a site on the chest. Examples of these devices are the Hickman, Groshong, and Cook catheters.

Another type of catheter for long-term use has an implantable infusion port that is inserted in the subcutaneous tissue under the skin. These devices are called *vascular access ports* and they have a larger drug port or

Figure 8•1

Central venous access site(s): (*A*) subclavian catheter; (*B*) peripherally inserted central catheter (PICC); (*C*) femoral catheter; (*D*) Hickman catheter; (*E*) subclavian catheter with implantable vascular access port; (*F*) implantable vascular access port. *F* redrawn from Winters, B. (1984). Implantable vascular access devices. *Oncology Nursing Forum, 11*(6), 25–30.

Figure 8•2

Infusion devices.

septum than other catheters. Care must be taken to use a noncoring needle that slices the port instead of making holes so that the septum will close instead of leak after the needle has been removed (Fig. 8–1).

Intermittent Infusion Devices

When IV access sites are used not for continuous infusion but rather for intermittent therapy, they must be irrigated periodically to maintain patency. An intermittent infusion device can be attached to the end of the IV catheter or needle to close the connection that was attached to the IV tubing (Fig. 8–2). These devices have ports (stoppers) where needles or IV tubing can be inserted when drug therapy is resumed. This practice can eliminate the need for a constant low-rate infusion to keep the vein open (KVO) and reduce excessive fluid intake. The use of intermittent infusion devices can allow the client more mobility and can be cost-effective because less IV tubing, IV solution, and regulating equipment is needed.

To maintain patency, IV sites, can be irrigated either every 8 hours or before and after each drug infusion, depending on each institution's policy. Peripheral sites are irrigated or flushed with 1 to 3 mL of normal saline. Central venous sites are flushed with a heparinized saline solution. The amount of heparin used varies; 10 U/1 mL to 100 U/1 mL is the dosage range commonly given, but each institution's policies and procedures should be followed. The volume of the flush solution can vary with the type of venous access device and the length of catheter tubing (Table 8–1).

DIRECT INTRAVENOUS INJECTIONS

Medications that are given by the IV injection route are calculated in the same manner as medications for intramuscular injection. This route often is referred to as *IV push*. Clinically, it is the preferred route for clients with poor muscle mass or decreased circulation, or for a drug that is poorly absorbed from the tissues. Medications administered by this route have a rapid onset of action, and calculation errors can have serious, even fatal consequences. Drug information inserts must be read carefully, and attention paid to the amount of drug that can be given per minute. If the drug is

t a b l e 8●1
VENOUS ACCESS DEVICES: FLUSHING GUIDELINES FOR INTERMITTENT USE

TYPE	LENGTH (inches)	FLUSH SOLUTION	VOLUME (mL)	FREQUENCY
Peripheral	1–2	Normal saline	1–3	After each use or q8h
Central Venous				
Single-lumen	8	Heparinized saline	1	After each use or q8h
Multi-lumen	8	Heparinized saline	1/port	After each use or q8h
External-tunneled Hickman, Cook, or Groshong	35	Heparinized saline	2–5	After each use or q8h
Peripherally inserted central catheter (PICC)	20	Normal saline	3–5	After each use or q12h
Implanted vascular access device	35	Heparinized saline	3–5	After each use; q5–7d when not in use

pushed into the bloodstream at a faster rate than specified in the drug literature, adverse reactions to the medication are likely to occur.

Calculating the amount of time needed to infuse a drug given by direct IV infusion can be determined by using ratio and proportion.

REMEMBER

When giving drugs by direct IV infusion, always verify the compatibility of the IV solution and the drug. Consider the length of the injection port on the tubing from the IV site, and that the tubing usually needs to be flushed after direct IV infusion to ensure that part of the drug has not been left in the tubing. Drug dose is not complete until the drug has entered the client.

e x a m p l e s

Set up a ratio and proportion using the recommended amount of drug per minute on one side of the equation; these are the known variables. On the other side of the equation are the desired amount of drug and unknown desired minutes.

PROBLEM 1: Order: Dilantin 200 mg, IV, STAT.
Drug available: Dilantin 250 mg/5 mL. IV infusion not to exceed 50 mg/minute.

known drug : known minutes : : desired drug : desired minutes

50 mg : 1 min : : 200 mg : X

50 X = 200

X = 4 min

PROBLEM 2: Order: Lasix 120 mg, IV, STAT.
Drug available: Lasix 10 mg/mL. IV infusion not to exceed 40 mg/minute.

known drug:known minutes : : desired drug:desired minutes

40 mg : 1 min : : 120 mg : X

40 X = 120

X = 3 min

When dosing instructions give the amount of drug and specify infusion time, the amount of drug can be divided by the number of minutes to give the per minute amount to be infused.

example

PROBLEM 3: Order: Amrinone (Inocor) 65 mg, IV bolus over 3 minutes.
Drug available: Inocor 100 mg/20 mL

H : V :: D :V

100 mg:20 mL : 65 mg:X

100 X = 1300

X = 13 mL

$$\frac{13 \text{ mL}}{3 \text{ min}} = 4.2 \text{ mL/min}$$

I Practice Problems: Direct IV Injection

Determine the number of minutes that are required for the direct IV drug dose to be administered for each of the practice problems.

1. Order: protamine sulfate 50 mg, IV, STAT.
Drug available:

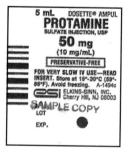

IV infusion not to exceed 5 mg/minute.

2. Order: dextrose 50% in 50 mL, IV, STAT.
Drug available: dextrose 50% in 50 mL.
IV infusion not to exceed 10 mL/minute.

3. Order: calcium gluconate 4.5 mEq, IV, STAT.
Drug available:

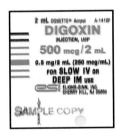

IV infusion not to exceed 1.5 mL/minute. **Note:** 4.65 mEq/10 mL.

4. Order: prednisolone 50 mg, IV, q12h.
Drug available: prednisolone 50 mg in 5 mL.
IV infusion not to exceed 10 mg/minute.

5. Order: morphine sulfate 6 mg, IV, q3h, PRN.
Drug available: morphine sulfate 10 mg/mL.
Infusion not to exceed 10 mg/4 minutes.

6. Order: digoxin 0.25 mg, IV, qd.
Drug available:

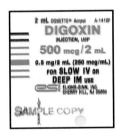

Infuse slowly over 5 minutes.
How many mL/min should be infused? _____

7. Order: Haldol 2 mg, IV, q4h, PRN.
Drug available: Haldol 5 mg/mL.
IV infusion not to exceed 1 mg/minute.

8. Order: Ativan 6 mg, IV, q6h, PRN.
Drug available: Ativan 4 mg/mL.
IV infusion not to exceed 2 mg/minute.

9. Order: diltiazem (Cardizem) 20 mg IV over 2 minutes.
Drug available:

    a. How many milliliters (mL) would you give? _____

    b. How many milliliters (mL) would you infuse per minute? _____

10. Order: granisetron (Kytril) 10 μg/kg, 30 minutes before chemotherapy.
Infuse 1 mg over 60 seconds.
Patient weighs 140 pounds.
Drug available:

    a. How many killigrams (kg) does the client weigh? _____

    b. How many milligrams (mg) should the client receive? _____

    c. For how many seconds should the drug dose be infused? _____

> **NOTE**
> When a drug is being pushed through IV tubing, the type of fluid used for infusion must be compatible with the drug or precipitation can result. Incompatibilities can be avoided if IV tubing is flushed with a drug-compatible solution, either sterile normal saline or sterile water, prior to and after administration.

CONTINUOUS INTRAVENOUS ADMINISTRATION

When IV solutions are required, the health care provider orders the amount of solution per liter or milliliter to be administered for a specific time, such as for 24 hours. The nurse calculates the IV flow rate according to the drop factor, the amount of fluids to be administered, and the infusion time.

Intravenous Sets

There are various IV infusion sets. The drop factor, or the number of drops per milliliter, is usually printed on the package. Sets that deliver large drops per milliliter (10–20 gtt/mL) are referred to as *macrodrip sets,* and those with small drops per milliliter (60 gtt/mL) are called *microdrip* or *minidrip sets.*

    Examples of sets that deliver macrodrip (large drops) or microdrip (small drops) are listed in Table 8–2. Figures 8–3, 8–4, and 8–5 illustrate sizes of IV drops, IV bags and bottles, and IV tubing.

    All microdrip sets deliver 60 gtt/mL. To determine the drop factor (gtt/mL), check the box or package of the IV set. This information is needed to calculate and regulate IV flow rate. In most instances, the nurse has a choice

table 8•2
INTRAVENOUS SETS

DROPS (gtt) PER MILLILITER	
Macrodrip Sets	**Microdrip Sets**
10 gtt/mL	60 gtt/mL
15 gtt/mL	
20 gtt/mL	

in using either a macrodrip or a microdrip set. If the IV rate is to infuse at 100 mL/hour or faster, a macrodrip set is generally used. If the infusion rate is slower than 100 mL/hour, the microdrip set is preferred. Slow drip rates of less than 100 mL/hour make macrodrip adjustment difficult. For example, at 50 mL/hour, the macrodrip rate would be 8 gtt/minute.

At times, IV fluids are given at a slow rate to *keep vein open* (KVO), also called *to keep open* (TKO). Reasons for ordering KVO include (1) a suspected or potential emergency situation requiring rapid administration of fluids and drugs and (2) maintaining an open line to give IV drugs at specified hours. For KVO, a microdrip set (60 gtt/mL) and a 250-mL IV bag can be used. KVO is usually regulated to deliver 10 mL/hour.

Macrodrip
10–20 gtt/ml

Microdrip
60 gtt/ml

Figure 8•3

Macrodrip and microdrip sizes.

Figure 8•4
Intravenous containers.

Calculation of Intravenous Flow Rate

Three different methods can be used to calculate IV flow rate (drops per minute or gtt/min). The nurse should select one of the methods, memorize it, and use it to calculate dosages.*

THREE-STEP METHOD

a. $\dfrac{\text{amount of solution}}{\text{hours to administer}} = \text{mL/hr}$

b. $\dfrac{\text{mL per hour}}{60\ \text{minutes}} = \text{mL/min}$

c. mL per minute $\times$ gtt per mL of IV set = gtt/min

_____

* The two-step method is the method most commonly used for calculating IV flow rate.

Spike end for
IV bag or bottle

Drop chamber

Adapter end of
tubing to needle

Roller clamp

Y-site

Figure 8•5
Intravenous tubing.

TWO-STEP METHOD

a. amount of fluid ÷ hours to administer = mL/hr

b. $\dfrac{\text{mL per hour} \times \text{gtt/mL (IV set)}}{60 \text{ minutes}} = \text{gtt/min}$

ONE-STEP METHOD

$$\dfrac{\text{amount of fluid} \times \text{gtt/mL (IV set)}}{\text{hours to administer} \times \text{minutes per hour (60)}} = \text{gtt/min}$$

Safety Considerations

All IV infusions should be checked every hour to ensure the rate of infusion and to assess for potential problems. Common problems associated with IV infusions are kinked tubing, extravasation of IV fluids, and "runaway" IV rates. IVs using electronic IV delivery devices also need to be monitored. Mechanical problems or incorrect settings can cause incorrect fluid administration. Fluid overload, thrombus formation, and infiltration at the IV site are complications of IV therapy that can be avoided with frequent monitoring of the IV infusion. See Appendix A for more detailed information on safe nursing practice for IV drug administration.

Mixing Drugs Used for Continuous Intravenous Administration

Drugs such as multiple vitamins and potassium chloride can be added to the IV solution bag for continuous IV infusion. It is suggested that the drug or drugs be added to the bag or bottle immediately before administering the IV fluid. Inject the drug into the rubber stopper on the IV bag or bottle and rotate several times to ensure dispersal of the drug. Do *not* add the drug while the infusion is running unless the bag is rotated. A drug solution injected into an upright infusing IV solution causes the drug to concentrate into the lower portion of the IV bag and not be dispersed. The client will receive a concentrated drug solution and this can be harmful (e.g., if the drug was potassium chloride). If drugs are injected into the IV bag prior to use, the bag should be refrigerated to maintain drug potency.

There are various nutrients (dextrose) and electrolytes in commercially prepared IV solutions. The commonly used solutions are dextrose in water, normal saline, one-half normal saline, and lactated Ringer's. These types of solutions are abbreviated as listed in Table 8–3.

examples

Two problems for determining IV flow rate are given. Each problem is solved using each of the three methods for calculating IV flow rate.

PROBLEM 1: Order: 1000 mL of $D_5\frac{1}{2}$ NSS (5% dextrose in ½ normal saline solution) in 6 hours.
Available: 1 L (1000 mL) of $D_5\frac{1}{2}$ NSS solution bag: IV set labeled 10 gtt/mL.
How many drops per minute (gtt/min) should the client receive?

table 8•3
ABBREVIATIONS FOR IV SOLUTIONS

IV SOLUTION	ABBREVIATION(S)
5% dextrose in water	D_5W, 5% D/W
10% dextrose in water	$D_{10}W$, 10% D/W
0.9% sodium chloride, normal saline solution	0.9% NaCl, NSS, PSS
0.45% sodium chloride, ½ normal saline solution	0.45% NaCl, ½ NSS, ½ PSS
5% dextrose in 0.9% sodium chloride	D_5NSS, 5% D/NSS, 5% D/0.9% NaCl, D_5 PSS
5% dextrose in 0.45% sodium chloride, 5% dextrose in ½ normal saline solution	$D_5\frac{1}{2}$ NSS, 5% D/½ NSS, ½ PSS
Lactated Ringer's solution	LRS

Three-Step Method: a. $\dfrac{1000 \text{ mL}}{6 \text{ hr}} = 166.6$ or 167 mL/hr

b. $\dfrac{167 \text{ mL}}{60 \text{ min}} = 2.7$ or 2.8 mL/min

c. $2.8 \text{ mL/min} \times 10 \text{ gtt/mL} = 28 \text{ gtt/min}$

Two-Step Method: a. $1000 \text{ mL} \div 6 \text{ hr} = 167 \text{ mL/hr}$

b. $\dfrac{167 \text{ mL/hr} \times \overset{1}{\cancel{10}} \text{ gtt/mL}}{\underset{6}{\cancel{60}} \text{ min}} = \dfrac{167}{6}$

$= 28 \text{ gtt/min}$

10 and 60 cancel to 1 and 6.

If mL/hr is given, use only part **b** of the two-step method for calculating IV flow rate.

One-Step Method: $\dfrac{1000 \text{ mL} \times \overset{1}{\cancel{10}} \text{ gtt/mL}}{6 \text{ hr} \times \underset{6}{\cancel{60}} \text{ min}} \times \dfrac{1000}{36}$

$= 27 - 28 \text{ gtt/min}$

10 and 60 cancel to 1 and 6.

To avoid errors, the use of a hand calculator is strongly suggested.

Answer: *28 gtt/minute.*

PROBLEM 2: Order: 1000 mL of D_5W (5% dextrose in water), 1 vial of MVI (multiple vitamin), and 20 mEq of KCl (potassium chloride) every 8 hours.
Available: 1000 mL D_5W solution bag
1 vial of MVI = 5 mL
40 mEq/20 mL of KCl in an ampule
IV set labeled 15 gtt/mL
How many milliliters (mL) of KCl would you withdraw as equivalent to 20 mEq of KCl?
How would you mix KCl in the IV bag?
How many drops per minute should the client receive?

Procedure: MVI: Inject 5 mL of MVI into the rubber stopper on the IV bag.
KCl: Calculate the prescribed dosage for KCl using the basic formula or ratio and proportion.

$\dfrac{D}{H} \times V = \dfrac{20}{40} \times 20$ **or** $\quad$ H : V :: D : X
$\qquad\qquad\qquad\qquad$ 40 mEq : 20 mL : : 20 mEq : X mL

$= \dfrac{400}{40} = 10 \text{ mL} \qquad\qquad$ 40 X $= 400$
$\qquad\qquad\qquad\qquad\qquad$ X $= 10 \text{ mL}$

Withdraw 10 mL of KCl and inject into the rubber stopper on the IV bag. Make sure the KCl solution is dispersed throughout the IV solution by rotating the IV bag.

Three-Step Method: a. $\dfrac{1000 \text{ mL}}{8 \text{ hr}} = 125 \text{ mL/hr}$

b. $\dfrac{125 \text{ mL}}{60 \text{ min}} = 2.0-2.1 \text{ mL/min}$

c. $2.1 \times 15 = 31-32 \text{ gtt/min}$

Two-Step Method: a. $1000 \div 8 = 125 \text{ mL/hr}$

b. $\dfrac{125 \text{ mL/hr} \times \overset{1}{\cancel{15}} \text{ gtt/mL}}{\underset{4}{\cancel{60}} \text{ min}} = \dfrac{125}{4}$

$= 31-32 \text{ gtt/min}$

15 and 60 cancel to 1 and 4.

IV flow rate should be 31 to 32 gtt/min.

One-Step Method: $\dfrac{1000 \text{ mL} \times \overset{1}{\cancel{15}} \text{ gtt/mL}}{8 \text{ hr} \times \underset{4}{\cancel{60}} \text{ min}} = \dfrac{1000}{32} = 32 \text{ gtt/min}$

15 and 60 cancel to 1 and 4.

IV flow rate should be 31 to 32 gtt/min.

NOTE Medication volume can be added to the total volume if strict intake and output are being recorded. In general, an IV bag contains more fluid than labeled on the bag; some estimates are as much as 50 mL. If an electric infusion device is used, the client will receive the amount programmed into the device. When the volume of the medication exceeds 20 mL, the amount should be added to the total volume to be infused. If the volume is less than 20 mL, it will not greatly change the hourly rate.

II Practice Problems: Continuous Intravenous Administration

Select *one* of the three methods for calculating IV flow rate. The two-step method is preferred by most nurses.

1. Order: 1000 L of D_5W to run for 12 hours.

    a. Would you use a macrodrip or microdrip IV set? _____

    b. Calculate the drops per minute (gtt/min) using one of the three

    methods. _____

2. Order: 3 L of IV solutions for 24 hours: 2 L of 5% D/½ NSS and 1 L of D_5W.

    a. One liter is equal to _____ mL.

b. Each liter should run for _____ hours.

c. The institution uses an IV set with a drop factor of 15 gtt/mL. How many drops per minute (gtt/min) should the client receive? _____

3. Order: 250 mL of D_5W for KVO.

a. What type of IV set would you use? _____

Why? _____

b. How many drops per minute should the client receive? _____

4. Order: 1000 mL of 5% D/0.2% NaCl with 10 mEq of KCl for 10 hours. Available: Macrodrop IV set with a drop factor of 20 gtt/mL and microdrip set; KCl 20 mEq/20 mL vial.

a. How many milliliters (mL) of KCl should be injected into the IV bag?

_____

b. How is KCl mixed in the IV solution? _____

c. How many drops per minute (gtt/min) should the client receive with both the macrodrip set and the microdrip set? _____

5. A liter (1000 mL) of IV fluid was started at 9 AM and was to run for 8 hours. The IV set delivers 15 gtt/mL. Four hours later, only 300 mL have been absorbed.

a. How much IV fluid is left? _____

b. Recalculate the flow rate for the remaining IV fluids. _____

6. The client is to receive 100 mL/hr of D_5W.
Available: Microdrip set (60 gtt/mL).

How many drops per minute should the client receive? _____

7. Order: 1000 D_5W with 40 mEq KCl at 125 mL/hr.
Drug available: potassium chloride

a. Which concentration of KCl would you choose? _____

b. How many milliliters (mL) of KCl should be injected into the IV bag?

_____

c. How many hours will the IV last? _____

8. Order: 1000 D_5/½ NSS with 20 mEq KCl at 100 mL/hr.
Available: Macrodrip set (10 gtt/mL)
Drug available: potassium chloride

a. Which concentration of KCl would you choose? _____

b. How many milliliters (mL) of KCl should be injected into the IV bag?

_____

c. How many hours will the IV last? _____

d. How many drops per minute (gtt/min) should the client receive?

_____

INTERMITTENT INTRAVENOUS ADMINISTRATION

Giving drugs via the intermittent IV route has many advantages. The IV route allows for rapid therapeutic concentration of the drug and control over the onset of action and peak concentrations. Blood serum concentrations can be achieved via the IV route if the oral route is unavailable because of the client's condition, such as gastrointestinal malabsorption or neurological deficits that prevent swallowing. The IV route can be used on an outpatient basis and can ensure compliance with drug therapy. The IV route also allows for the rapid correction of electrolyte imbalances. IV medications can be given at intervals within a 24-hour period for days or weeks. These medications are administered in a small volume of fluid (50 to 250 mL of D_5W or saline). The drug solution is usually delivered to the client in 15 minutes to 1 hour, depending on the medication. A separate delivery set or secondary set is used for intermittent therapy if the client is also receiving continuous infusion through the same IV site.

Secondary Intravenous Sets

Two sets available for administering IV drugs are (1) the calibrated cylinder (chamber) with tubing, such as Buretrol, Volutrol, and Soluset, and (2) the secondary set, which is similar to a regular IV set except that the tubing is shorter (Fig. 8–6). The secondary set is primarily used for infusing small volumes, such as 50-, 100-, and 250-mL bags or bottles. The chambers of the Buretrol, Volutrol, and Soluset devices each hold 150 mL of solution. Medication is injected into the chamber and diluted with solution. These methods for administering IV drugs are referred to as *IV piggyback* (IVPB). Usually,

Figure 8•6

Secondary intravenous sets.

drugs administered by Buretrol, Volutrol, or Soluset are prepared by the nurse.

Normally, drugs for IV infusion are diluted prior to infusion. Clinical agencies frequently have their own protocols for dilutions; if not, the drug information insert should have infusion guidelines. If the information is not available, the hospital pharmacy should be contacted. Guidelines and protocols help in preventing drug and fluid incompatibility.

The current trend in IV medication administration is the use of premixed IV drugs in 50- to 500-mL bags. These premixed IV medications can be prepared by the manufacturer or by the hospital pharmacy. The problems of contamination and drug errors are decreased with the use of premixed IV medication. Each IV drug bag has its separate tubing to avoid admixture. Cost is higher but risk is lower with the use of premixed IV drug bags. Because not all medication can be premixed in the solution, nurses will continue to prepare some drugs for IV administration.

> **NOTE:** When using a calibrated cylinder such as the Buretrol, add 15 mL of IV solution to flush the drug out of the IV line after the drug infusion is completed. The flush volume is added to the client's intake.

Electronic Intravenous Delivery Devices

Controllers and pumps are the two basic types of electronic IV delivery devices. Controllers (Fig. 8–7A) work by the pressure that gravity exerts on the fluid in the IV container, bag, or bottle. They have an electronically controlled clamp that adjusts the flow by clamping and releasing the IV tubing. The controller's drop sensor on the drip chamber detects any increase or decrease of drops and automatically adjusts the clamp. Controllers are sensitive to any restrictions, such as infiltrations, and an alarm is sounded when the set rate cannot be maintained. Controllers are not accurate for volumes less than 5 mL/hr. To ensure the correct rate of infusion, the IV bag or bottle must be 3 feet above the IV site, and the tubing must be free of occlusions.

IV DELIVERY PUMPS

An IV delivery pump pushes with pressure to infuse the fluid. The two types of IV delivery pumps are the peristaltic pump and the volumetric pump (Fig. 8–7B). The peristaltic pump and the volumetric pump have different pushing mechanisms. With the peristaltic pump, ridges move in wavelike motion against the IV tubing. The pressure on the IV tubing moves the fluid along.

The volumetric pump is more accurate. It requires a specific administration set that functions as a reservoir. The pump fills the reservoir and empties every cycle to deliver the programmed fluid rate. The increments of fluid delivered can be as low as one tenth to one hundredth of a milliliter with micropumps.

Figure 8•7

(*A*) Infusion controller. (*B*) Infusion pump.

Pumps have safety features such as air-in-line, occlusion, and infusion complete alarms as well as low battery or low power alerts. IV pumps are recommended for use with all central venous lines, arterial lines, and hyperalimentation. For clients who need multiple infusions, multichanneled pumps are available that have two or more programmable pumps, each of which can be set for a different infusion rate (Fig. 8–8*A* and *B*). Every model pump has different features and parameters, and nurses must be familiar with capabilities of the infusion devices they use.

SYRINGE PUMPS

Syringe pumps are primarily used when a small volume of medication is given. The syringe with medication is fitted into the pump, and the plunger is pushed by a piston-controlled mechanism, which delivers the medication at a controlled rate (Fig. 8–8*C*). Some pumps can operate with syringes of various sizes, from 5 mL to a 60 mL. Syringe pumps are therapy-specific and are used in oncology, obstetrics, and anesthesia. Syringe pumps usually do not have the same alarms as the IV delivery pumps and require closer monitoring.

PATIENT-CONTROLLED ANALGESIA (PCA)

Patient-controlled analgesia (PCA) devices enable the client to self-administer IV analgesics (Fig. 8–8*D*). These programmable pumps are designed to deliver the analgesic at a loading dose or a continual dose, and allow a client to administer a bolus dose at set intervals. The pump can be programmed to lock out bolus doses that are not within the preset time frame in order to prevent overdose. Morphine is commonly used as the analgesic with a dilution of 1 mg/mL. Clients' therapy is documented every 2 to 4 hours, with assessments and recordings of the amount of drug infused.

Flow Rates for Infusion Devices

Determining the flow rates for electronic delivery devices depends on whether the type of flow control is controller or pump. Pump delivery devices deliver a specific volume of fluid at a specific rate, measured in milliliters per hour (mL/hr). Controller delivery devices are designed to infuse at a drop rate (gtt/min). Distinguishing between these types of delivery devices involves checking the calibration on the machine display for rate units (mL/hr or gtt/min).

Calculating Flow Rates for Intravenous Drugs and Electrolytes

Drugs that are given by intermittent infusion must be diluted and infused slowly. The pH and the osmolality determine the dilution. A slower infusion time allows for the medication to be diluted in the blood vessel, thereby preventing phlebitis and high concentrations of drug in plasma and tissues that might cause time-related overdose, toxicity, or allergic reaction. Drug-dosing instructions indicate the amount and type of solution and the length of infusion time. The nurse must calculate the drug dose from the physician's order, then calculate the flow rate from the drug-dosing information.

Figure 8•8

(*A*) Dual-channel infusion pump. (*B*) Single infusion pump. (*C*) Syringe pump. (*D*) Patient-controlled analgesia (PCA) pump. (*A* courtesy of IMED Corp., San Diego, CA; *B* courtesy of Baxter Healthcare Corp., Round Lake, IL; *C*, from Bowden, V., Dickey, S., & Greenberg, C. (1998). *Children and Their Families: The Continuum of Care.* Philadelphia: W.B. Saunders: *D* courtesy of Baxter Healthcare Corp., Round Lake, IL.)

When calibrated cylinders, such as Voltrol, Buretrol, or Soluset, are used for drug infusion, the tubing must be flushed after each infusion to make sure the entire drug dose was given. The rinse can range from 10 to 25 mL and is added to the IV intake. When a minibag is used, the IV tubing should be drained so the client receives the complete dose.

SECONDARY SETS

Secondary sets (calibrated cylinders and 50- to 250-mL IV bags) use drops per minute (gtt/min). The one-step method for calculating drops per minute (gtt/min) is used when IV drugs are administered with secondary sets.

One-Step Method for IV Drug Calculation with Secondary Set

$$\frac{\text{amount of solution} \times \text{gtt/mL of the set}}{\text{minutes to administer}} = \text{gtt/min}$$

INFUSION PUMPS

Infusion pumps use units of milliliters per hour. Use the following method to calculate milliliters per hour.

$$\text{Amount of solution} \div \frac{\text{minutes to administer}}{60 \text{ minutes/hour}} = \text{mL/hr}$$

> **NOTE**
>
> Medication volume that exceeds 5 mL should be added to the dilution volume in intermittent drug therapy. Because smaller volumes of fluid are used for IV infusion, drug dosage may be decreased if the volume of medication is not included in the dilution volume. The amount of solution in the formula should include both volumes.

examples

PROBLEM 1: Order: Tagamet 200 mg, IV, q6h.
Drug available:

Set and solution: Buretrol set with drop factor of 60 gtt/mL; 500 mL of D_5W.

Instruction: Dilute drug in 100 mL of D_5W and infuse over 20 minutes.

Drug Calculation:

$$\frac{D}{H} \times V = \frac{200}{300} \times 2 \quad \textbf{or} \qquad H \ : \ V \ :: \ D \ : \ X$$
$$300 \text{ mg} : 2 \text{ mL} :: 200 \text{ mg} : X \text{ mL}$$
$$= \frac{400}{300} \qquad\qquad 300 X = 400$$
$$X = \frac{400}{300} = 300\overline{)400.0}^{\,1.3}$$
$$X = 1.3 \text{ mL of Tagamet} \qquad X = 1.3 \text{ mL of Tagamet}$$

Flow Rate Calculation:

$$\frac{\text{amount of solution} \times \text{gtt/mL}}{\text{minutes to administer}} = \frac{100 \text{ mL} \times \overset{3}{\cancel{60}} \text{ gtt}}{\underset{1}{\cancel{20}}} = 300 \text{ gtt/min}$$

Answer: Inject 1.3 mL of Tagamet into 100 mL of D_5W in the Buretrol chamber.
Regulate IV flow rate to 300 gtt/min.
It would be impossible to count 300 gtt/min. Instead of using the Buretrol, the nurse could use a secondary set with a larger drop factor or a regulator. If the Buretrol is the only available secondary IV set, the 300 gtt/min rate should be approximated.

PROBLEM 2: Order: Mandol 500 mg, IV, q6h.
Drug available: cefamandole (Mandol) 2 g vial in powdered form. Add 6.6 mL of diluent = 8 mL of drug solution (2g = 8 mL).

Set and solution: secondary set with 100 mL D_5W and a drop factor of 15 gtt/mL.
Instruction: Dilute in 100 mL of D_5W and infuse over 30 minutes.

Drug Calculation: (2.0 g = 2.000 mg).

$$\frac{D}{H} \times V = \frac{500}{2000} \times 8 \quad \textbf{or} \qquad H \ : \ V \ :: \ D \ : \ X$$
$$2000 \text{ mg} : 8 \text{ mL} :: 500 \text{ mg} : X \text{ mL}$$
$$= \frac{4000}{2000} = 2 \text{ mL of Mandol} \qquad 2000 X = 4000$$
$$X = 2 \text{ mL of Mandol}$$

Flow Rate Calculation:

$$\frac{\text{amount of solution} \times \text{gtt/mL}}{\text{minutes to administer}} = \frac{100 \text{ mL} \times \overset{1}{\cancel{15}}}{\underset{2}{\cancel{30}}} = \frac{100}{2} = 50 \text{ gtt/min}$$

Answer: Inject 2 mL of Mandol into the 100 mL D$_5$W bag.
Regulate IV flow rate at 50 gtt/min.

PROBLEM 3: Order: oxacillin 1 g, IV, q6h.
Drug available:

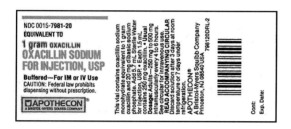

Add 5.7 mL of diluent = 6 mL per 1 g.
Set: Use an infusion pump.
Instruction: Dilute in 50 mL of D$_5$W and infuse over 15 minutes.

Drug Calculation: oxacillin 1 g = 6 mL of drug solution

Infusion Pump Rate: amount of solution $\div \dfrac{\text{minutes to administer}}{60 \text{ minutes}} = \text{mL/hr}$

$$56 \text{ mL} \div \frac{15 \text{ min}}{60 \text{ min}} = 56 \times \frac{\overset{4}{\cancel{60}}}{\underset{1}{\cancel{15}}} = 224 \text{ mL/hr}$$

Note: Amount of solution is 50 mL of D$_5$W + 6 mL medication = 56 mL.

Answer: Rate on infusion pump should be set at 224 mL/hr to deliver oxacillin 1 g in 15 minutes.

PROBLEM 4: Order: albumin 25 g, IV.
Available: albumin 25 g in 50 mL.
Set: Use an infusion pump.
Instruction: Administer over 25 minutes, or 2 mL/min.

Drug Calculation: Not applicable.

Infusion Pump Rate:

$$50 \text{ mL} \div \frac{25 \text{ min}}{60 \text{ min}} = 50 \times \frac{60}{25} = \frac{3000}{25} = 120 \text{ mL/hr}$$

Answer: Infusion rate should be set at 120 mL/hr.

PROBLEM 5: Order: potassium phosphate 10 mM IV in 100 mL NSS over 90 minutes.
Drug available:

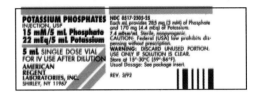

Set: Use infusion pump.

Drug Calculation:

$$\frac{D}{H} \times V = \frac{10}{15} \times 5 \quad \textbf{or} \quad \begin{array}{c} H : V :: D : X \\ 15\ \text{mM} : 5\ \text{mL} :: 10\ \text{mM} : X\ \text{mL} \end{array}$$

$$= \frac{50}{15} \qquad\qquad 15\ X = 50$$

$$\qquad\qquad\qquad X = 3.3\ \text{mL or potassium phosphate}$$

$$= 3.3\ \text{mL of potassium phosphate}$$

Infusion Pump Rate:

$$\text{amount of solution} \div \frac{\text{minutes to administer}}{60\ \text{minutes}} = \text{mL/hr}$$

$$100\ \text{mL} \div \frac{90\ \text{min}}{60\ \text{min}} = 100 \times \frac{60}{90} = 66.6\ \text{or}\ 67\ \text{mL/hr}$$

Answer: Rate on the infusion pump should be 67 mL/hr to deliver potassium phosphate 10 mM in 90 minutes.

NOTE When the electrolyte potassium is administered, the maximum infusion rate is 10 mEq/hr.

III Practice Problems: Intermittent Intravenous Administration

Calculate the fluid rate by using a calibrated cylinder (Buretrol), secondary set, or an infusion pump, as indicated in each question.

1. Order: cephapirin (Cefadyl) 500 mg, IV, q6h.
Drug available:

Drug label: add _____ mL of diluent _____;

1 g = _____ mL; 100 mg = 1 mL.

What type of syringe should be used? _____

Set and solution: Buretrol set with a drop factor of 60 gtt/mL; 500 mL of D₅W.

Instruction: Dilute drug in 75 mL of D₅W and infuse over 30 minutes.

Drug calculation:

_____

Flow rate calculation:

_____

2. Order: oxacillin 400 mg, IV, q6h.
Drug available:

Drug label: add _____ mL of diluent _____;

250 mg = _____ mL; 1 g = _____ mL.

Set and solution: secondary set with a drop factor of 15 gtt/mL; 500 mL of D₅W.

Instruction: Dilute drug in 100 mL of D₅W and infuse over 40 minutes.

Drug calculation:

_____

Flow rate calculation:

_____

3. Order: ticarcillin (Ticar) 500 mg, IV, q6h.
Drug available:

Set and solution: Buretrol set with a drop factor of 60 gtt/mL; infusion pump; 500 mL of D₅W.

Instruction: Dilute drug in 75 mL of D₅W and infuse over 40 minutes.

Drug calculation: Add _____ mL to ticarcillin vial (see drug label).

Flow rate calculation (gtt/min):
How many drops per minute should the client receive with use of the Buretrol set?

Infusion pump rate (mL/hr):
With an infusion pump, how many mL/hr should be administered?

---

4. Order: piperacillin 2.5 g, IV, q6h.
   Drug available: piperacillin 4 g vial in powdered form; add 7.8 mL of diluent to yield 10 mL of drug solution (4 g = 10 mL).
   Set and solution: Buretrol set with a drop factor of 60 gtt/mL; infusion pump; 500 mL of D₅W.
   Instruction: Dilute drug in 100 mL of D₅W and infuse over 30 minutes.

   Drug calculation:

Flow rate calculation (gtt/min):
How many drops per minute should the client receive with use of the Buretrol set?

Infusion pump rate (mL/hr):
With an infusion pump, how many mL/hr should be administered?

---

5. Order: methicillin (Staphcillin) 1 g, IV, q6h.
   Drug available: Staphcillin 4 g in powdered form in vial; add 5.7 mL of diluent to yield 8 mL.
   Set and solution: secondary set with a drop factor of 15 gtt/mL; 100 mL bag of D₅W; infusion pump.
   Instruction: Dilute drug in 100 mL of D₅W and infuse over 40 minutes.

   Drug calculation:

Explain the procedure for diluting the drug and adding it to the IV bag.

Flow rate calculation (gtt/min):
How many drops per minute should the client receive with use of a secondary set?

_____

Infusion pump rate (mL/hr):
With an infusion pump, how many mL/hr should be administered?

_____

6. Order: Vibramycin 100 mg, IV, q12h.
   Drug available: doxycycline (Vibramycin) 100-mg vial in powdered form; add 10 mL of diluent.

   Set and solution: secondary set with a drop factor of 15 gtt/mL; 100 mL of D_5W; infusion pump.
   Instruction: Dilute 10 mL in 90 mL of D_5W and infuse over 60 minutes. Dilution should be 1 mg = 1 mL.

   Drug calculation:

   _____

   Flow rate calculation (gtt/min):
   How many drops per minute should the client receive with use of the Buretrol set?

   _____

   Infusion pump rate (mL/hr):
   With an infusion pump, how many mL/hr should be administered?

   _____

7. Order: potassium chloride 20 mEq in 150 mL D_5W infused over 2 hours.
   Drug available:

   Set and solution: secondary set with drop factor 15 gtt/mL; 150 mL bottle D_5W; infusion pump.

   Drug calculation:

   _____

   Infusion pump rate (mL/hr):
   How many mL/hr should be administered?

   _____

8. Order: magnesium sulfate 5 g in 100 mL D_5W infused over 3 hours.
   Drug available:

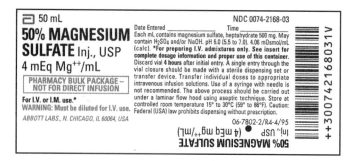

Set and solution: secondary set with drip factor of 15 gtt/mL; 10 mL bag D₅W; infusion pump.

Drug calculation:

a. 1 mL = _____ mg (see drug label).

b. 5 g = _____ mL.

Infusion pump rate (mL/hr):
How many mL/hr should be administered?

---

9. Order: calcium gluconate 10%, 16 mEq in 100 mL D₅W infused over 30 minutes.
Drug available:

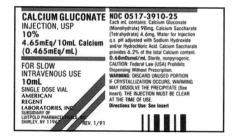

Set and solution: secondary set with a drip factor of 15 gtt/mL; 100 mL bag D₅W; infusion pump.

Drug calculation:

Infusion pump rate (mL/hr):
How many mL/hr should be administered?

---

10. Order: ranitidine (Zantac) 50 mg, IV, q6h.
Set: infusion pump.
Drug available: premixed drug in bag (Zantac 50 mg in 0.45% NaCl [½ NSS]).

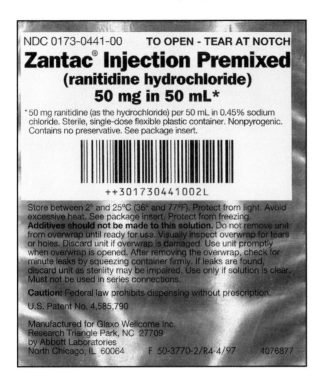

Instruction: Infuse over 15 minutes.

Infusion pump rate:
How many mL/hr should be administered?

---

11. Order: cefepime (Maxipime) 750 mg, IV, q12h.
Set and solution: Infusion pump; 100 mL D₅W.
Drug available:

Instruction: Add 8.7 mL of diluent to Maxipime to yield 10 mL of drug solution. Dilute in 100 mL of D₅W; infuse over 30 minutes.

Drug calculations:

Infusion pump rate (mL/hr):

---

12. Order: rifampin (Rifadin) 600 mg, IV, qd.
Set and solution: Infusion pump; 500 mL D$_5$W.
Drug available: Rifadin 600 mg sterile powder
Instruction: Add 10 mL of diluent to the rifampin vial. Dilute rifampin in 500 mL of D$_5$W; infuse over 3 hours.

Infusion pump rate (mL/hr):

ANSWERS

I. Direct IV Injection

1. known drug : known minutes : : desired drug : desired minutes
5 mg : 1 min : : 50 mg : X
$$5 X = 50$$
$$X = 10 \text{ minutes}$$

2. known drug : known minutes : : desired drug : desired minutes
10 mL : 1 min : : 50 mL : X
$$10 X = 50$$
$$X = 5 \text{ minutes}$$

3. known drug : known minutes : : desired drug : desired minutes
1.5 mL : 1 min : : 10 mL : X
$$1.5 X = 10$$
$$X = 6.6 \text{ minutes or 7 minutes}$$

4. known drug : known minutes : : desired drug : desired minutes
10 mg : 1 min : : 50 mg : X
$$10 X = 50$$
$$X = 5 \text{ minutes}$$

5. known drug : known minutes : : desired drug : desired minutes
10 mg : 4 min : : 6 mg : X
$$10 X = 24$$
$$X = 2.4 \text{ minutes}$$

6. known drug : known minutes : : desired drug : desired minutes
1 mL : 5 min : : X mL : 1 min
$$5 X = 1$$
$$X = 0.2 \text{ mL/minutes}$$

7. known drug : known minutes : : desired drug : desired minutes
1 mg : 1 min : : 2 mg : X
$$X = 2 \text{ minutes}$$

8. known drug : known minutes : : desired drug : desired minutes
2 mg : 1 min : : 6 mg : X
$$2 X = 6$$
$$X = 3 \text{ minutes}$$

9. H : V : : D : V

    25 mg : 5 mL : : 20 mg : X mL

        25 X = 100

          X = 4 mL

$$\frac{\text{amount of drug}}{\text{number of minutes}} = \frac{4\ mL}{2\ min} = 2\ mL/min$$

Answer: Infuse 2 mL of cardizem per minute.

10. **a.** 140 lb ÷ 2.2 = 64 kg

   b. 10 μg × 64 kg = 640 μg

   c. Change micrograms (μg) to milligrams by moving the decimal point three spaces to the *left:* 640 μg = 0.640 mg or 0.6 mg.

        known drug : known seconds : : desired drug : desired seconds

          1 mg   : 60 seconds : :   .6 mg   :   X

                        X = 36 seconds

Answer: Infuse 0.6 mg of granisetron (Kytril) over 36 seconds.

II. Continuous Intravenous Administration

1. **a.** Microdrip set, because the patient is to receive 83 mL/hr

   b. Three-step method: (a) $\dfrac{1000}{12}$ = 83 mL/hr

                    (b) $\dfrac{83}{60}$ = 1.38 mL/min

                    (c) 1.4 mL/min × 60 gtt/mL = 84 gtt/min

   Using a microdrip set (60 gtt/mL); IV should run at 84 gtt/min.

2. **a.** 1 L = 1000 mL

   b. Each liter should run for 8 hours.

   c. Two-step method: 1000 ÷ 8 = 125 mL/hr

$$\frac{125 \times \overset{1}{\cancel{15}}}{\underset{4}{\cancel{60}}} = \frac{125}{4} = 31{-}32\ gtt/min$$

   With a 15 gtt/mL drop set, IV should run at 31−32 gtt/min.

3. **a.** Microdrip set with drop factor of 60 gtt/mL

   b. One-step method: $\dfrac{250 \times \overset{1}{\cancel{60}}}{24 \times \underset{1}{\cancel{60}}}$ = 10 gtt/min

   With a microdrip set, IV should run at 10 gtt/min. KVO usually means 24 hours.

4. **a.** 10 mL of KCl

   b. Use a 10-mL syringe; withdraw 10 mL of KCl and inject into the rubber part stopper of the IV bag.

   c. Microdrip set: 100 gtt/min
      Macrodrip set: drop factor of 20 gtt/mL; 34 gtt/min

5. a. 700 mL of IV fluid is left and 4 hours are left.

   b. Recalculate using 700 mL and 4 hours to run.

Three-step method: (a) $\dfrac{700}{4} = 175$ mL/hr

(b) $\dfrac{175}{60} = 2.9$ mL/min

(c) $2.9 \times 15 = 44$ gtt/min

6. 100 gtt/min

Two-step method: $\dfrac{100 \times \overset{1}{\cancel{60}} \text{ gtt/mL}}{\underset{1}{\cancel{60}} \text{ min}} = 100$ gtt/min

7. a. KCl 40 mEq/20 mL

   b. 20 mL

   c. $\dfrac{1000 \text{ mL}}{125 \text{ mL/hr}} = 8$ hours

8. a. KCl 20 mEq/10mL

   b. 10 mL

   c. $\dfrac{1000 \text{ mL}}{100 \text{ mL/hr}} = 10$ hours

   d. $\dfrac{100 \text{ mL} \times \overset{1}{\cancel{10}} \text{ gtt/mL}}{\underset{6}{\cancel{60}} \text{ min}} = \dfrac{100}{6} = 16-17$ gtt/min

or

$\dfrac{1000 \text{ mL} \times \overset{1}{\cancel{10}} \text{ gtt/mL}}{\underset{1}{\cancel{10}} \text{ hr} \times 60 \text{ min}} = \dfrac{1000}{60} = 16-17$ gtt/min

III. Intermittent Intravenous Administration

   1. Add 10 mL of sterile or bacteriostatic water (1 g = 10 mL).

Drug calculation: Change 500 mg to grams because the drug label is in grams. Move the decimal point three spaces to the *left:* 500. mg = 0.5 g.

$\dfrac{D}{H} \times V = \dfrac{0.5}{1} \times 10 \text{ mL}$ **or**   H : V :: D : X
                                           1 g : 10 mL :: 0.5 g : X mL

$= \dfrac{5}{1} = 5 \text{ mL Cefadyl}$ 1 X = 10 × 0.5
                                                 X = 5 mL Cefadyl

Use a 10-mL syringe to reconstitute the drug.

Flow rate calculation:

$$\dfrac{\text{amount of solution} \times \text{gtt/mL (set)}}{\text{minutes to administer}} = \dfrac{75 \text{ mL} \times \overset{2}{\cancel{60}} \text{ gtt/mL}}{\underset{1}{\cancel{30}} \text{ minutes}} = 150 \text{ gtt/min}$$

Regulate flow rate for 150 gtt/min.

2. Add 5.7 mL of sterile water.
   250 mg = 1.5 mL; 1 g = 6 mL (250 mg is ¼ of a gram; 4 × 1.5 = 6 mL)

   Drug calculation: Change 400 mg to grams because the drug label is in grams. Move the decimal point three spaces to the *left:*
   400. mg = 0.4 g.

   $$\frac{0.4}{1} \times 6 \text{ mL} = 2.4 \text{ mL of oxacillin} \quad \textbf{or} \quad 1 \text{ g} : 6 \text{ mL} : : 0.4 \text{ g} : X \text{ mL}$$

   $$1 X = 6 \times 0.4$$
   $$X = 2.4 \text{ mL of oxacillin}$$

   Flow rate calculation:

   $$\frac{100 \text{ mL} \times 15 \text{ gtt/mL (set)}}{40 \text{ minutes}} = 37.5 \text{ or } 38 \text{ gtt/min}$$

   Regulate flow rate for 38 gtt/min.

3. *Drug calculation:* ticarcillin 500 mg = 2 mL
   Flow rate calculation: total solution: 75 mL D_5W + 2 mL of drug solution = 77 mL

   For Buretrol set:

   $$\frac{77 \text{ mL} \times \overset{3}{\cancel{60}} \text{ gtt/mL (set)}}{\underset{2}{\cancel{40}} \text{ minutes}} = \frac{231}{2} = 115.5 \text{ or } 116 \text{ gtt/min}$$

   Infusion pump rate:

   $$\text{amount of solution} \div \frac{\text{minutes to administer}}{60 \text{ min/hr}} = \text{mL/hr}$$

   $$77 \text{ mL} \div \frac{\overset{2}{\cancel{40}} \text{ min to administer}}{\underset{3}{\cancel{60}} \text{ min/hr}} = 77 \times \frac{3}{2} = \frac{231}{2} = 116 \text{ mL/hr}$$

   Set pump rate at 119 mL/hr to deliver Ticar 500 mg in 40 minutes.

4. *Drug calculation:*

   $$\frac{D}{H} \times V = \frac{2.5 \text{ g}}{\underset{2}{\cancel{4} \text{ g}}} \times \overset{5}{\cancel{10}} \text{ mL} \quad \textbf{or} \quad \begin{array}{c} H : \quad V \quad : : \quad D \quad : \quad X \\ 4 \text{ g} : 10 \text{ mL} : : 2.5 \text{ g} : X \text{ mL} \end{array}$$

   $$= \frac{12.5}{2} = 6.25 \text{ mL} \qquad\qquad \begin{array}{c} 4 X = 25 \\ X = 6.25 \text{ mL} \end{array}$$

   piperacillin 2.5 g = 6.25 mL

   Flow rate calculation for Buretrol set:

   $$\frac{100 \text{ mL} \times \overset{2}{\cancel{60}} \text{ gtt/mL}}{\underset{1}{\cancel{30}} \text{ min/hr}} = 200 \text{ gtt/minute}$$

Infusion pump rate: 100 mL + 6 mL medication = 106 mL

$$106 \text{ mL} \div \frac{\overset{1}{\cancel{30}} \text{ min to administer}}{\underset{2}{\cancel{60}} \text{ min/hr}} = 106 \times \frac{2}{1} = 212 \text{ mL/hr}$$

Set pump rate at 212 mL/hr to deliver piperacillin 2.5 g in 30 minutes.

5. *Drug calculation:* Staphcillin 4 g = 8 mL. Withdraw 2 mL from vial to yield Staphcillin 1 g.

Flow rate calculation for secondary set:

$$\frac{\overset{5}{\cancel{100}} \text{ mL} \times 15 \text{ gtt/mL (set)}}{\underset{2}{\cancel{40}} \text{ minutes}} = \frac{75}{2} = 37.5 \text{ or } 38 \text{ gtt/min}$$

Infusion pump rate:

$$100 \text{ mL} \times \frac{\overset{2}{\cancel{40}} \text{ min to administer}}{\underset{3}{\cancel{60}} \text{ min/hr}} = 100 \times \frac{3}{2} = \frac{300}{2} = 150 \text{ mL/hr}$$

Set pump rate at 150 mL/hr to deliver Staphcillin 1 g in 40 minutes.

6. *Drug calculation:* Mix 10 mL of diluent with Vibramycin 100 mg in vial.

Flow rate calculation: Expel 10 mL of IV solution. Inject 10 mL of drug solution into 90 mL of IV solution.

For secondary set:

$$\frac{100 \text{ mL} \times \overset{1}{\cancel{15}} \text{ gtt/mL}}{\underset{4}{\cancel{60}} \text{ minutes}} = \frac{100}{4} = 25 \text{ gtt/min}$$

Infusion pump rate:

$$100 \text{ mL} \div \frac{\overset{1}{\cancel{60}} \text{ minutes to administer}}{\underset{1}{\cancel{60}} \text{ min/hr}} = 100 \text{ mL/hr}$$

Set pump rate at 100 mL/hr to deliver Vibramycin 100 mg in 60 minutes.

7. *Drug calculation:*

$$\frac{D}{H} \times V = \frac{20}{40} \times 20 \quad \textbf{or} \quad \begin{array}{c} H : V :: D : X \\ 40 : 20 :: 20 : X \end{array}$$

$$= \frac{400}{40} \qquad\qquad 40 \, X = 400$$
$$\qquad\qquad\qquad X = 10 \text{ mL KCl}$$
$$= 10 \text{ mL KCl}$$

Amount of solution: 150 mL + 10 mL = 160 mL

Infusion pump rate:

$$160 \text{ mL} \div \frac{120 \text{ min to administer}}{60 \text{ min/hr}} = 160 \times \frac{1}{2} = 80 \text{ mL/hr}$$

Set pump rate at 80 mL/hr to deliver KCl 20 mEq in 2 hr.

8. *Drug calculation:*

a. 1 mL = 500 mg and 2 mL = 1 g.

b. $\dfrac{D}{H} \times V = \dfrac{5}{1} \times 2$ **or**
$\begin{array}{l} H:V::D:X \\ 1:2::5:X \end{array}$

= 10 mL of MgSO$_4$ X = 10

X = 10 mL MgSO$_4$

Amount of solution: 10 mL + 100 mL = 110 mL

Infusion pump rate:

$$110 \text{ mL} \div \frac{\overset{3}{\cancel{180}} \text{ min to administer}}{\underset{1}{\cancel{60}} \text{ min/hr}} (3 \text{ hr}) = 110 \times \frac{1}{3} = 36.6 \text{ or } 37 \text{ mL/hr}$$

Set pump rate at 37 mL/hr to deliver MgSO$_4$ 5 g in 3 hr.

9. *Drug calculation:*

$$\frac{D}{H} \times V = \frac{16}{23.25} \times 50 \quad \textbf{or} \quad \begin{array}{l} H \;:V::\,D\,:X \\ 23.25:50::16:X \end{array}$$

$$= \frac{800}{23.25} \qquad\qquad 23.25 \, X = 800$$

$$\qquad\qquad\qquad\qquad\qquad X = 34.4 \text{ mL calcium}$$

$$= 34.4 \text{ mL calcium gluconate} \qquad \text{gluconate}$$

Amount of solution: 34.4 mL + 100 mL = 134.4 mL

Infusion pump rate:

$$134.4 \text{ mL} \div \frac{30 \text{ min to administer}}{60 \text{ min/hr}} = 134.4 \times \frac{2}{1} = 268.8 \text{ or } 269 \text{ mL/hr}$$

10. *Amount of solution:* $\div \dfrac{\text{min to administer}}{60 \text{ mL/hr}}$

$$50 \text{ mL} \div \frac{15 \text{ min}}{60 \text{ min}} = 50 \text{ mL} \times \frac{\overset{4}{\cancel{60} \text{ min}}}{\underset{1}{\cancel{15} \text{ min}}} = 200 \text{ mL/hr}$$

Infusion pump rate: 200 mL/hr

11. 1 g = 1000 mg (use conversion table as needed) of Maxipime

a. $\dfrac{D}{H} \times V = \dfrac{\overset{3}{\cancel{750} \text{ mL}}}{\underset{4}{\cancel{1000} \text{ mL}}} \times 10 \text{ mL} = \dfrac{30}{4} = 7.5 \text{ mL drug solution}$

b. *Pump rate:*

$$7.5 \text{ drug sol} + 100 \text{ mL} \div \frac{30 \text{ min to administer}}{60 \text{ min/hr}} = 107.5 \text{ mL} \times \frac{\overset{2}{\cancel{60}}}{\underset{1}{\cancel{30}}}$$

$$= 215 \text{ mL/hr pump rate}$$

12. $10 \text{ mL of drug sol} + 500 \text{ mL} \div \dfrac{180 \text{ min (3 hrs)}}{60 \text{ min/hr}} = 510 \text{ mL} \times \dfrac{\overset{1}{\cancel{60}}}{\underset{3}{\cancel{180}}}$

$$= \frac{510}{3} = 170 \text{ mL/hr}$$

Infusion pump rate: 170 mL/hr for 3 hr

part
four

calculations for
specialty areas

pediatrics

bjectives

- Utilize the two primary methods in determining pediatric drug dosages.
- State the reason for checking pediatric dosages prior to administration.
- Describe the dosage inaccuracies that can occur with pediatric drug formulas.
- Identify the steps in determining body surface area from a pediatric nomogram.

utline

FACTORS INFLUENCING PEDIATRIC DRUG ADMINISTRATION

Drug dosages for children differ greatly from those for adults because of the physiological differences between the two. Neonates and infants have immature kidney and liver function, which delays metabolism and elimination of many drugs. Drug absorption in neonates is different as a result of slow gastric emptying time. Decreased gastric acid secretion in children younger than 3 years contributes to altered drug absorption. Neonates and infants have a lower concentration of plasma proteins, which can cause toxicity with drugs that are highly bound to proteins. They have less total body fat and more total body water. Therefore, lipid-soluble drugs require smaller doses because less than normal fat is present, and water-soluble drugs can require larger doses because of a greater percentage of body water. As children grow, changes in fat, muscle, body water, and organ maturity can alter the pharmacokinetic effects of drugs. It is the nurse's responsibility to ensure that a safe drug dosage is given and to closely monitor signs and symptoms of adverse reactions to drugs. The purpose of learning how to calculate pediatric drug doses is to ensure that the child receives the correct dose within the therapeutic range.

Oral

Oral pediatric drug delivery often requires the use of a calibrated measuring device, because most drugs for small children are in liquid form. The measuring device can be a small plastic cup, an oral dropper, a measuring spoon, or an oral syringe (Fig. 9–1). Some liquid medications come with their own calibrated droppers. The type of measuring device chosen depends on the developmental level of the child. For infants and toddlers, the oral syringe and dropper provide better drug delivery than a small cup. A

FIGURE 9•1

Calibrated measuring devices. From Kee, J., & Hayes, E. (2000). *Pharmacology: A Nursing Process Approach* (3rd ed.). Philadelphia: W. B. Saunders.

young child who is cooperative is able to use a small cup or measuring spoon. All liquid medications can be drawn up with a syringe to ensure accuracy and then transferred to a small cup or measuring spoon. It may be necessary to rinse the cup or spoon with water or juice to ensure that the child has received all of the prescribed medication. Avoid giving oral medications to a crying child or infant, who could easily aspirate the medication. Some chewable medications are available for use in the older child. Because many drugs are enteric coated or in time-release form, the child must be told which medications are to be swallowed and not chewed.

Intramuscular

Intramuscular sites are chosen on the basis of the age and muscle development of the child (Table 9–1). All injections should be given in a manner that minimizes physical and psychosocial trauma. The child must be adequately restrained, if necessary, and provided with a momentary distraction. The procedure must be performed quickly, with comfort measures immediately following.

> The usual needle length and gauge for pediatric clients are ½ to 1 inch long and 22 to 25 gauge. Another method of estimating needle length is to grasp the muscle for injection between the thumb and the forefinger; half the distance would be the needle length.
>
> **NOTE**

Intravenous

For children, the maximum amount of IV fluids varies with body weight. Their 24-hour fluid status must be monitored closely to prevent overhydration. The amount of fluid given with IV medication must be considered in the planning of their 24-hour intake (Table 9–2). After the correct dosage of drug is obtained, it may need further dilution and to be given over a specified time, as mentioned in Chapter 8. Usually, the drug is diluted with 5 to 60 mL of IV fluid, depending on the drug or dosage, placed in a calibrated cylinder, and infused over 20 to 60 minutes, depending on the type of drug. After the drug has infused, the cylinder is flushed with 3 to

table 9•1
PEDIATRIC GUIDELINES FOR INTRAMUSCULAR INJECTIONS ACCORDING TO MUSCLE GROUP*

AGE (yr)	AMOUNT BY MUSCLE GROUP (mL)				
	Rectus	Vastus Lateralis	Gluteus Maximus	Ventrogluteal	Deltoid
Birth to 2	0.5–1	0.5–1	Not safe	Not safe	Not safe
2 to 3	1	1	1	1	0.5
3 to 7	1.5	1.5	1.5	1.5	0.5
7 to 16	1.5–2	1.5–2	1.5–2	1.5–2	0.5–1
16 to adult	2–2.5	2–2.5	2–3	2–3	1–2

*The safe use of all sites is based on normal muscle development and size of the child.

table 9•2

PEDIATRIC GUIDELINES FOR 24-HOUR INTRAVENOUS FLUID THERAPY

100 mL/kg up to 10 kg body weight
50 mL/kg for the next 5 kg body weight
10 mL/kg after 15 kg body weight

Example: Child's weight 25 kg

$$100 \text{ mL/kg} \times 10 \text{ kg} = 1000 \text{ mL}$$
$$50 \text{ mL/kg} \times 5 \text{ kg} = 250 \text{ mL}$$
$$10 \text{ mL/kg} \times 10 \text{ kg} = \underline{100 \text{ mL}}$$
$$1350 \text{ mL for 24 hours}$$

20 mL of IV fluid to ensure that the child has received all of the medication and to prevent admixture. Refer to Chapter 8 for methods of calculating IV infusion rates.

The safety factors that must be considered when administering medications to children are similar to those for adults. See Appendix A for more detailed information on safe nursing practice for drug administration.

PEDIATRIC DRUG CALCULATIONS

The two main methods in determining drug dosages for pediatric drug administration are body weight and body surface area. The first method uses a specific number of milligrams, micrograms, or units for each kilogram of body weight (mg/kg, mcg/kg, U/kg). Usually, drug data for pediatric dosage (mg/kg) are supplied by manufacturers in a drug information insert. Body surface area (BSA), measured by m^2, is considered a more accurate method than body weight. BSA takes into consideration the relation between basal metabolic rate and surface area, which correlates with blood volume, cardiac output, and organ growth and development. Although BSA has primarily been used to calculate the dosage of antineoplastic agents, manufacturers are beginning to include body surface area parameters (mg/m^2, mcg/m^2, U/m^2) in drug information.

If the manufacturer does not supply data for pediatric dosing, the child's dosage can be determined from the adult dose. The body surface area formula is used to calculate the pediatric dose. The BSA is considered more accurate than previously used formulas, such as Clark's, Young's, and Fried's rules. Drug calculations according to the BSA are safer than formulas that rely solely on the child's age or weight. Although the BSA formula has improved the accuracy of drug dosing in infants and children, calculation of drug doses for neonates and preterm infants with this method does not guarantee complete accuracy.

NOTE If the manufacturer states in the drug information insert that the medication is not for pediatric use, the alternative formulas should not be used for dosage calculation.

Dosage per Kilogram Body Weight

The following information is needed to calculate the dosage.

a. Physician's order with the name of the drug, the dosage, and the frequency of administration.

b. The child's weight in kilograms:

$$1 \text{ kg} = 2.2 \text{ lb}$$

c. The pediatric dosage as listed by the manufacturer or hospital formulary.

d. Information on how the drug is supplied.

· ·

e x a m p l e s

PROBLEM 1: **a.** Order: amoxicillin (Amoxil) 60 mg, po, tid.
Child's weight: 12½ lb.

b. Change pounds to kilograms.

$$\frac{12.5}{2.2} = 5.7 \text{ kg}$$

c. Pediatric dosage for children who weigh 20 kg: 20–40 mg/kg/day in three equal doses.

Step 1: Check dosing parameters by multiplying the child's weight by the minimum and maximum daily dose of the drug.

$$20 \text{ mg/kg/day} \times 5.7 \text{ kg} = 114 \text{ mg/day}$$

$$40 \text{ mg/kg/day} \times 5.7 \text{ kg} = 228 \text{ mg/day}$$

Step 2: Multiply the dosage by the frequency to determine the daily dose.
The order for amoxicillin 60 mg, po, tid means that three doses will be given per day.

$$60 \text{ mg} \times 3 = 180 \text{ mg}$$

Because the daily dose of amoxicillin 180 mg falls within the recommended range, it is considered a safe dose.

d. Drug preparation:

Use either the basic formula, ratio and proportion, or fraction equation.

Basic formula	**or**	*Ratio and proportion*

$$\frac{D}{H} \times V = \frac{60 \text{ mg}}{125 \text{ mg}} \times 5 \text{ mL} \qquad 125 \text{ mg} : 5 \text{ mL} : : 60 \text{ mg} : X \text{ mL}$$

$$= 2.4 \text{ mL} \qquad\qquad\qquad 125 X = 300$$
$$X = 2.4 \text{ mL}$$

Answer: amoxicillin 60 mg, po = 2.4 mL

PROBLEM 2: a. Order: ampicillin 350 mg, IV, q6h. Mix with 20 mL D$_5$/¼ NSS, infuse over 20 minutes. Flush with 15 mL. Child weighs 61.5 lb.

b. Change pounds to kilograms.

$$\frac{61.5}{2.2} = 27.95 \text{ or } 28 \text{ kg}$$

c. Pediatric dose is 25–50 mg/kg/day in divided doses.

Step 1: Multiply weight by minimum and maximum daily dose:

$$25 \text{ mg} \times 28 \text{ kg} = 700 \text{ mg/day}$$

$$50 \text{ mg} \times 28 \text{ kg} = 1400 \text{ mg/day}$$

Step 2: Multiply the dose by the frequency:

$$350 \text{ mg} \times 4 = 1400 \text{ mg/day}$$

The dose is considered safe because it does not exceed the therapeutic range.

d. Drug available: When diluted, 500 mg = 2 mL. Use your selected formula to calculate the dosage.

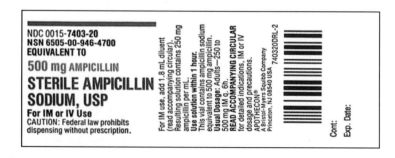

$$\frac{D}{H} \times V = \frac{350 \text{ mg}}{500 \text{ mg}} \times 2 \text{ mL} \quad \textbf{or} \quad 500 \text{ mg} : 2 \text{ mL} :: 350 \text{ mg} : X \text{ mL}$$

$$= 1.4 \text{ mL} \qquad\qquad\qquad 500 \text{ X} = 700$$
$$X = 1.4 \text{ mL}$$

Answer: Each dose is 1.4 mL.

e. Amount of fluid to infuse medication:

$$1.4 \text{ mL} + 20 \text{ mL (dilution)} = 21.4 \text{ mL}$$

f. Flow rate calculation (60 gtt/mL set):

$$\frac{\text{amount of solution} \times \text{gtt/mL (set)}}{\text{minutes to administer}} = \text{gtt/min}$$

$$\frac{21.4 \text{ mL} \times \overset{3}{\cancel{60}} \text{ gtt/mL}}{\underset{1}{\cancel{20}} \text{ minutes}} = 64.2 \text{ gtt/min}$$

g. Total fluid for medication infusion: 21.4 mL + 15 mL (flush) = 36.4 mL

REMEMBER

- The IV flush (3–20 mL) is part of the total IV fluids necessary for medication administration and must be included in client intake. The flush is started after IV medication infusion is completed, and it is infused at the same rate.
- For a 60 gtt/mL set, the drop per minute rate is the same as the milliliter per minute rate.

Dosage per Body Surface Area

The following information is needed to calculate the dosage:

a. Physician's order with name of drug, dosage, and time frame or frequency.

b. Child's height, weight in kilograms, and age.

c. Information on how the drug is supplied.

d. Pediatric dosage (in m²) as listed by manufacturer or hospital formulary.

e. Body surface area (BSA) nomogram for children (Fig. 9–2).

. . . .

example

PROBLEM 1: a. Order: methotrexate 50 mg, IV, × 1.

b. Child's height, weight, age: 134 cm, 32.5 kg, 9 yr.

c. Pediatric dose: 25–75 mg/m² wk.

d. Drug preparation: 2.5 mg/mL, 25 mg/mL.

FIGURE 9•2

West nomogram for infants and children. *Directions:* (1) Find height; (2) find weight; (3) draw a straight line connecting the height and weight. Where the line intersects on the SA column is the body surface area (m²). Modified from data of E. Boyd and C. D. West, in Behrman, R. E., Kliegman, R. M., and Arvin, A. M. (1996). *Nelson Textbook of Pediatrics* (15th ed.). Philadelphia: W. B. Saunders.

e. Body surface area nomogram for children: The child's height (134 cm) and weight (32.5 kg) intersect at 1.11 m² BSA.

Multiply the BSA, 1.11 m², by the minimum and maximum dose. (Substitute BSA for weight.)

$$25 \text{ mg/m}^2 \times 1.11 \text{ m}^2 = 28.0 \text{ mg}$$

$$75 \text{ mg/m}^2 \times 1.11 \text{ m}^2 = 83.0 \text{ mg}$$

This dose is considered safe because it is within the therapeutic range for the child's body surface area.

f. Calculate drug dose: to determine the amount of drug to be administered, either formula can be used:

$$\frac{D}{H} \times V = \frac{50 \text{ mg}}{25 \text{ mg}} \times 1 \text{ mL} \quad \textbf{or} \quad 25 \text{ mg} : 1 \text{ mL} : : = 50 \text{ mg} : X \text{ mL}$$

$$= 2 \text{ mL} \qquad\qquad\qquad 25 X = 50$$
$$X = 2 \text{ mL}$$

Answer: methotrexate 50 mg = 2 mL

Practice Problems

With the following dosage problems for oral, IM, and IV administration, determine whether the ordered dose is safe and how much of the drug should be given.

I. Oral

1. Child with rheumatic fever.
Order: penicillin V potassium 250 mg, po, q8h.
Child's weight: 45 lb.
Pediatric dose: 25–50 mg/kg/day.
Drug available:

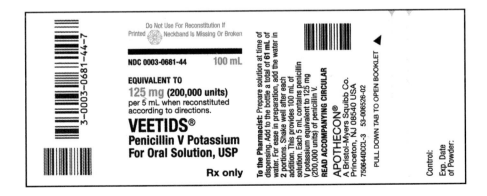

2. Child with seizures.
Order: Phenobarbital 25 mg, po, bid.
Child's weight: 7.2 kg.

Pediatric dose: 5–7 mg/kg/day.
Drug available: phenobarbital 20 mg/5 mL.

3. Child with lower respiratory tract infection.
Order: cefprozil (Cefzil) 100 mg, po, q12h.
Child's weight: 17 lb.; age: 6 months.
Pediatric dose > mo: 15 mg/kg/q12h.
Drug available:

4. Child with pain.
Order: codeine 7.5 mg, po, q4h, PRN × 6 doses/day.
Child's height and weight: 43 inches, 50 lb.
Pediatric dose: 100 mg/m^2/day (see Fig. 9–1).
Drug available: codeine 15-mg tablets.

5. Child with seizures.
Order: Zarontin 125 mg, po, bid.
Child's weight: 13 kg.
Pediatric dose: 20 mg/kg/day.
Drug available:

6. Child with seizures.
Order: Dilantin 40 mg, po, bid.
Child's weight: 6.7 kg.
Pediatric dose: 5–7 mg/kg/day.
Drug available: Dilantin 125 mg/5 mL.

7. Child with a urinary tract infection.
Order: Gantrisin 1.5 g, po, qid.
Child's weight: 30.4 kg.
Pediatric dose: 150–200 mg/kg/day.
Drug available: Gantrisin 500 mg tablets.

8. Infant with upper respiratory tract infection.
Order: Augmentin oral suspension 75 mg, po, q8h.
Child's weight: 8 kg.
Pediatric dose: 20–40 mg/kg/day.
Drug available:

9. Child with poison ivy.
Order: Benadryl 25 mg, po, q6h.
Child's weight: 25 kg.
Pediatric dose: 5 mg/kg/day.
Drug available: Benadryl 12.5 mg/5 mL.

10. Child with cystic fibrosis exposed to influenza A.
Order: Symmetrel 25 mg, po, tid.
Child's weight: 14 kg.
Pediatric dose: 4–8 mg/kg/day.
Drug available: Symmetrel 50 mg/5 mL.

11. Order: cefaclor (Ceclor) 50 mg, qid.
Child's weight: 15 lb.
Pediatric dose: 20–40 mg/kg/day in three to four divided doses.
Drug available:

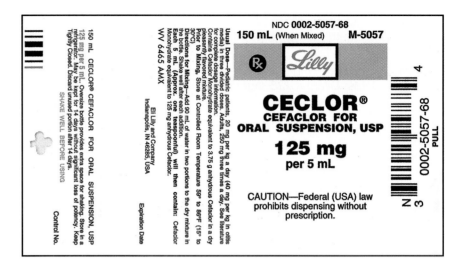

Is the prescribed dose safe?

II. Intramuscular

12. Child with nausea after surgery.
Order: Phenergan 20 mg, IM, q6h.
Child's weight: 45 kg.
Pediatric dose: 0.25–0.5 mg/kg/dose, repeat 4–6 hr.
Drug available: Phenergan 25 mg/mL.

13. Child has strep throat (Streptococcal pharyngitis).
Order: Bicillin C-R, 1,000,000 U, IM, × 1.
Child's weight: 44 lb.
Pediatric dose: 30–60 lb: 900,000–1,200,000 U daily.
Drug available: Bicillin C-R 1,200,000 U/2 mL.

14. Child receiving preoperative medication.
Order: hydroxyzine (Vistaril) 25 mg, IM.
Child's height and weight: 47 inches, 45 lb.
Pediatric dose: 30 mg/m^2.
Drug available: Vistaril 25 mg/mL.

15. Child receiving preoperative medication.
Order: atropine 0.2 mg, IM.
Child's weight: 12 kg.
Pediatric dose: 24–40 lb/0.2 mg.
Drug available:

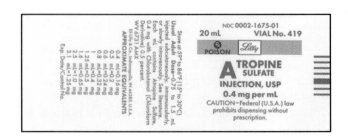

16. Child with cancer.
    Order: methotrexate 50 mg, IM, q weekly.
    Child's height and weight: 56 inches, 100 lb.
    Pediatric dose: 25–75 mg/m²/wk.
    Drug available: methotrexate 2.5 mg/mL; 25 mg/mL; 100 mg/mL.

17. Order: A newborn is to receive AquaMEPHYTON (Vitamin K) 0.5 mg,
    IM, immediately after delivery.
    Pediatric dose: 0.5–1 mg per dose.
    Drug available:

    a. Which AquaMEPHYTON container would you select?

    b. How many milliliters (mL) should the newborn receive?

    c. Is drug dose within safe parameters?

III. Intravenous

18. Adolescent with progressive hip pain secondary to rheumatoid arthritis.
    Order: morphine sulfate 2.5 mg, IV piggyback, in 10 mL NSS over 5
    minutes. Flush with 5 mL.
    Child's weight: 50 kg.
    Pediatric dose: 50–100 mcg/kg/dose for IV.
    Drug available:

19. Treatment to reverse postoperative narcotic depression.
    Order: Narcan (Naloxone) 0.3 mg, IV push.
    Child's weight: 32 kg.
    Pediatric dose: 0.005–0.01 mg/kg.
    Drug available:

20. Infant with sepsis.
    Order: Amikin 40 mg, IV, q12h, in D₅W 5 mL, over 20 minutes. Flush
    with 3 mL.
    Child's weight: 5.3 kg.
    Pediatric dose: 15 mg/kg/day.
    Drug available:

21. Child with head trauma.
    Order: Decadron 2 mg, IV, q6h, in D₅W 10 mL, over 15 minutes. Flush
    with 5 mL.
    Child's weight and age: 10.1 kg, 16 months.
    Pediatric dose: 0.4 mg/kg/day in divided doses.
    Drug available:

22. Child with pneumonia.
    Order: cefazolin (Ancef) 500 mg, IV, q6h, in D₅W 20 mL, over 30
    minutes.
    Flush with 10 mL.
    Child's weight: 5.6 kg.
    Pediatric dose: 25–100 mg/kg/day in three divided doses.
    Drug available:

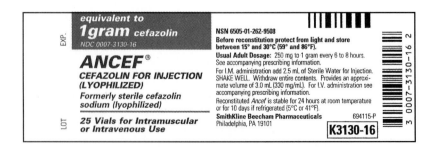

23. Child with sepsis.
    Order: gentamicin 10 mg, IV, q8h, in D_5W, 4 mL over 30 minutes. Flush with 3 mL.
    Child's height, weight, age: 21 inches, 4 kg, 1 month.
    Pediatric dose: >7 days old: 5–7.5 mg/kg/day, three divided doses.
    Drug available: gentamicin 10 mg/mL.

24. Child with postoperative wound infection.
    Order: cefazolin 185 mg, IV, q6h, in D_5W 20 mL, over 20 minutes. Flush with 15 mL.
    Child's weight: 15 kg.
    Pediatric dose: 25–50 mg/kg/day.
    Drug available:

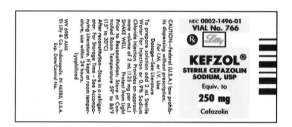

25. Child with wound infection after spinal fusion.
    Order: nafcillin 250 mg, IV, q6h, in D_5W 20 mL, over 30 minutes. Flush with 15 mL.
    Child's weight: 40 kg
    Pediatric dose: 25 mg/kg/day.
    Drug available:

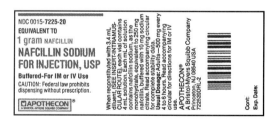

26. Child with congestive heart failure.
    Order: digoxin 40 mcg, IV, bid, in NSS 2 mL, over 1 minute.
    Child's weight and age: 6 lb, 1 month.
    Pediatric dose: 2 weeks to 2 years: 25–50 mcg(μg)/kg.
    Drug available: digoxin 0.1 mg/mL.

27. Child with lymphoma.
    Order: Cytoxan 180 mg, IV, in $D_5\frac{1}{2}$ NSS, 300 mL over 3 hours, no flush to follow.
    Child's weight and height: 16 kg, 75 cm.

Pediatric dose: 300 mg/m²/day.
Drug available:

28. Child with severe respiratory infection.
Order: kanamycin (Kantrex) 60 mg, IV, q8h.
Child's weight and age: 26 lb, 12 months.
Pediatric dose parameters: 15 mg/kg/day q8−12h, not to exceed 1.5 g per day.
Drug available:

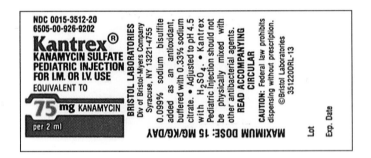

a. How many mL of kanamycin will the child receive per q8h?

_____

b. How many mL of kanamycin will the child receive per day?

_____

c. Is the drug dose within safe parameters? _____

29. Child with severe systemic infection.
Order: tobramycin (Nebcin) 15 mg, IV, q6h.
Drug available:

Child's weight and age: 10 kg, 18 months.
Pediatric dose parameters: 6−7.5 mg/kg/day in four divided doses.

a. How many mL of tobramycin would you give?

_____

b. Is the drug dose within safe parameters?

_____

30. Child with acute lymphocytic leukemia.
Order: daunorubicin HCl 40 mg, IV, qd.
Pediatric dose parameters: >2 yr: 25−45 mg/m²/d.
Child's age, weight, and height: 10 years, 72 lb, 60 inches.
Drug available: daunorubicin 20 mg/4 mL.
Instruction: Mix in 100 mL D_5W; infuse in 45 minutes.

a. The BSA is _____ .

b. How many milliliters should be mixed in the D_5W? _____

c. Is the drug dose within safe parameters? _____

PEDIATRIC DOSAGE FROM ADULT DOSAGE

Body Surface Area Formula

The following information is needed to calculate the pediatric dosage using the BSA formula:

a. Physician's order with the name of the drug, the dosage, and the time frame or frequency.

b. The child's height and weight.

c. A body surface area nomogram for children.

d. The adult drug dosage.

e. The body surface area formula:

$$\frac{\text{surface area (m}^2)}{1.73 \text{ m}^2} \times \text{adult dose} = \text{child's dose}$$

example

PROBLEM 1: a. erythromycin 80 mg, po, qid.

b. Child's height is 34 inches and weight is 28.5 lb.

Note: _Height and weight do not have to be converted to the metric system._

c. Height (34 inches) and weight (28.5 lb) intersect the nomogram at 0.57 m². See BSA nomogram, Figure 9−1.

d. The adult drug dosage is 1000 mg/24 hr.

e. Body surface area formula:

$$\frac{\text{surface area (m}^2)}{1.73 \text{ m}^2} \times \text{adult dose} = \frac{0.57 \text{ m}^2}{1.73 \text{ m}^2} \times 100$$
$$= 0.33 \times 1000$$
$$= 330 \text{ mg/24 hr}$$

Dose frequency:

$$330 \text{ mg} \div 4 \text{ doses} = 82.5$$

or

80 mg per dose

Dosage is safe.

$$80 \text{ mg} \times 4 \text{ times per day} = 320 \text{ mg/day}$$

Age Rules

Fried's rule and Young's rule are two methods for determining pediatric drug doses based on the child's age. Fried's rule is primarily used for children younger than 1 year of age, whereas Young's rule is used for children between 2 and 12 years of age. In current practice, these rules are infrequently used. Because the maturational development of infants and children is variable, age cannot be an accurate basis for drug dosing.

Fried's Rule:

$$\frac{\text{age in months}}{150} \times \text{adult dose} = \text{infant dose}$$

Young's Rule:

$$\frac{\text{child's age in years}}{\text{age in years} + 12} \times \text{adult dose} = \text{child dose}$$

Body Weight Rule

Clark's rule is another method to derive a pediatric dosage based on the child's weight in pounds and the average adult weight of 150 lb. Population studies have shown an increase in the average weight of adults; therefore, 150 lb is not an accurate constant. Using the fixed constant in Clark's rule can lead to the underdosing of infants. Clark's rule is being phased out as a method for determining drug dosage in children.

Clark's Rule:

$$\frac{\text{child's weight in pounds}}{150 \text{ lb}} \times \text{adult dose} = \text{child dose}$$

NOTE The age and weight rules should not be used if a pediatric dose is provided by the manufacturer.

ANSWERS

I. Oral

1. Pounds to kilograms: $\dfrac{45 \text{ lb}}{2.2 \text{ lb/kg}} = 20.4$ kg

   Dosage parameters: 25 mg/kg/day $\times$ 20.4 kg = 510 mg/day
   50 mg/kg/day $\times$ 20.4 kg = 1020 mg/day
   Dosage frequency: 250 mg $\times$ 3 = 750 mg
   Dosage is safe.

   $$\frac{D}{H} \times V = \frac{250 \text{ mg}}{125 \text{ mg}} \times 5 \text{ mL} = 10 \text{ mL}$$

2. Dosage parameters: 5 mg/kg/day $\times$ 7.2 kg = 36 mg/day
   7 mg/kg/day $\times$ 7.2 kg = 50.4 mg/day
   Dose frequency: 25 mg $\times$ 2 = 50 mg
   Dosage is safe.

   $$\frac{D}{H} \times V = \frac{25 \text{ mg}}{20 \text{ mg}} \times 5 \text{ mL} = 6.25 \text{ mL/dose}$$

3. Dosage parameters: 15 mg/kg, q12h $\times$ 8 kg = 120 mg, q12h
   Dosage frequency: 100 mg, q12h.
   Dosage is safe.

   $$\frac{D}{H} \times V = \frac{100 \text{ mg}}{125 \text{ mg}} \times 5 \text{ mL} = 4 \text{ mL/dose}$$

4. Height and weight intersect at 0.84 m^2.
   Dosage parameters: 100 mg/0.84 m^2/day = 84 mg/day
   Dose frequency: 84 mg/day $\div$ 6 = 14 mg/dose
   Dosage is safe.

   $$\frac{D}{H} \times V = \frac{7.5 \text{ mg}}{15 \text{ mg}} \times 1 = 0.50 \text{ or } \tfrac{1}{2} \text{ tablet}$$

5. Dosage parameters: 20 mg/kg/day $\times$ 13 kg = 260 mg/day
   Dose frequency: 125 mg $\times$ 2 = 250 mg/day
   Dosage is safe.

   $$\frac{D}{H} \times V = \frac{125 \text{ mg}}{250 \text{ mg}} \times 5 \text{ mL} = 2.5 \text{ mL}$$

6. Dosage parameters: 5 mg/kg/day $\times$ 6.7 kg = 33.5 mg/day
   7 mg/kg/day $\times$ 6.7 kg = 46.9 mg/day
   Dose frequency: 40 mg $\times$ 2 = 80 mg/d
   Dosage exceeds the therapeutic range. Dosage is *not safe.*

7. Dosage parameters: 150 mg/kg/day $\times$ 30.4 = 4560 mg or 4.5 g
   200 mg/kg/day $\times$ 30.4 = 6080 mg or 6.1 g
   Dose frequency: 1.5 g $\times$ 4 = 6.0 g or 6000 mg
   Dosage is safe.

   $$\frac{D}{H} = \frac{1500 \text{ mg}}{500 \text{ mg}} = 3 \text{ tablets/dose}$$

8. Dosage parameters: 20 mg/kg/day × 8 kg = 160 mg/day
 40 mg/kg/day × 8 kg = 320 mg/day
Dosage frequency: 75 mg × 3 = 225 mg
Dosage is safe.

$$\frac{D}{H} \times V = \frac{75 \text{ mg}}{125 \text{ mg}} \times 5 \text{ mL} = 3 \text{ mL}$$

9. Dosage parameters: 5 mg/kg/day × 25 kg = 125 mg/day
Dosage frequency: 25 mg × 4 = 100 mg/day
Dosage is safe.

$$\frac{D}{H} \times V = \frac{25 \text{ mg}}{12.5 \text{ mg}} \times 5 \text{ mL} = 10 \text{ mL}$$

10. Dosage parameters: 4 mg/kg/day × 14 kg = 56 mg/day
 8 mg/kg/day × 14 kg = 112 mg/day
Dose frequency: 25 mg × 3 = 75 mg
Dosage is safe.

$$\frac{D}{H} \times V = \frac{25 \text{ mg}}{50 \text{ mg}} \times 5 \text{ mL} = 2.5 \text{ mL/dose}$$

11. a. 15 lb ÷ 2.2 = 6.8 kg
Drug parameters: 20 mg × 6.8 kg = 136 mg/day
 40 mg × 6.8 kg = 272 mg/day
Dose frequency: 50 mg × 4 = 200 mg/day
Dosage is within safe parameters.

b. $\dfrac{D}{H} \times V = \dfrac{50}{125} \times 5 = \dfrac{250}{125} = 2 \text{ mL}$

$$\text{H} \quad : \quad \text{V} \quad :: \quad \text{D} \quad : \quad \text{X}$$
$$125 \text{ mg} : 5 \text{ mL} :: 50 \text{ mg} : \text{X mL}$$

$$125 \text{ X} = 250$$
$$\text{X} = 2 \text{ mL}$$

II. Intramuscular

12. Dosage parameters: 0.25/kg/dose × 45 kg = 11.25 mg/dose
 0.5/kg/dose × 45 kg = 22.5 mg/dose
Dose frequency: 20 mg IM/dose
Dosage is safe.

$$\frac{D}{H} \times V = \frac{20 \text{ mg}}{25 \text{ mg}} \times 1 = 0.8 \text{ mL}$$

13. Dosage parameters: Child's weight is 44 lb, which falls in the 30–60 lb pediatric dose range.
Dose frequency: The one-time dose of 1,000,000 U falls within the pediatric dose range.
Dosage is safe.

$$\frac{D}{H} \times V = \frac{1,000,000 \text{ U}}{1,200,000 \text{ U}} \times 2 = 1.6 \text{ mL}$$

14. Height and weight intersect at 0.82 m².
    Dosage parameters: 30 mg/m² × 0.82 m² = 24.6 mg or 25 mg
    Dose frequency: 25 mg IM
    Dosage is safe.

$$\frac{D}{H} \times V = \frac{25 \text{ mg}}{25 \text{ mg}} \times 1 = 1.0 \text{ mL}$$

15. Kilograms to pounds: 12 kg × 2.2 lb/kg = 26.4 lb
    Dosage is safe.

$$\frac{D}{H} \times V = \frac{0.2}{0.4} \times 1 = 0.5 \text{ mL}$$

16. Height and weight intersect at 1.38 m².
    Dosage parameters: 25 mg/m²/wk × 1.38 m² = 34.5 mg/wk
    75 mg/m²/wk × 1.38 m² = 103.5 mg/wk
    Dose frequency: 50 mg/wk IM
    Dosage is safe.

$$\frac{D}{H} \times V = \frac{50}{100} \text{ mg} \times 1 = 0.5 \text{ mL}$$

17. **a.** Preferred selection is AquaMEPHYTON 1 mg = 0.5 mL

    b. *AquaMEPHYTON 1 mg = 0.5 mL:*

$$\frac{D}{H} \times V = \frac{0.5 \text{ mg}}{1.0 \text{ mg}} \times 0.5 \text{ mL} = \frac{0.25}{1.0} = 0.25 \text{ mL}$$

   AquaMEPHYTON 10 mg = 1 mL:

$$\frac{D}{H} \times V = \frac{0.5 \text{ mg}}{10 \text{ mg}} \times 1.0 \text{ mL} = \frac{0.5}{10} = 0.05 \text{ mL}$$

   For AquaMEPHYTON 1 mg = 0.5 mL, give 0.25 mL (use a tuberculin syringe).
   For AquaMEPHYTON 10 mg = 1 mL, give 0.05 mL (use a tuberculin syringe; however, it would be difficult to give this small amount.)

   c. Drug dose is within the safe parameters.

III. Intravenous

18. Dosage parameters: 50 mcg/kg/dose × 50 kg = 2500 mcg/dose or
    2.5 mg/dose
    100 mcg/kg/dose × 50 kg = 5000 mcg/dose or
    5 mg/dose
    Dosage is safe.

$$\frac{D}{H} \times V = \frac{2.5}{4} \times 1 = 0.62 \text{ or } 0.6 \text{ mL}$$

Amount of fluid to infuse: 0.6 mL + 10 mL = 10.6 mL

$$\frac{10.6 \text{ mL} \times \overset{12}{\cancel{60}} \text{ gtt/mL}}{\underset{1}{\cancel{5} \text{ minutes}}} = 127.2 \text{ gtt/min}$$

Total fluid for medication infusion: 10.6 mL + 5 mL = 15.6 mL.

19. Dosage parameters: 0.005 mg/kg/dose × 32 kg = 0.16 mg
0.01 mg/kg/dose × 32 kg = 0.32 mg
Dosage is safe.

$$\frac{D}{H} \times V = \frac{0.3}{0.4} \times 1 = 0.75 \text{ mL}$$

20. Dosage parameters: 15 mg/kg/day × 5.3 = 79.5 mg/day
Dosage frequency: 40 mg IV × 2 = 80 mg
79.5 mg is rounded off to 80 mg. The dosage is safe.

$$\frac{D}{H} \times V = \frac{40 \text{ mg}}{100 \text{ mg}} \times 2 = 0.8 \text{ mL}$$

Amount of fluid to infuse: 0.8 mL + 5 mL = 5.8 mL

$$\frac{5.8 \text{ mL} \times \overset{3}{\cancel{60}} \text{ gtt/mL}}{\underset{1}{\cancel{20}} \text{ minutes}} = 17.4 \text{ gtt/min}$$

Total fluid for medication infusion: 5.8 mL + 3 mL = 8.8 mL.

21. Dosage parameters: 0.4 mg/kg/day × 10.1 kg = 4 mg/day
4 mg ÷ 4 doses = 1 mg per dose
Dose frequency: 2 mg × 4 times/day = 8 mg per day
Dose exceeds therapeutic range of 1 mg per dose. Dosage is *not safe.*

22. Dosage parameters: 25−100 mg/kg/day in four divided doses.

25 mg × 5.6 kg = 140 mg/day

100 mg × 5.6 kg = 560 mg/day

560 mg ÷ 4 = 140 mg/dose

Dose frequency: 500 mg × 4 = 2000 mg/day
Dose exceeds therapeutic range of 140 mg/dose. Dosage is *not safe.*

23. Dosage parameters: 5 mg/kg/day × 4 kg = 20 mg/day
7.5 mg/kg/day × 4 kg = 30 mg/day
Dose frequency: 10 mg × 3 times/day = 30 mg
Dosage is safe.

$$\frac{D}{H} \times V = \frac{10 \text{ mg}}{10 \text{ mg}} \times 1 \text{ mL} = 1 \text{ mL}$$

Amount of fluid to infuse: 1 mL + 4 mL = 5 mL

$$\frac{5 \text{ mL} \times \overset{2}{\cancel{60}} \text{ gtt/mL}}{\underset{1}{\cancel{30}} \text{ minutes}} = 10 \text{ gtt/min}$$

Total fluid for medication infusion: 5 mL + 3 mL = 8 mL

24. Dosage parameters: 25 mg/kg/day × 15 kg = 375 mg/day
50 mg/kg/day × 15 kg = 750 mg/day

Dosage frequency: 185 mg × 4 = 740 mg/day
Dosage is safe.

$$\frac{D}{H} \times V = \frac{185 \text{ mg}}{125 \text{ mg}} \times 1 \text{ mL} = 1.48 \text{ or } 1.5 \text{ mL}$$

Amount of fluid to infuse: 1.5 mL + 20 mL = 21.5 mL

$$\frac{21.5 \text{ mL} \times \overset{3}{\cancel{60}} \text{ gtt/mL}}{\underset{1}{\cancel{20} \text{ minutes}}} = 64.5 \text{ gtt/min}$$

Total fluid for medication infusion: 21.5 mL + 15 mL = 36.5 mL

25. Dosage parameters: 25 mg/kg/day × 40 kg = 1000 mg
Dosage frequency: 250 mg × 4 = 1000 mg/day
Dosage is safe.

$$\frac{D}{H} \times V = \frac{250}{1000} \times 4 = 1 \text{ mL}$$

Amount of fluid to infuse: 1 mL + 20 mL = 21 mL

$$\frac{21 \text{ mL} \times \overset{2}{\cancel{60}} \text{ gtt/mL (set)}}{\underset{1}{\cancel{30} \text{ minutes}}} = 42 \text{ gtt/min}$$

Total fluid for medication infusion: 21 mL + 15 mL = 36 mL

26. Dosage parameters: 25 mcg/kg/day × 2.72 kg = 68 mcg
                              50 mcg/kg/day × 2.72 kg = 136 mcg
Dosage frequency: 40 mcg × 2 = 80 mcg
0.1 mg = 100 mcg(μg)
Dosage is safe.

$$\frac{D}{H} \times V = \frac{40 \text{ mcg}}{100 \text{ mcg}} \times 1 = 0.4 \text{ mL}$$

27. Height and weight intersect at 0.6 m².
Dosage parameters: 300 mg/m²/day × 0.6 m² = 180 mg/day
Dosage is safe.

$$\frac{D}{H} \times V = \frac{180 \text{ mg}}{200 \text{ mg}} \times 10 \text{ mL} = 9 \text{ mL}$$

Total amount of fluid to infuse: 9 mL + 300 mL = 309 mL

$$\frac{309 \text{ mL}}{3 \text{ hr}} = 103 \text{ mL/hr or 103 gtt/min with a 60 gtt/mL set}$$

28. a. $\frac{60}{75} \times 2 \text{ mL} = \frac{120}{75} = 1.6 \text{ mL}$ **or** 75 mg : 2 mL : : 60 mg : X

$$75 X = 120$$
$$X = 1.6 \text{ mL of}$$
kanamycin

b. 4.8 mL/day

    c. Dosage parameters: 15 mg $\times$ 12 kg = 180 mg/day

                              60 mg $\times$ 3 (q8h) = 180 mg/day

    Drug dose per day is within safe parameters.

29. a. $\dfrac{15}{\overset{20}{\underset{10}{}}} \times \overset{1}{2} \text{ mL} = \dfrac{15}{10}$ **or**   20 mg : 2 mL : : 15 mg : X

                = 1.5 mL of Nebcin   20 X = 30

                                      X = 1.5 mL of Nebcin

    b. Pediatric dose parameters: 6 mg/10 kg/day = 60 mg/day

                               7.5 mg/10 kg/day = 75 mg/day

                             15 mg $\times$ 4 (q6h) = 60 mg/day

    Drug dose per day is within safe parameters.

30. a. The BSA is 1.16.

    b. 8 mL of daunorubicin HCl mixed in 100 mL D_5W.

    c. 25 mg $\times$ 1.16 m² = 29 mg/day

    45 mg $\times$ 1.16 m² = 52.2 mg/day

    Child is to receive 40 mg/day of daunorubicin HCl

    Drug dose is within safe parameters.

$$\dfrac{108 \text{ mL} \times \overset{1}{\cancel{15}} \text{ gtt/min (secondary set)}}{\underset{3}{\cancel{45}} \text{ min}} = 36 \text{ gtt/min}$$

critical care

objectives

- Calculate the prescribed concentration of a drug in solution.
- Identify the units of measure designated for the amount of drug in solution.
- Describe the four determinants of infusion rates.
- Calculate the concentration of drug per unit time for a specific body weight.
- Recognize the variables needed for the basic fractional formula.
- Describe how the titration factor is used when infusion rates are changed.
- Recognize the methods of determining the total amount of drug infused over time.

outline

Medication administration has become increasing individualized for critically ill clients. Nurses are responsible for safe and accurate delivery of these drugs. Administration of potent drugs in milligrams, micrograms, or units per body weight or unit time requires extreme accuracy in calculations. Physicians determine the amount of drug to be mixed in the intravenous solution and designate infusion rates or the dosage per kilogram of body weight per unit time. Some institutions have their own guidelines for preparation of medication in the critical care areas. Research studies have shown a high incidence of error in drug calculations among nurses and physicians. Many institutions have initiated policies of drug infusion standardization, especially for the concentration of solution, to limit infusion errors.

Because some institutions have their own guidelines for preparations and medication in the critical care areas, the medication often comes in premixed bags or bottles from the pharmacy ready for infusion. Still, in some facilities, these drugs are prepared by the nurse. The nurse must know what data are needed for each drug and apply those parameters to whatever intravenous (IV) equipment is available. Wide use of volumetric intravenous infusion pumps has improved the safety of individualized drug administration. The accuracy of the infusion rate with the pump has almost eliminated the need for drop counting, but nurses are still responsible for all other infusion rates. Each drug has its own dosing parameters. Some drugs are dosed in the concentration per hour or minute and others are administered in micrograms, milligrams, or units per kilogram body weight. The nurse must be familiar with the specific dosing parameters to ensure the accuracy of infusion rates.

The mathematical skills needed to solve problems in this chapter include the knowledge of proper and improper fractions, cancellation of units, ratio and proportion, and conversion to the metric system.

CALCULATING AMOUNT OF DRUG OR CONCENTRATION OF A SOLUTION

The first step in administering a medication is to determine the concentration of the solution, which is the amount of drug in each milliliter of solution. This is written as units per milliliter, milligrams per milliliter, or micrograms per milliliter and must be calculated for each problem. For all problems, remember to convert to like units before solving.

Calculating Units per Milliliter

. . . .

example

PROBLEM: Infuse heparin 5000 U in D_5W 250 mL at 30 mL/hr. What will be the concentration of heparin in each milliliter of D_5W?

Method: units/mL

Set up a ratio and proportion. Solve for X.	5000 U : 250 mL : : X U : mL

$$250 X = 5000$$
$$X = 20 U$$

Answer: The D_5W with heparin will have a concentration of 20 U/mL of solution.

Calculating Milligrams per Milliliter

e x a m p l e

PROBLEM: Infuse lidocaine 2 g in 500 mL D_5W at 2 mg/min. What will be the concentration of lidocaine in each milliliter of D_5W?

Method: mg/mL

Convert grams to milligrams. Set up a ratio and proportion and solve for X.	2 g = 2000 mg 2000 mg : 500 mL : : X mg : mL

$$500 X = 2000$$
$$X = 4 mg$$

Answer: The D_5W with lidocaine has a concentration of 4 mg/mL of solution.

Calculating Micrograms per Milliliter

e x a m p l e

PROBLEM: Infuse dobutamine 250 mg in 500 mL D_5W at 650 mcg/min. What is the concentration of dobutamine in each milliliter of D_5W?

Method: mcg/mL

Convert milligrams to micrograms. Set up a ratio and proportion and solve for X.	250 mg = 250,000 mcg 250,000 mcg : 500 mL : : X mcg : mL

$$500 X = 250,000$$
$$X = 500 mcg/mL$$

Answer: The D_5W with dobutamine will have a concentration of 500 mcg/mL of solution.

I Practice Problems: Calculating Concentration of a Solution

1. Infuse heparin 10,000 U in 250 mL D_5W at 30 mL/hr.

2. Infuse aminophylline 250 mg in 500 mL D_5W at 50 mL/hr.

3. Order: regular insulin 100 U in 500 mL NSS at 30 mL/hr.

4. Order: lidocaine 1 g in 100 mL D_5W at 30 mL/hr.

5. Order: norepinephrine 4 mg in 500 mL D_5W at 15 mL/hr.

6. Order: dopamine 500 mg in 250 mL D_5W at 10 mL/hr.

7. Order: dobutamine 400 mg in 250 mL D_5W at 20 mL/hr.

8. Order: Isuprel 2 mg in 250 mL D_5W at 10 mL/hr.

9. Order: streptokinase 750,000 U in 50 mL D_5W over 30 minutes.

10. Order: nitroprusside 50 mg in 500 mL D_5W at 50 mcg/min.

11. Order: aminophylline 1 g in 250 mL D_5W at 20 mL/hr.

12. Order: Pronestyl 2 g in 250 mL D_5W at 16 mL/hr.

13. Order: heparin 25,000 U in 250 mL D_5W at 5 mL/hr.

14. Order: aminophylline 1 g in 500 mL at 40 cc/hr.

15. Order: nitroglycerin 50 mg in 250 mL D_5W at 50 mcg/min.

16. Order: alteplase 100 mg in NSS 100 mL over 2 hours.

_____

17. Order: theophylline 800 mg in D_5W 500 mL at 0.5 mg/kg.

_____

18. Order: milrinone 20 mg in D_5W 100 mL at 0.50 mcg/kg/min.

_____

19. Order: streptokinase 1.5 million units in D_5W 100 mL over 60 minutes.

_____

20. Order: amiodarone 150 mg in D_5W 100 mL over 10 minutes.

CALCULATING INFUSION RATE FOR CONCENTRATION AND VOLUME PER UNIT TIME

The second step for administering medication is to calculate the _infusion rate_ of drug per _unit time_. Infusion rates can mean two things: the rate of volume (mL) given or the rate of concentration (units, mg, mcg) administered. _Unit time_ means per hour or per minute. For drugs administered by continuous infusion, the four most important determinants are the concentration per hour and minute and the volume per hour and minute. Infusion rates of potent drugs are usually part of the physician's order and may be stated in concentration or volume per unit time.

Many hospitals have policies requiring that all potent drugs be delivered via volumetric infusion pump. New technology has produced pumps that are programmable and calculate the drug dosage. The information entered in the pump's control panel is (1) the name of the drug, (2) the amount of the drug, (3) the amount of the solution, and (4) the client's weight in kilograms. The nurse enters the ordered dose and the correct dosage parameters, i.e., mg/min, U/hr, mcg/min. The pump automatically delivers the appropriate dosage.

Not all facilities have infusion pumps with advanced technology; therefore, the nurse must be able to calculate the infusion rates. For infusion pumps that deliver mL/hr, the volume per hour of the drug must be known. _Remember:_ If an infusion device is unavailable, a microdrip IV administration set is the appropriate set to use because the drops per minute rate (gtt/min) corresponds to the volume per hour rate (mL/hr).

Complete infusion rates for volume and concentration are given in the examples and practice problems. In clinical practice, not all the data are needed for each drug. For heparin, the concentration per minute is not as vital as the concentration per hour, whereas for vasoactive drugs such as dobutamine, the concentration per minute is essential information and the concentration per hour is not. The same methods of calculation are used for both drugs, and the same information can be obtained. The nurse must have knowledge of pharmacology and clinical practice to determine what are the most useful data.

Concentration and Volume per Hour and Minute with a Drug in Units

example

PROBLEM: Infuse heparin 5000 U in D_5W 250 mL at 30 mL/hr.
Concentration of solution is 20 units/mL. (Also note that volume/hr is given.)
How many milliliters will infuse per minute?

Find volume per minute:

Method: mL/min

Set up a ratio and proportion. Use volume/hour, 30 mL/hr, or 30 mL/60 min as the known variable.	30 mL : 60 min : : X mL : min 60 X = 30 X = 0.5 mL

Answer: The infusion rate for volume per minute is 0.5 mL/min and the hourly rate is 30 mL/hr.

What is the concentration per minute and hour?
Find concentration per minute:

Method: U/min

Multiply the concentration of solution by the volume per minute.	20 U/mL × 0.5 mL/min = 10 U/min

Find concentration per hour:

Method: U/hr

Multiply the volume per minute by 60 min/hr.	10 U/min × 60 min/hr = 600 U/hr

Answer: The concentration per minute of heparin is 10 U/min and the concentration per hour is 600 U/hr.

Concentration and Volume per Hour and Minute with a Drug in Milligrams

example

PROBLEM: Infuse lidocaine 2 g in D_5W 500 mL at 2 mg/min.
Concentration of solution is 4 mg/mL. (Also note that concentration/min is given.)
How many milligrams will be infused per hour?

Find concentration per hour:

Method: mg/hr

| Find the concentration/minute. Multiply concentration/min × 60 min/hr. | lidocaine 2 mg/min

2 mg/min × 60 min = 120 mg/hr |

Answer: The amount of lidocaine infused per hour is 120 mg/hr.

How many milliliters of lidocaine will be infused in 1 hour?
Find volume per hour:

Method: mL/hr

| Calculate concentration of solution. Divide the concentration/hr by the concentration of solution. | lidocaine 4 mg/mL

$\dfrac{120 \text{ mg/hr}}{4 \text{ mg/mL}} = 30 \text{ mL/hr}$ |

Answer: The infusion rate in milliliters for lidocaine 2 mg/min is 30 mL/hr.

How many milliliters of lidocaine will be infused in 1 minute?
Find volume per minute:

Method: mL/min

| Divide the concentration/min by the concentration of solution. | $\dfrac{2 \text{ mg/min}}{4 \text{ mg/mL}} = 0.5 \text{ mL/min}$ |

Answer: The infusion rate for lidocaine 2 mg/min is 0.5 mL/min.

Concentration and Volume per Minute and Hour with a Drug in Micrograms

example

PROBLEM: Infuse dobutamine 250 mg in D_5W 500 mL at 650 mcg/min.
Concentration of solution is 500 mcg/mL. (Also note that concentration/min is given in the order.)
How many micrograms will be infused in 1 hour?

Find concentration per hour:

Method: mcg/hr

| Find the concentration/min. Multiply concentration/min by 60 min/hr. | dobutamine 650 mcg/min

650 mcg/min × 60 min/hr = 39,000 mcg/hr |

Answer: The concentration of dobutamine infused per hour is 39,000 mcg/hr.

How many milliliters of dobutamine will be infused in 1 hour?

Find volume per hour:

Method: mL/hr

Calculate concentration of solution. Divide the concentration/hr by the concentration of solution.	dobutamine 500 mcg/mL $\dfrac{39{,}000 \text{ mcg/hr}}{500 \text{ mcg/mL}} = 78 \text{ mL/hr}$

Answer: The infusion rate for dobutamine 650 mcg/min is 78 mL/hr.

How many milliliters of dobutamine should be infused in 1 minute? Find volume per minute:

Method: mL/min

Divide concentration/min by concentration of solution.	$\dfrac{650 \text{ mcg/min}}{500 \text{ mcg/mL}} = 1.3 \text{ mL/min}$

Answer: The infusion rate for dobutamine is 1.3 mL/min.

II Practice Problems: Calculating Infusion Rate

Use the examples to find the following information:

● Concentration of the solution
● Infusion rates per unit time:

    a. Volume per minute
    b. Volume per hour
    c. Concentration per minute
    d. Concentration per hour

1. Order: heparin 1000 U in D_5W 500 mL at 50 mL/hr.

_____

2. Order: nitroprusside 100 mg in D_5W 500 mL at 60 mL/hr.

_____

3. Order: nitroprusside 25 mg in D_5W 250 mL at 50 mcg/min.

_____

4. Order: dopamine 800 mg in D_5W 500 mL at 400 mcg/min.

_____

5. Order: norepinephrine 2 mg in D_5W 250 mL at 45 mL/hr.

_____

6. Order: dobutamine 1000 mg in D_5W 500 mL at 12 mL/hr.

_____

7. Order: dobutamine 250 mg in D_5W 250 mL at 10 mL/hr.

_____

8. Order: lidocaine 2 g in D_5W 500 mL at 4 mg/min.

_____

9. Order: dopamine 400 mg in D_5W 250 mL at 60 mL/hr.

_____

10. Order: isoproterenol 4 mg in D_5W 500 mL at 65 mL/hr.

_____

11. Order: morphine sulfate 50 mg in 150 mL NSS at 3 mg/hr.

_____

12. Order: regular Humulin insulin 50 U in 250 mL NSS at 4 U/hr.

_____

13. Order: aminophylline 2 g in 250 mL D_5W at 20 mL/hr.

_____

14. Order: nitroglycerin 50 mg in 250 mL D_5W at 24 mL/hr.

_____

15. Order: heparin 25,000 U in 500 mL D_5W at 10 mL/hr.

_____

16. Order: amiodarone 900 mg in D_5W 500 mL at 33.3 mL/hr.

_____

17. Order: procainamide 1 g in D_5W 250 mL at 4 mg/min.

_____

18. Order: diltiazem 100 mg in 100 mL NSS at 10 mg/hr.

_____

19. Order: streptokinase 750,000 U in 250 mL/NSS at 100,000 U/hr.

_____

20. Order: bretylium 1 g in 250 mL D_5W at 1 mg/min.

_____

CALCULATING INFUSION RATES OF A DRUG FOR SPECIFIC BODY WEIGHT PER UNIT TIME

The last method is calculating infusion rates for the amount of drug per unit time for a specific body weight. The weight parameter is an accurate means of dosing for a therapeutic effect. The metric system is used for all drug dosing, so pounds must be changed to kilograms. The physician orders the *desired dose per kilogram of body weight* and the *concentration of the solution.* From this information, infusion rates can be calculated for administering an individualized dose. Accurate daily weights are essential for the correct dosage.

The previous methods for calculating *concentration of solution* and *infusion rates* for concentration and volume are used, with one addition. The *concentration per minute* is obtained by multiplying the *body weight* by the *desired dose per kilogram per minute,* which must be done before the other infusion rates can be calculated. For many vasoactive drugs given as examples in this chapter, the most useful information clinically is the concentration per minute for the specific body weight, volume per minute, and volume per hour, because these parameters determine the infusion pump settings.

New volumetric infusion pumps now can deliver fractional portions of a milliliter from tenths to hundreths in addition to calculating dosages for infusion rates. If the infusion pumps available do not have this feature and the volume per hour is a fractional amount, it must be rounded off to a whole number (1.8 mL/hr = 2 mL/hr). When calculating concentration per minute and hour and volume per minute, carry out the problem to three decimal places, if necessary, before rounding off. The volume per hour, if fractional, can then be rounded off, making the volume per hour as accurate as possible. There are two exceptions to rounding off fractional infusion rates:

1. If the client's condition is labile, the difference between 1 or 2 mL could be important.

2. Because physicians order the medication, they must be consulted if rounding off would significantly change the drug dosage.

Micrograms per Kilogram Body Weight

example

PROBLEM: Infuse dobutamine 250 mg in 500 mL D$_5$W at 10 mcg/kg/min.
Patient weighs 143 lb.
Concentration of solution is 500 mcg/mL.
How many micrograms of dobutamine would be infused per minute? Per hour?

Convert pounds to kilograms:

Divide pounds by 2.2.	$\dfrac{143 \text{ lb}}{2.2 \text{ lb/kg}} = \text{kg}$

Find concentration per minute:

Method: mcg/min

Multiply client's weight by the desired dose of mcg/kg/min.	65 kg × 10 mcg/kg/min = 650 mcg/min

Find concentration per hour:

Method: mcg/hr

Multiply concentration/min by 60 min/hr.	650 mcg/min × 60 min/hr = 39,000 mcg/hr

Answer: The concentration of dobutamine infused per minute and per hour is 650 mcg/min and 39,000 mcg/hr for the patient's body weight.

How many milliliters of dobutamine will infuse per minute? Per hour? Find volume per minute:

Method: mL/min

Divide the concentration/min by the concentration of the solution.	$\dfrac{650 \text{ mcg/min}}{500 \text{ mcg/mL}} = 1.241$ mL/min

Find volume per hour:

Method: mL/hr

Multiply volume/min by 60 min/hr.	1.241 mL/min × 60 min/hr = 74.46 or 74 mL/hr

Answer: The volume of dobutamine infused per minute is 1.241 mL/min, and the infusion rate per hour is 74 mL/hr.

BASIC FRACTIONAL FORMULA

A fractional equation can create a basic formula that can be used as another quick method to determine any one of the following quantities: concentration of solution, volume per hour, and desired concentration per minute (× kilogram of body weight, if required). The equation has one constant, the drop rate of the IV set, 60 gtt/mL. The unknown quantity can be represented by X. (See Chapter 3 for fractional equations.) The basic formula is not accurate to the nearest hundredth, as are the other methods in this section:

$$\frac{\text{concentration of solution (U, mg, mcg/mL)}}{\text{drop rate of set (60 gtt/mL)}} = \frac{\text{desired concentration/min} \times \text{kg body weight}}{\text{volume/hr (mL/hr or gtt/min)}}$$

Using Basic Formula to Find Volume per Hour or Drops per Minute

....

example

PROBLEM: Infuse heparin 5000 U in 250 mL D_5W at 0.15 U/kg/min.

Client weighs 70 kg. The concentration of solution is 20 U/mL.

Desired concentration/minute: 0.15 U/kg/min × 70 kg = 10.5 U/min

$$\frac{20 \text{ U/mL}}{60 \text{ gtt/mL}} = \frac{10.5 \text{ U/min}}{X \text{ (mL/hr or gtt/min)}}$$

20 X = 630

X = 31 mL/hr or 31 gtt/min

Using Basic Formula to Find Desired Concentration per Minute

> **example**

PROBLEM: Infuse lidocaine 2 g in 500 mL D_5W at 30 mL/hr. The concentration of the solution is 4 mg/mL.

$$\frac{4 \text{ mg/mL}}{60 \text{ gtt/mL}} = \frac{X}{30 \text{ mL/hr}}$$

60 X = 120

X = 2 mg/min

Using Basic Formula to Find Concentration of Solution

> **example**

PROBLEM: Infuse dobutamine 250 mg in D_5W 500 mL at 10 mcg/kg/min with rate of 74 mL/hr. Client weighs 65 kg.

Desired concentration per minute = 10 mcg/kg/min × 65 kg
= 650 mcg/min

$$\frac{X}{60 \text{ gtt/mL}} = \frac{650 \text{ mcg/min}}{74 \text{ mL/hr}}$$

74 X = 39,000

X = 527 mcg/mL

III Practice Problems: Calculating Infusion Rate for Specific Body Weight

Determine the infusion rates for specific body weight by calculating the following:

- Concentration of the solution
- Weight in kilograms
- Infusion rates:

   a. Concentration per minute

   b. Concentration per hour (not always measured)

   c. Volume per minute

d. Volume per hour

You can use the basic fractional formula and compare answers.

1. Infuse dobutamine 500 mg in 250 mL D_5W at 5 mcg/kg/min. Client weighs 182 lb.

_____

2. Infuse amrinone 250 mg in 250 mL NSS at 5 mcg/kg/min. Client weighs 165 lb.

_____

3. Infuse dopamine 400 mg in 250 mL D_5W at 10 mcg/kg/min. Client weighs 140 lb.

_____

4. Infuse nitroprusside 100 mg in 500 mL D_5W at 3 mcg/kg/min. Client weighs 55 kg.

_____

5. Infuse dobutamine 1000 mg in 500 mL D_5W at 15 mcg/kg/min. Client weighs 110 lb.

_____

6. Infuse propofol (Diprivan) 500 mg/50 ml infusion bottle at 10 mcg/kg/min. Client weighs 187 lb.

_____

7. Infuse alfentanil (Alfenta) 10,000 mcg in D_5W 250 mL at 0.5 mcg/kg/min. Client weighs 175 lb.

_____

8. Infuse milrinone (Primacor) 20 mg in D_5W 100 mL at 0.375 mcg/kg/min. Client weighs 160 lb.

_____

9. Infuse theophylline 400 mg in D_5W 500 mL at 0.55 mg/kg/hr. Client weighs 70 kg.

_____

10. Infuse esmolol 2.5 g in NSS 250 mL at 150 mcg/kg/min. Client weighs 148 lb.

_____

TITRATION OF INFUSION RATE

Drugs administered by titration are based on (1) _concentration of solution,_ (2) _infusion rates,_ (3) _specific concentration per kilogram of body weight,_ and (4) _titration factor._ The _titration factor_ is the concentration of drug per drop in

U/gtt, mg/gtt, or mcg/gtt. For the programmable volumetric infusion pump, the titration factor is the increment of increase or decrease in units, mcg, or mg. If the only IV equipment available has the mL/hr feature, the titration factor of concentration per drop can be used. The titration factor can be added to or subtracted from the baseline infusion rate to determine the exact concentration of an infusion. Because the titration method of drug administration is primarily used when a client's condition is labile, calculating the titration factor gives the nurse the means of determining the exact amount of drug being infused.

Charts for drug infusion, developed by drug manufacturers, can be used to adjust infusion rates for drug titrations. Often, the amount of drug being infused falls between calibrations on the charts. When this occurs, the titration factor can be used to determine the exact concentration of drug being administered. The titration factor can also be used to verify the correct selection from the chart.

example

PROBLEM: Infuse Isuprel 2 mg in 250 mL D$_5$W.
Titrate 1–3 mcg/min to maintain heart rate > 50 and < 130 and blood pressure > 90 systolic.

a. Find concentration of solution:

Convert mg to mcg. Set up ratio and proportion.	$2 \text{ mg} = 2000 \text{ mcg}$
	$2000 \text{ mcg} : 250 \text{ mL} :: X \text{ mcg} : \text{mL}$
	$250 \, X = 2000$
	$X = 8 \text{ mcg}$
	8 mcg/mL

b. Infusion rate by volume per unit time:
Desired infusion rate by concentration is stated in the problem.
Note that the upper dosage and lower dosage must be determined.

REMEMBER Hourly rate and the number of drops per minute are the same with a microdrip administration set.

Find volume rate per minute: mL/min:

Divide concentration/min by concentration of solution.	*Lower*	*Upper*
	$\dfrac{1 \text{ mcg/min}}{8 \text{ mcg/mL}}$	$\dfrac{3 \text{ mcg/min}}{8 \text{ mcg/mL}}$
	$= 0.125 \text{ mL/min}$	$= 0.375 \text{ mL/min}$

Find volume rate per hour: mL/hr (equivalent to gtt/min):

| Multiply volume rate/min by 60 min. | *Lower*
0.125 mL/min × 60 min/hr
= 7.5 mL/hr (7.5 gtt/min)

Upper
0.375 mL/hr × 60 min/hr
= 22.5 mL/hr (22.5 gtt/min) |

c. Determine the titration factor:

| Find rate in gtt/min.
Divide concentration/min by gtt/min. | 7.5 gtt/min

$\dfrac{1 \text{ mcg/min}}{7.5 \text{ gtt/min}} = 0.133 \text{ mcg/gtt}$ |

The *titration factor* is 0.133 mcg/gtt in a solution of Isuprel 2 mg in 250 mL D₅W. To repeat, changing drops per minute results in a corresponding change in milliliters per hour. If the baseline infusion rates are **1 mcg/min** for concentration and **7.5 mL/hr** for volume, increasing the infusion rate by **1 gtt/min** changes the concentration/minute by **0.133 mcg** and increases the hourly volume by **1 mL** to give a rate of **8.5 mL/hr.**

d. Increasing or decreasing infusion rates.
To increase the infusion rate by 5 gtt/min from a baseline rate of 1 mcg/min, set up a ratio and proportion or multiply the titration factor (mcg/gtt) by 5 to obtain the increment of increase.

example

| Set up a ratio and proportion with rate in gtt/min as the known variables. | 7.5 gtt : 1 mcg : : 5 gtt : X mcg
7.5 X = 5
X = 0.666 mcg
5 gtt/0.66 mcg |

or

| Multiply titration factor in mcg/gtt by 5. | 0.133 mcg/gtt × 5 gtt = 0.665 mcg |

Adding 5 gtt/min increases the volume infusion rate by 5 mL/hr, from 7.5 to 12.5 mL/hr. The concentration of drug delivered is increased by 0.665 mcg/min to 1.665 mcg/min. For example,

   1.000 mcg/min baseline rate
+ 0.665 mcg/min increment of rate increased
   1.665 mcg/min adjusted infusion rate

Suppose the infusion rate was 3 mcg/min and a decrease was needed. To decrease the infusion rate by 10 gtt, set up another ratio and proportion or multiply the titration factor (mcg/gtt) by 10.

example

| Set up a ratio and proportion with rate in gtt/mcg as the known variable. | 7.5 gtt : 1 mcg : : 10 gtt : X mcg
7.5 X = 10
X = 1.33 mcg
1.33 mcg/10 gtt |

or

| Multiply titration factor in mcg/gtt by 10. | 0.133 mcg/gtt $\times$ 10 gtt = 1.33 mcg |

Subtracting 10 gtt/min decreases the infusion rate by 10 mL/hr, from 22.5 to 12.5 mL/hr. The amount of drug delivered is decreased by 1.33 mcg/min to 1.67 mcg/min. For example,

3.00 mcg/min	baseline infusion rate
− 1.33 mcg/min	increment of rate decreased
1.67 mcg/min	adjusted infusion rate

IV Practice Problems: Titration of Infusion Rate

1. What are the units of measure for the following terms?
    a. Concentration of solution per minute for specific body weight

    b. Concentration of solution

    c. Volume per hour

    d. Concentration per minute

    e. Volume per minute

    f. Concentration per minute

2. Order: nitroprusside 50 mg in 250 mL D₅W. Titrate 0.5–1.5 mcg/kg/min to maintain mean systolic blood pressure at 100 mm Hg. Client weighs 70 kg.
    Find the following:
    a. Concentration of solution

b. Concentration per minute

_____

c. Volume per minute and hour

_____

d. Titration factor

_____

e. Increase the infusion rate of 11 gtt/min by 5 gtt. What is the concentration per minute? What is the volume per hour?

_____

f. Increase the infusion rate of 16 gtt/mL by 13 gtt. What is the concentration per minute? What is the volume per hour?

_____

3. Order: dopamine 400 mg in 250 mL D_5W. Titrate beginning at 4 mcg/kg/min to maintain a mean systolic blood pressure of 100 to 120 mm Hg. Client weighs 75 kg.

Find the following:

a. Concentration of solution

_____

b. Concentration per minute

_____

c. Volume per minute and hour

_____

d. Titration factor

_____

e. Increase the infusion rate of 113 gtt/min by 7 gtt. What is the concentration per minute? What is the volume per hour?

_____

f. Decrease the infusion rate of 120 mL/hr (120 gtt/min) by 5 gtt. What is the concentration per minute? What is the volume per hour?

_____

TOTAL AMOUNT OF DRUG INFUSED OVER TIME

Determining the total amount of drug infused over time is useful when changes in drug therapy occur. If adverse effects, toxic levels, therapeutic failure, or discontinuance of a drug occurs, knowing the amount that was administered can be important for charting and for determining future therapies.

For this calculation, the concentration of the drug in solution must be known, as must the time that drug therapy began to the nearest minute. Again, with 60-gtt sets, the hourly rate is the same as the drip rate per minute.

example

PROBLEM: Heparin 10,000 U in 250 mL D$_5$W at 30 mL/hr has been infusing for 3 hours. The drug is discontinued.

How much heparin did the client receive?

Find concentration of solution:

Set up a ratio and proportion. Solve for X.	10,000 U : 250 mL : : X U : mL
	250 X = 10,000
	X = 40 U
	40 U/mL

Find concentration per hour:

Multiply concentration of solution by volume/hr.	40 U/mL × 30 mL/hr = 1200 U/hr

Calculate total amount of drug infused:

Multiply concentration/hr by length of administration.	1200 U/hr × 3 hr = 3600 U/hr

Answer: The total amount of heparin infused over 3 hours was 3600 U.

V Practice Problems: Total Amount of Drug Infused Over Time

Solve for the amount of drug infused over time.

1. In 1 hour, a client received two boluses of lidocaine 100 mg and an IV infusion of 4 mg/mL at 40 mL/hr for 30 minutes. How many milligrams have been infused?

   Note: Do not exceed 300 mg/hr of lidocaine.

2. Heparin 20,000 U in 500 mL D$_5$W at 50 mL/hr has been infused for 5½ hours. The drug is discontinued. How much heparin has been given?

ANSWERS

I. Calculating Concentration of a Solution

1. 10,000 U : 250 mL : : X U : mL
   250 X = 10,000
   X = 40 U
   The concentration of solution is 40 U/mL.

2. 250 mg : 500 mL : : X mg : mL
   500 X = 250
   X = 0.5 mg
   The concentration of solution is 0.5 mg/mL.

3. 100 U : 500 mL : : X U : mL
   500 X = 100
   X = 0.2 U
   The concentration of solution is 0.2 U/mL.

4.   1 g = 1000 mg
   1000 mg : 1000 mL : : X mg : mL
        1000 X = 1000
        X = 1 mg
   The concentration of solution is 1 mg/mL.

5.   4 mg = 4000 mcg
   4000 mcg : 500 mL : : X mcg : mL
        500 X = 4000
        X = 8 mcg
   The concentration of solution is 8 mcg/mL.

6. 500 mg : 250 mL : : X mcg : mL
   250 X = 500
   X = 2 mg
   The concentration of solution is 2 mg/mL.

7. 400 mg : 250 mL : : X mg : mL
   250 X = 400
   X = 1.6 mg
   The concentration of solution is 1.6 mg/mL.

8.   2 mg = 2000 mcg
   2000 mcg : 250 mL : : X mcg : mL
        250 X = 2000
        X = 8 mcg
   The concentration of solution is 8 mcg/mL.

9. 750,000 U : 50 mL : : X U : mL
   50 X = 750,000
   X = 15,000 U
   The concentration of solution is 15,000 U/mL.

10.   50 mg = 50,000 mcg
    50,000 mcg : 500 mL : : X mcg : mL
         500 X = 50,000
         X = 100 mcg
    The concentration of solution is 100 mcg/mL.

11.
$$1 \text{ g} = 1000 \text{ mg}$$
$$1000 \text{ mg} : 250 \text{ mL} : : X \text{ mg} : \text{mL}$$
$$250 \text{ X} = 1000$$
$$X = 4 \text{ mg}$$
The concentration of solution is 4 mg/mL.

12.
$$2 \text{ g} = 2000 \text{ mg}$$
$$2000 \text{ mg} : 250 \text{ mL} : : X \text{ mg} : \text{mL}$$
$$250 \text{ X} = 2000$$
$$X = 8 \text{ mg}$$
The concentration of solution is 8 mg/mL.

13. $25,000 \text{ U} : 250 \text{ mL} : : X \text{ mg} : \text{mL}$
$$250 \text{ X} = 25,000$$
$$X = 100 \text{ U}$$
The concentration of solution is 100 U/mL.

14.
$$1 \text{ g} = 1000 \text{ mg}$$
$$1000 \text{ mg} : 500 \text{ mL} : : X \text{ mg} : \text{mL}$$
$$500 \text{ X} = 1000$$
$$X = 2 \text{ mg}$$
The concentration of solution is 2 mg/mL.

15.
$$50 \text{ mg} = 50,000 \text{ mcg}$$
$$50,000 \text{ mcg} : 250 \text{ mL} : : X \text{ mcg} : \text{mL}$$
$$250 \text{ X} = 50,000 \text{ mcg}$$
$$X = 200 \text{ mcg}$$
The concentration of solution is 200 mcg/mL.

16. $100 \text{ mg} : 100 \text{ mL} : : X \text{ mg} : \text{mL}$
$$100 \text{ X} = 100$$
$$X = 1 \text{ mg/mL}$$
The concentration of solution is 1 mg/mL.

17. $800 \text{ mg} : 500 \text{ mL} : : X \text{ mg} : \text{mL}$
$$500 \text{ X} = 800$$
$$X = 1.6 \text{ mg/mL}$$
The concentration of solution is 1.6 mg/mL.

18. $20 \text{ mg} : 100 \text{ mL} : : X \text{ mg} : \text{mL}$
$$100 \text{ X} = 20$$
$$X = .2 \text{ mg/mL}$$
The concentration of solution is 0.2 mg/mL.

19. $1,500,000 \text{ U} : 100 \text{ mL} : : X \text{ mg} : \text{mL}$
$$100 \text{ X} = 1,500,000$$
$$X = 15,000 \text{ U/mL}$$
The concentration of solution is 15,000 U/mL.

20. $150 \text{ mg} : 100 \text{ mL} : : X \text{ mg} : \text{mL}$
$$100 \text{ X} = 150$$
$$= 1.5 \text{ mg/mL}$$
The concentration of solution is 1.5 mg/mL.

II. Calculating Infusion Rate

1. *Concentration of solution:*

$$1000 \text{ U} : 500 \text{ mL} = \text{X U} : \text{mL}$$
$$500 \text{ X} = 1000$$
$$\text{X} = 2 \text{ U}$$

The concentration of solution is 2 U/mL.

Infusion rates:

a. Volume/min:

$$50 \text{ mL} : 60 \text{ min} : : \text{X mL} : \text{min}$$
$$60 \text{ X} = 50$$
$$\text{X} = 0.833 \text{ mL or } 0.83 \text{ mL}$$
$$0.83 \text{ mL/min}$$

b. Volume/hr:

$$50 \text{ mL/hr}$$

c. Concentration/min:

$$2 \text{ U/mL} \times 0.83 \text{ mL/min} = 1.66 \text{ U/min}$$

d. Concentration/hr:

$$1.66 \text{ U/min} \times 60 \text{ min/hr} = 99.6 \text{ U/hr or } 100 \text{ U/hr}$$

2. *Concentration of solution:*

$$100 \text{ mg} : 500 \text{ mL} : : \text{X mg} : \text{mL}$$
$$500 \text{ X} = 100$$
$$\text{X} = 0.2 \text{ mg}$$

The concentration of solution is 0.2 mg/mL.

Infusion rates:

a. Volume/min.

$$60 \text{ mL} : 60 \text{ min} : : \text{X mL} : \text{min}$$
$$60 \text{ X} = 60$$
$$\text{X} = 1 \text{ mL}$$
$$1 \text{ mL/min}$$

b. Volume/hr:

$$60 \text{ mL/hr}$$

c. Concentration/min:

$$0.2 \text{ mg/mL} \times 1 \text{ mL/min} = 0.2 \text{ mg/min}$$

d. Concentration/hr:

$$0.2 \text{ mg/min} \times 60 \text{ min/hr} = 12 \text{ mg/hr}$$

3. *Concentration of solution:*

$$25 \text{ mg} = 25,000 \text{ mcg}$$
$$25,000 \text{ mcg} : 250 \text{ mL} : : \text{X mcg} : \text{mL}$$
$$250 \text{ X} = 25,000$$
$$\text{X} = 100 \text{ mcg}$$

The concentration of solution is 100 mcg/mL.

Infusion rates:

a. Volume/min:

$$\frac{50 \text{ mcg/min}}{100 \text{ mcg/mL}} = 0.5 \text{ mL/min}$$

b. Volume/hr:

$$0.5 \text{ mL/min} \times 60 \text{ min/hr} = 30 \text{ mL/hr}$$

c. Concentration/min:

$$50 \text{ mcg/min}$$

d. Concentration/hr:

$$50 \text{ mcg/min} \times 60 \text{ min/hr} = 3000 \text{ mcg/hr}$$

4. *Concentration of solution:*

$$800 \text{ mg} = 800,000 \text{ mcg}$$
$$800,000 \text{ mcg} : 500 \text{ mL} : : X \text{ mcg} : \text{mL}$$
$$500 X = 800,000$$
$$X = 1600 \text{ mcg}$$

The concentration of solution is 1600 mcg/mL.

Infusion rates:

a. Volume/min:

$$\frac{400 \text{ mcg/min}}{1600 \text{ mcg/mL}} = 0.25 \text{ mL/min}$$

b. Volume/hr:

$$0.25 \text{ mL/min} \times 60 \text{ min/hr} = 15 \text{ mL/hr}$$

c. Concentration/min:

$$400 \text{ mcg/min}$$

d. Concentration/hr:

$$400 \text{ mcg/min} \times 60 \text{ min/hr} = 24,000 \text{ mcg/hr}$$

5. *Concentration of solution:*

$$2 \text{ mg} = 2000 \text{ mcg}$$
$$2000 \text{ mcg} : 250 \text{ mL} : : X \text{ mcg} : \text{mL}$$
$$250 X = 2000$$
$$X = 8 \text{ mcg}$$

The concentration of solution is 8 mcg/mL.

Infusion rates:

a. Volume/min:

$$45 \text{ mL} : 60 \text{ min} : : X \text{ mL} : \text{min}$$
$$60 X = 45$$
$$X = 0.75 \text{ mL/min}$$

b. Volume/hr:

45 mL/hr

c. Concentration/min:

8 mcg/mL $\times$ 0.75 mL/min = 6 mcg/min

d. Concentration/hr:

6 mcg/min $\times$ 60 min/hr = 360 mcg/hr

6. *Concentration of solution:*

1000 mg = 1,000,000 mcg
1,000,000 mcg : 500 mL : : X mcg : mL
500 X = 1,000,000
X = 2000 mcg

The concentration of solution is 2000 mcg/mL.

Infusion rates:

a. Volume/min:

12 mL : 60 min : : X mL : min
60 X = 12
X = 0.2 mL
0.2 mL/min

b. Volume/hr:

12 mL/hr

c. Concentration/min:

2000 mcg/mL $\times$ 0.2 mL/min = 400 mcg/min

d. Concentration/hr:

400 mcg/min $\times$ 60 min/hr = 24,000 mcg/hr

7. *Concentration of solution:*

250 mg = 250,000 mcg
250,000 mcg : 250 mL : : X mcg : mL
250 X = 250,000
X = 1000 mcg

The concentration of solution is 1000 mcg/mL.

Infusion rates:

a. Volume/min:

60 mL : 60 min : : X mL : 1 min
60 X = 10 mL
X = 0.1666 mL or 0.167 mL
0.167 mL/min

b. Volume/hr:

10 mL/hr

c. Concentration/min:

$$1000 \text{ mcg/mL} \times 0.167 \text{ mL/min} = 167 \text{ mcg/min}$$

d. Concentration/hr:

$$167 \text{ mcg/min} \times 60 \text{ min/hr} = 10,020 \text{ mcg/hr or } 10,000 \text{ mcg/hr}$$

8. *Concentration of solution:*

$$2 \text{ g} = 2000 \text{ mg}$$
$$2000 \text{ mg}:500 \text{ mL}::X \text{ mg}:\text{mL}$$
$$500 \text{ X} = 2000$$
$$X = 4 \text{ mg}$$

The concentration of solution is 4 mg/mL.

Infusion rates:

a. Volume/min:

$$\frac{4 \text{ mg/mL}}{4 \text{ mg/min}} = 1 \text{ mL/min}$$

b. Volume/hr:

$$1 \text{ mL/min} \times 60 \text{ min/hr} = 60 \text{ mL/hr}$$

c. Concentration/min:

$$4 \text{ mg/min}$$

d. Concentration/hr:

$$4 \text{ mg/min} \times 60 \text{ min/hr} = 240 \text{ mg/hr}$$

9. *Concentration of solution:*

$$400 \text{ mg}:250 \text{ mL}::X \text{ mg}:\text{mL}$$
$$250 \text{ X} = 400$$
$$X = 1.6 \text{ mg}$$

The concentration of solution is 1.6 mg/mL.

Infusion rates:

a. Volume/min:

$$60 \text{ mL}:60 \text{ min}::X \text{ mL}:\text{min}$$
$$60 \text{ X} = 60$$
$$X = 1 \text{ mL}$$
$$1 \text{ mL/min}$$

b. Volume/hr:

$$60 \text{ mL/hr}$$

c. Concentration/min:

$$1.6 \text{ mg/mL} \times 1 \text{ mL/min} = 1.6 \text{ mg/min}$$

d. Concentration/hr:

$$1.6 \text{ mg/min} \times 60 \text{ min/hr} = 96 \text{ mg/hr}$$

10. *Concentration of solution:*

$$4 \text{ mg} = 4000 \text{ mcg}$$
$$4000 \text{ mcg} : 500 \text{ mL} :: X \text{ mcg} : \text{mL}$$
$$500 \text{ X} = 4000$$
$$X = 8 \text{ mcg}$$

The concentration of solution is 8 mcg/mL.

Infusion rates:

a. Volume/min:

$$65 \text{ mL} : 60 \text{ min} :: X \text{ mL} : \text{min}$$
$$60 \text{ X} = 65$$
$$X = 1.083 \text{ mL}$$
$$1.08 \text{ mL/min}$$

b. Volume/hr:

$$65 \text{ mL/hr}$$

c. Concentration/min:

$$8 \text{ mcg/mL} \times 1.08 \text{ mL/min} = 8.64 \text{ mcg/min}$$

d. Concentration/hr:

$$8.64 \text{ mcg/min} \times 60 \text{ min/hr} = 518.4 \text{ mcg/hr}$$

11. *Concentration of solution:*

$$50 \text{ mg} : 150 \text{ mL} :: X \text{ mg} : \text{mL}$$
$$150 \text{ X} = 50$$
$$X = 0.33 \text{ mg}$$

The concentration of solution is 0.33 mg/mL.

Infusion rates:

a. Concentration/min:

$$3 \text{ mg} : 60 \text{ min} :: X \text{ mg} : \text{min}$$
$$60 \text{ X} = 3$$
$$X = 0.05 \text{ mg/min}$$

b. Concentration/hr:

$$3 \text{ mg/hr}$$

c. Volume/min:

$$\frac{0.05 \text{ mg/min}}{0.33 \text{ mg/mL}} = 0.15 \text{ mL/min}$$

d. Volume/hr:

$$\frac{3 \text{ mg/hr}}{0.33 \text{ mg/mL}} = 9.09 \text{ or } 9 \text{ mL/hr}$$

12. *Concentration of solution:*

$$50 \text{ U} : 250 \text{ mL} :: X \text{ mg} : \text{mL}$$
$$250 \text{ X} = 50$$
$$X = 0.2 \text{ U}$$

The concentration of solution is 0.2 U/mL.

Infusion rates:

a. Concentration/min:

$$4\ U:60\ min::X\ U:min$$
$$60\ X = 4$$
$$X = 0.066\ U/min$$

b. Concentration/hr:

$$4\ U/hr$$

c. Volume/min:

$$\frac{0.66\ U/min}{0.2\ U/mL} = 0.33\ mL/min$$

d. Volume/hr:

$$\frac{4\ U/hr}{0.2\ U/mL} = 20\ mL/hr$$

13. *Concentration of solution:*

$$2\ g = 2000\ mg$$
$$2000\ mg:250\ mL::X\ mg:mL$$
$$250\ X = 2000$$
$$X = 8\ mg$$

The concentration of solution is 8 mg/mL.

Infusion rates:

a. Volume/hr = 20 mL/hr

b. Volume/min:

$$20\ mL:60\ min/hr::X\ mL:min$$
$$60\ X = 20$$
$$X = 0.3\ mL/min$$

c. Concentration/min:

$$8\ mg/mL \times 0.3\ mL/min = 2.4\ mg/min$$

d. Concentration/hr:

$$2.4\ mg/min \times 60\ min/hr = 360\ mg/hr$$

14. *Concentration of solution:*

$$50\ mg = 50{,}000\ mcg$$
$$50{,}000\ mcg:250\ mL::X\ mg:mL$$
$$250\ X = 50{,}000$$
$$X = 200\ mcg$$

The concentration of solution is 200 mcg/mL.

Infusion rates:

a. Volume/hr = 24 mL/hr

b. Volume/min:

$$24 \text{ mL/hr} : 60 \text{ min/hr} :: X \text{ mL} : \text{min}$$
$$60 X = 24$$
$$X = 0.4 \text{ mL/min}$$

c. Concentration/min:

$$200 \text{ mcg/mL} \times 0.4 \text{ mL/min} = 80 \text{ mcg/min}$$

d. Concentration/hr:

$$80 \text{ mcg/min} \times 60 \text{ min} = 4800 \text{ mcg/hr}$$

15. *Concentration of solution:*

$$25,000 \text{ U} : 500 \text{ mL} :: X \text{ U} : \text{mL}$$
$$500 X = 25,000$$
$$X = 50 \text{ U}$$

The concentration of solution is 50 U/mL.

Infusion rates:

a. Volume/hr:

$$10 \text{ mL/hr}$$

b. Volume/min:

$$10 \text{ mL} : 60 \text{ min/hr} :: X \text{ mL} : \text{min}$$
$$60 X = 10$$
$$X = 0.165 \text{ mL/min}$$

c. Concentration/hr:

$$50 \text{ U/mL} \times 10 \text{ mL/hr} = 500 \text{ U/hr}$$

d. Concentration/min:

$$50 \text{ U/mL} \times 0.165 \text{ mL/min} = 8.25 \text{ U/min}$$

16. *Concentration of solution:*

$$900 \text{ mg} : 500 \text{ mL} :: X \text{ mg} : \text{mL}$$
$$500 X = 900$$
$$X = 1.8 \text{ mg/mL}$$

The concentration of solution is 1.8 mg/mL.

Infusion rates:

a. Volume/hr:

$$33.3 \text{ mL/hr}$$

b. Volume/min:

$$33.3 \text{ mL} : 60 \text{ min} :: X \text{ mL} : \text{min}$$
$$60 X = 33.3$$
$$X = 0.55 \text{ mL/min}$$

c. Concentration/hr:

$$1.8 \text{ mg/mL} \times 60 \text{ min/hr} = 108 \text{ mg/hr}$$

d. Concentration/min:

$$1.8 \text{ mg/mL} \times 0.55 \text{ mL/min} = 0.99 \text{ mg/mL}$$

17. *Concentration of solution:*

$$1 \text{ g} = 1000 \text{ mg}$$
$$1000 \text{ mg}:250 \text{ mL}::X \text{ mg}:\text{mL}$$
$$250 \text{ X} = 1000$$
$$X = 4 \text{ mg/mL}$$

The concentration of solution is 4 mg/mL.

Infusion rates:

a. Volume/min:

$$\frac{4 \text{ mg/min}}{4 \text{ mg/mL}} = 1 \text{ mL/min}$$

b. Volume/hr:

$$1 \text{ mL/min} \times 60 \text{ min/hr} = 60 \text{ mL/hr}$$

c. Concentration/hr:

$$4 \text{ mg/min} \times 60 \text{ min/hr} = 240 \text{ mg/hr}$$

d. Concentration/min:

$$4 \text{ mg/min}$$

18. *Concentration of solution:*

$$100 \text{ mg}:100 \text{ mL}::X \text{ mg}:\text{mL}$$
$$100 \text{ X} = 100$$
$$X = 1 \text{ mg/mL}$$

The concentration of solution is 1 mg/mL.

Infusion rates:

a. Volume/hr:

$$\frac{10 \text{ mg/hr}}{1 \text{ mg/mL}} = 10 \text{ mL/hr}$$

b. Volume/min:

$$\frac{10 \text{ mL/hr}}{60 \text{ min/hr}} = 0.166 \text{ mL/min}$$

c. Concentration/hr:

$$10 \text{ mg/hr}$$

d. Concentration/min:

$$1 \text{ mg/mL} \times 0.166 \text{ mL/min} = 0.166 \text{ mg/min}$$

19. *Concentration of solution:*

$$750,000 \text{ U}:250 \text{ mL}::X \text{ U}:\text{mL}$$
$$250 \text{ X} = 750,000$$
$$X = 3000 \text{ U/mL}$$

The concentration of solution is 3000 U/mL.

Infusion rates:

a. Volume/hr:

$$\frac{100,000 \text{ U/hr}}{3000 \text{ U/mL}} = 33.3 \text{ mL/hr}$$

b. Volume/min:

$$\frac{33.3 \text{ mL/hr}}{60 \text{ min/hr}} = 0.55 \text{ mL/min}$$

c. Concentration/hr:

$$100,000 \text{ U/hr}$$

d. Concentration/min:

$$\frac{100,000 \text{ U/hr}}{60 \text{ min/hr}} = 166.6 \text{ U/min}$$

20. *Concentration of solution:*

$$1 \text{ g} = 1000 \text{ mg}$$
$$1000 \text{ mg} : 250 \text{ mL} :: X \text{ mg} : \text{mL}$$
$$250 \text{ X} = 1000$$
$$X = 4 \text{ mg/mL}$$

The concentration of solution is 4 mg/mL.

Infusion rates:

a. Volume/min:

$$\frac{1 \text{ mg/min}}{4 \text{ mg/mL}} = 0.25 \text{ mL/min}$$

b. Volume/hr:

$$0.25 \text{ mL/min} \times 60 \text{ min/hr} = 15 \text{ mL/hr}$$

c. Concentration/hr:

$$4 \text{ mg/mL} \times 15 \text{ mL/hr} = 60 \text{ mg/hr}$$

d. Concentration/min:

$$1 \text{ mg/min}$$

III. Calculating Infusion Rate for Specific Body Weight

1. *Concentration of solution:*

lb to kg

$$500 \text{ mg} = 500,000 \text{ mcg}$$
$$500,000 : 250 \text{ mL} :: X \text{ mcg} : \text{mL}$$
$$250 \text{ X} = 500,000$$
$$X = 2000 \text{ mcg}$$

$$\frac{182}{2.2} = 82.7 \text{ kg}$$

The concentration of solution is 2000 mcg/mL.

Infusion rates:

a. Concentration/min:

$$\text{body weight} \times \text{desired dose/kg/min}$$
$$82.7 \text{ kg} \times 5 \text{ mcg/kg/min}$$
$$= 413.4 \text{ mcg/min}$$

b. Concentration/hr:

$$413.5 \text{ mcg/min} \times 60 \text{ min/hr} = 24,810 \text{ mcg/hr}$$

c. Volume/min:

$$\frac{413.5 \text{ mcg/min}}{2000 \text{ mcg/mL}} = 0.206 \text{ mL/min}$$

d. Volume/hr:

$$0.206 \text{ mL/min} \times 60 \text{ min/hr} = 12.36 \text{ or } 12 \text{ mL/hr}$$

2. *Concentration of solution:*

lb to kg

$$250 \text{ mg} = 250,000 \text{ mcg}$$
$$250,000 \text{ mcg}:250 \text{ mL}::X \text{ mcg}:mL$$
$$250 X = 250,000$$
$$X = 1000 \text{ mcg}$$

$$\frac{165}{2.2} = 75 \text{ kg}$$

The concentration of solution is 1000 mcg/mL.

Infusion rates:

a. Concentration/min:

$$\text{body weight} \times \text{desired dose/kg/min}$$
$$75 \text{ kg} \times 5 \text{ mcg/kg/min} = 375 \text{ mcg/min}$$

b. Concentration/hr:

$$375 \text{ mcg/min} \times 60 \text{ min/hr} = 22,500 \text{ mcg/hr}$$

c. Volume/min:

$$\frac{375 \text{ mcg/min}}{1000 \text{ mcg/mL}} = 0.375 \text{ mL/min}$$

d. Volume/hr:

$$0.375 \text{ mL/min} \times 60 \text{ min/hr} = 22.5 \text{ mL/hr or } 23 \text{ mL/hr}$$

3. *Concentration of solution:*

lb to kg

$$400 \text{ mg} = 400,000 \text{ mcg}$$
$$400,000 \text{ mg}:250 \text{ mL}::X \text{ mg}:mL$$
$$250 X = 400,000$$
$$X = 1600 \text{ mcg}$$

$$\frac{140}{2.2} = 63.6 \text{ kg}$$

The concentration of solution is 1600 mcg/mL.

Infusion rates:

a. Concentration/min:

$$\text{body weight} \times \text{desired dose/kg/min}$$
$$63.6 \text{ kg} \times 10 \text{ mcg/kg/min}$$
$$= 636 \text{ mcg/min}$$

b. Concentration/hr:

$$636 \text{ mcg/min} \times 60 \text{ min/hr} = 38{,}160 \text{ mcg/hr}$$

c. Volume/min:

$$\frac{636 \text{ mcg/min}}{1600 \text{ mcg/mL}} = 0.39 \text{ mL/min}$$

d. Volume/hr:

$$0.39 \text{ mL/min} \times 60 \text{ min/hr} = 23.4 \text{ mL/hr or } 23 \text{ mL/hr}$$

4. *Concentration of solution:*

Patient weight
55 kg

$$100 \text{ mg} = 100{,}000 \text{ mcg}$$
$$100{,}000 \text{ mcg} : 500 \text{ mL} : : X \text{ mg} : \text{mL}$$
$$500 \text{ X} = 100{,}000$$
$$X = 200 \text{ mcg}$$

The concentration of solution is 200 mcg/mL.

Infusion rates:

a. Concentration/min:

$$3 \text{ mcg/kg/min} \times 55 \text{ kg} = 165 \text{ mcg/min}$$

b. Concentration/hr:

$$165 \text{ mcg/min} \times 60 \text{ min/hr} = 9900 \text{ mcg/hr}$$

c. Volume/min:

$$\frac{165 \text{ mcg/min}}{200 \text{ mcg/mL}} = 0.825 \text{ mL/min}$$

d. Volume/hr:

$$0.825 \text{ mL/min} \times 60 \text{ min/hr} = 49.5 \text{ mL/hr or } 50 \text{ mL/hr}$$

5. *Concentration of solution:*

lb to kg

$$1000 \text{ mg} = 1{,}000{,}000 \text{ mcg}$$
$$1{,}000{,}000 \text{ mcg} : 500 \text{ mL} : : X \text{ mcg} : \text{mL}$$
$$\frac{110}{2.2} = 50 \text{ kg}$$
$$500 \text{ X} = 1{,}000{,}000$$
$$X = 2000 \text{ mcg}$$

The concentration of solution is 2000 mcg/mL.

Infusion rates:

a. Concentration/min:

$$\text{body weight} \times \text{desired dose/kg/min}$$
$$50 \text{ kg} \times 15 \text{ mcg/kg/min}$$
$$= 750 \text{ mcg/min}$$

b. Concentration/hr:

$$750 \text{ mcg/min} \times 60 \text{ min/hr} = 45,000 \text{ mcg/hr}$$

c. Volume/min:

$$\frac{750 \text{ mcg/min}}{2000 \text{ mcg/mL}} = 0.375 \text{ mL/min}$$

d. Volume/hr:

$$0.375 \text{ mL/min} \times 60 \text{ min/hr} = 22.5 \text{ mL/hr or } 23 \text{ mL/hr}$$

6. *Concentration of solution:*

lb to kg

$$500 \text{ mg} : 50 \text{ mL} : : X \text{ mg} : \text{mL} \qquad \frac{187}{2.2} = 85 \text{ kg}$$
$$50 X = 500$$
$$X = 10 \text{ mg/mL}$$

The concentration of solution is 10 mg/mL or 10,000 mcg/mL.

Infusion rates:

a. Concentration/min:

$$\text{body weight} \times \text{desired dose/kg/min}$$
$$85 \text{ kg} \times 10 \text{ mcg/kg/min}$$
$$= 850 \text{ mcg/min}$$

b. Concentration/hr:

$$850 \text{ mcg/min} \times 60 \text{ min/hr} = 51,000 \text{ mcg/hr or } 51 \text{ mg/hr}$$

c. Volume/min:

$$\frac{850 \text{ mcg/min}}{10,000 \text{ mcg/mL}} = 0.085 \text{ mL/min}$$

d. Volume/hr:

$$0.085 \text{ mL/min} \times 60 \text{ min/hr} = 5.1 \text{ mL/hr}$$

7. *Concentration of solution:*

lb to kg

$$10,000 \text{ mcg} : 250 \text{ mL} : : X \text{ mcg} : \text{mL} \qquad \frac{175}{2.2} = 79.5 \text{ kg}$$
$$250 X = 10,000$$
$$X = 40 \text{ mcg/mL}$$

Infusion rates:

a. Concentration/min:

$$\text{body weight} \times \text{desired dose/kg/min}$$
$$79.5 \text{ kg} \times 0.5 \text{ mcg/kg/min}$$
$$= 39.75 \text{ mcg/min}$$

b. Concentration/hr:

$$39.75 \text{ mcg/min} \times 60 \text{ min/hr} = 2385 \text{ mcg/hr or 2.4 mg/hr}$$

c. Volume/min:

$$\frac{39.75 \text{ mcg/min}}{40 \text{ mcg/mL}} = 0.99 \text{ mL/min or 1 mL/min}$$

d. Volume/hr:

$$0.99 \text{ mL/min} \times 60 \text{ min/hr} = 59.6 \text{ mL/hr}$$

8. *Concentration of solution:*

lb to kg

$$20 \text{ mg} : 100 \text{ mL} : : X \text{ mg} : \text{mL} \qquad \frac{160}{2.2} = 72.70 \text{ kg}$$
$$100 \text{ X} = 20$$
$$X = 0.2 \text{ mg/mL}$$
$$\text{or } 200 \text{ mcg/mL}$$

Infusion rates:

a. Concentration/min:

body weight × desired dose/kg/min
72.7 kg × 0.375 mcg/kg/min
= 27.2 mcg/min

b. Concentration/hr:

$$27.2 \text{ mcg/min} \times 60 \text{ min/hr} = 1635 \text{ mcg/hr or 1.6 mg/hr}$$

c. Volume/min:

$$\frac{27.2 \text{ mcg/min}}{200 \text{ mcg/mL}} = 0.136 \text{ mL/min}$$

d. Volume/hr:

$$0.136 \text{ mL/min} \times 60 \text{ min/hr} = 8.16 \text{ mL/hr}$$

9. *Concentration of solution:*

Client weight

$$400 \text{ mg} : 500 \text{ mL} : : X \text{ mg} : \text{mL} \qquad 70 \text{ kg}$$
$$500 \text{ X} = 400$$
$$X = 0.8 \text{ mg/mL}$$

Infusion rates:

a. Concentration/hr:

body weight × desired dose/kg/min
70 kg × 0.55 mg/kg/min
= 38.5 mg/hr

b. Volume/hr:

$$\frac{38.5 \text{ mg/hr}}{0.8 \text{ mg/mL}} = 48.125 \text{ mL/hr}$$

10. *Concentration of solution:*

lb to kg

2500 mg : 250 mL : : X mg : mL $\dfrac{148}{2.2} = 67.2$ kg

250 X = 2500

X = 10 mg/mL

Infusion rates:

a. Concentration/min:

body weight × desired dose/kg/min

67.2 × 150 mcg/kg/min

= 10,080 mcg/min or 10 mg/min

b. Concentration/hr:

10 mg/min × 60 min/hr = 600 mg/hr

c. Volume/min:

$$\frac{10 \text{ mg/min}}{10 \text{ mg/mL}} = 1 \text{ mL/min}$$

d. Volume/hr:

1 mL/min × 60 min/hr = 60 mL

IV. Titration of Infusion Rate

1. a. (U, mg, mcg)/kg/min

   b. (U, mg, mcg)/mL

   c. mL/hr

   d. (U, mg, mcg)/min

   e. mL/min

   f. (U, mg, mcg)/min

2. a. Concentration of solution:

50 mg = 50,000 mcg

50,000 mcg : 250 mL : : X mcg : 1 mL

250 X = 50,000

X = 200 mcg

The concentration of solution is 200 mcg/mL

b. Concentration/min:

Lower: 0.5 mcg/kg/min × 70 kg = 35 mcg/min

Upper: 1.5 mcg/kg/min × 70 kg = 105 mcg/min

c. Volume/min and volume/hr:

Lower

$$\frac{35 \text{ mcg/min}}{200 \text{ mcg/mL}} = 0.175 \text{ mL/min} \times 60 \text{ min/hr} = 10.5 \text{ or } 11 \text{ mL/hr}$$

Upper

$$\frac{105 \text{ mcg/min}}{200 \text{ mcg/mL}} = 0.525 \text{ mL/min} \times 60 \text{ min/hr} = 31.5 \text{ or } 32 \text{ mL/hr}$$

d. Titration factor:

$$11 \text{ mL/hr} = 11 \text{ gtt/min} \frac{35 \text{ mcg/min}}{11 \text{ gtt/min}} = 3.18 \text{ or } 3 \text{ mcg/gtt}$$

e. Concentration/min and volume/hr:

$$5 \text{ gtt} \times 3 \text{ mcg/gtt} = 15 \text{ mcg}$$
$$15 \text{ mcg} + 35 \text{ mcg/min} = 50 \text{ mcg/min}$$
$$5 \text{ gtt} + 11 \text{ gtt/min} = 16 \text{ gtt/min or } 16 \text{ mL/hr}$$

f. Concentration/min and volume/hr:

$$13 \text{ gtt} \times 3 \text{ mcg/gtt} = 39 \text{ mcg}$$
$$39 \text{ mcg} + 50 \text{ mcg} = 89 \text{ mcg/min}$$
$$13 \text{ gtt} + 16 \text{ gtt} = 29 \text{ gtt/mL or } 29 \text{ mL/hr}$$

3. a. Concentration of solution:

$$400 \text{ mg} = 40,000 \text{ mcg}$$
$$40,000 \text{ mcg} : 250 \text{ mL} : : X \text{ mcg} : 1 \text{ mL}$$
$$250 \text{ X} = 40,000 \text{ mcg}$$
$$X = 160 \text{ mcg}$$

The concentration of solution is 160 mcg/mL.

b. Concentration/min:

$$4 \text{ mcg/kg/min} \times 75 \text{ kg} = 300 \text{ mcg/min}$$

c. Volume/min and volume/hr:

$$\frac{300 \text{ mcg/min}}{160 \text{ mcg/mL}} = 1.875 \text{ mL/min} \times 60 \text{ min/hr} = 112.5 \text{ or } 113 \text{ mL/hr}$$

d. Titration factor:

$$113 \text{ mL/hr} = 113 \text{ gtt/min}$$

$$\frac{300 \text{ mcg/min}}{113 \text{ gtt/min}} = 2.65 \text{ or } 3 \text{ mcg/gtt}$$

e. Concentration/min and volume/hr:

$$7 \text{ gtt} \times 3 \text{ mcg/gtt} = 21 \text{ mcg}$$
$$21 \text{ mcg} + 300 \text{ mcg/min} = 321 \text{ mcg/min}$$
$$7 \text{ gtt} + 113 \text{ gtt/min} = 120 \text{ gtt/min or } 120 \text{ mL/hr}$$

f. Concentration/min and volume/h:

$$5 \text{ gtt} \times 3 \text{ mcg/gtt} = 15 \text{ mcg}$$
$$321 \text{ mcg/min} - 15 \text{ mcg} = 306 \text{ mcg/min}$$
$$120 \text{ gtt/min} - 5 \text{ gtt} = 115 \text{ gtt/min or } 115 \text{ mL/hr}$$

V. Total Amount of Drug Infused Over Time

1. Lidocaine bolus:

$$\begin{array}{r} 100 \text{ mg} \\ + 100 \text{ mg} \\ \hline 200 \text{ mg} \end{array}$$

Lidocaine IV infusion:

a. Concentration of solution: given as 4 mg/mL in problem.

b. Concentration/hr:

$$4 \text{ mg/mL} \times 40 \text{ mL/hr} = 160 \text{ mg/hr}$$

c. Concentration over ½ hr:

$$160 \text{ mg/hr} \times \frac{30 \text{ min}}{60 \text{ min/hr}} = 80 \text{ mg over 30 min}$$

d. Amount of IV drug infused:

Lidocaine per two boluses: 200 mg
Lidocaine per IV infusion: + 80 mg
                           280 mg total amount infused over 1 hr

Note: The infusion rate is close to exceeding the maximum therapeutic range, which is 200–300 mg/hr.

2. Concentration of solution:

$$20,000 \text{ U} : 500 \text{ mL} :: X \text{ U} : 1 \text{ mL}$$
$$500 \text{ X} = 20,000$$
$$X = 40 \text{ U}$$

a. The concentration of solution is 40 U/mL.

b. Concentration/hr:

$$40 \text{ U/mL} \times 50 \text{ mL/hr} = 2000 \text{ U/hr}$$

c. Amount of IV drug infused over 5½ hours:

$$2000 \text{ U} \times \frac{30 \text{ min}}{60 \text{ min/hr}} = 1000 \text{ U over ½ hr}$$

$$200 \text{ U} \times 5 \text{ hr} = 10,000 \text{ U/5 hr}$$

       10,000 U
+ 1,000 U
       11,000 U over 5½ hr

pediatric critical care

objectives

- Recognize factors that contribute to errors in drug and fluid administration.
- Identify the steps in calculating dilution parameters.
- Determine the accuracy of the dilution parameters in a drug order.

outline

In delivery of emergency drugs with complex dilution calculations, it is important for the nurse to evaluate the accuracy of the physician's order and to ensure that a child does not receive excessive fluids. Many institutions are attempting to standardize the concentration of the solution for various pediatric intravenous dosages to decrease the occurrence of miscalculations.

As noted in Chapter 10, the concepts of concentration of the solution, infusion rates for concentration and volume, and concentration of a drug for specific body weight per unit time are employed in adult critical care also used to prepare pediatric doses.

FACTORS INFLUENCING INTRAVENOUS ADMINISTRATION

Excess fluid can be given when the fluid volume of the emergency drug is not considered in the 24-hour fluid intake. Long intravenous (IV) tubing can be another source of fluid excess and can cause errors in drug delivery. When the priming or filling volume of the IV tubing is not considered, the child may receive extra fluid, especially if medication is added to the primary IV set via a secondary IV set. IV medication may not reach the child if the IV infusion rate is low, such as 1 mL/hr, or if the IV tubing has not been primed or filled with the medication prior to infusion. most pediatric departments are developing protocols for safe and consistent IV drug delivery.

CALCULATING ACCURACY OF DILUTION PARAMETERS

The nurse may find it necessary to calculate the dilution parameters of a drug order that specifies the concentration/kg/min and the volume/hr infusion rate. The physician should determine all drug dose parameters, including concentration/kg/min, volume/hr, and dilution parameters. The nurse should check the accuracy of the dilution parameters to ensure that the correct drug dosage is given. These methods are also used to prepare the pediatric dose. In many pediatric critical care areas, intravenous fluids for drug administration are limited to prevent fluid overload. If the physician changes the drug dosage, rather than increasing the volume (mL), the concentration of the solution will be changed.

....

examples

PROBLEM 1: A 6-day-old infant, weight 3.5 kg, is in septic shock.
Order: dopamine 5 mcg/kg/min at 1 mL/hr and dilute as follows: 100 mg in 100 mL D$_5$½ NSS.
Dosage: 2–5 mcg/kg/min.
Drug available: dopamine 40 mg/mL.

The following steps are needed to determine whether dilution orders will give the correct concentration of solution to deliver 5 mcg/kg/min at 1 mL/hr:

Step 1: Determine infusion rates for concentration per unit time.

1. Find the concentration per minute.

$$\text{infant weight} \times \text{concentration/kg/min} =$$
$$3.5 \text{ kg} \quad \times \quad 5 \text{ mcg/kg/min} \quad = 17.5 \text{ mcg/min}$$

2. Calculate the concentration per hour.

$$17.5 \text{ mcg/min} \times 60 \text{ min/hr} = 1050 \text{ mcg/hr}$$

Step 2: Determine concentration of solution.
Divide the concentration per hr by volume per hr.

$$\frac{1050 \text{ mcg/hr}}{1 \text{ mL/hr}} = 1050 \text{ mcg/mL} \quad \text{or} \quad 1 \text{ mg/mL}$$

Step 3: Determine the accuracy of the dilution order.
Find how much dopamine must be added to 100 mL
Set up a ratio and proportion.

$$1 \text{ mg} : 1 \text{ mL} :: X : 100 \text{ mL}$$
$$X = 100 \text{ mg}$$

Dilution order is correct.

Preparation of Drug Dosage

$$\frac{D}{H} \times V = \frac{100}{40} \times 1 = 2.5 \text{ mL} \quad \textbf{or}$$

$$H \quad : \quad V \quad :: \quad D \quad : \quad V$$
$$40 \text{ mg} : 1 \text{ mL} :: 100 \text{ mg} : X \text{ mL}$$
$$40 X = 100$$
$$X = 2.5 \text{ mL}$$

Answer: Add 2.5 mL of dopamine 40 mg/mL to 100 mL D$_5$½ NSS.

PROBLEM 2: A 3-week-old infant, weight 1.6 kg, is in septic shock.
Order: dobutamine 2.5 mcg/kg/min by a syringe pump with a 35-mL syringe at 1 mL/hr.
Dilution: dobutamine 8.4 mg with D$_5$¼ NSS to equal 35 mL.
Dosage: 2.5−40 mcg/kg/min.
Drug available: dobutamine 250 mg/20 mL.
Determine accuracy of dilution order to deliver 2.5 mcg/kg/min at 1 mL/hr.

Step 1: Find the infusion rates for concentration per unit time.

1. Determine the concentration per minute.

$$\text{Infant weight} \times \text{concentration/kg/min} =$$
$$1.6 \text{ kg} \quad \times \quad 2.5 \text{ mcg/kg/min} \quad = 4 \text{ mcg/min}$$

2. Determine the concentration per hour.

$$4 \text{ mcg/min} \times 60 \text{ min/hr} = 240 \text{ mcg/hr}$$

Step 2: Determine the concentration of solution.

Divide the concentration per hr by volume per hr.

$$\frac{240 \text{ mcg/hr}}{1 \text{ mL/hr}} = 240 \text{ mcg/mL}$$

Step 3: Determine the accuracy of the dilution order.
Find how much dobutamine must be added to make 35 mL.

$$240 \text{ mcg} : 1 \text{ mL} \; : : \; X \text{ mcg} : 35 \text{ mL}$$
$$X = 8400 \text{ mcg or } 8.4 \text{ mg}$$

Dilution order is correct.

Preparation of Drug Dosage

$$\frac{D}{H} \times V = \frac{8.4 \text{ mg}}{250 \text{ mg}} \times 20 \text{ mL} = 0.672 \text{ mL}$$

or

$$\begin{array}{cccc} \text{H} & : \text{V} & \text{D} & : \text{V} \\ 250 \text{ mg} : 20 \text{ mL} & : : & 8.4 \text{ mg} : X \text{ mL} \end{array}$$
$$250 \text{ X} = 168$$
$$X = 0.67 \text{ mL}$$

Answer: Add 0.67 mL of dobutamine 250 mg/20 mL to 34.33 mL $D_5\frac{1}{4}$ NSS.

PROBLEM 3: For the same infant, the physician increases the dose of dobutamine. Again, fluids must be limited, and another concentration must be prepared.
Order: 15 mcg/kg/min by a syringe pump. Dilute 40.5 mg in 35 mL $D_5\frac{1}{4}$ NSS and administer 1 mL/hr.
Determine the accuracy of dilution order to deliver 15 mcg/kg/min at 1 mL/hr.

Step 1: Determine the infusion rates for concentration per unit time.

1. Find the concentration per minute.

$$\begin{array}{ccc} \text{infant weight} & \times & \text{concentration/kg/min} = \\ 1.6 \text{ kg} & \times & 15 \text{ mcg/kg/min} & = 24 \text{ mcg/min} \end{array}$$

2. Find the concentration per hour.

$$24 \text{ mcg/min} \times 60 \text{ min/hr} = 1440 \text{ mcg/hr}$$

Step 2: Calculate the concentration of solution.
Divide the concentration per hr by volume per hr.

$$\frac{1440 \text{ mcg/hr}}{1 \text{ mL/hr}} = 1440 \text{ mcg/mL}$$

Step 3: Determine the accuracy of the dilution order.

$$1440 \text{ mcg} : 1 \text{ mL} \; : : \; X \text{ mcg} : 35 \text{ mL}$$
$$X = 50,400 \text{ mcg}$$

$$50,400 \text{ mcg} = 50.4 \text{ mg} \quad \text{or} \quad 50 \text{ mg}$$

Answer: The dilution order is *incorrect:* 50 mg of dobutamine is needed to deliver 15 mcg/kg/min.

Summary Practice Problems

Determine whether dilution orders will yield the correct concentration of solution.

1. A 2-year-old child with acute status asthmaticus.
   Child weighs 10.5 kg.
   Order: aminophylline 110 mg in 500 mL of D_5W at 40 mL/hr.
   Pediatric dose: 0.85 mg/kg/hr.
   Drug available: aminophylline 250 mg/10 mL.

2. A 9-year-old child with supraventricular tachycardia.
   Child weighs 30 kg.
   Order: lidocaine 20 mcg/kg/min.
   Dilute: 300 mg in 250 mL of D_5W at 30 mL/hr.
   Pediatric dose: 20–40 mcg/kg/min.
   Drug available: lidocaine 1 g/25 mL.

3. A 1-year-old child with septic shock.
   Child weighs 9 kg.
   Order: dopamine 5 mcg/kg/min.
   Dilute: 100 mg in 200 mL of D_5¼ NSS at 6.75 mL/hr.
   Pediatric dose: 2–5 mcg/kg/min.
   Drug available: dopamine 400 mg/5 mL.

4. A 3-year-old child in shock.
   Child weighs 16 kg.
   Order: sodium nitroprusside 2 mcg/kg/min.
   Dilute: 25.25 mg in 250 mL of D_5W at 19 mL/hr.
   Pediatric dose: 200–500 mcg/kg/hr.
   Drug available: sodium nitroprusside 50 mg/5 mL.

5. A 10-year-old child with diabetic ketoacidosis.
   Child weighs 32 kg.
   Order: regular Humulin insulin 50 U in 500 mL of normal saline at 32 mL/hr.
   Pediatric dose: 0.1 U/kg/hr.
   Drug available: 100 U/mL.

6. A 2-day-old infant with patent ductus arteriosus.
   Child weighs 3.4 kg.
   Order: alprostadil 0.1 mcg/kg/min.
   Dilute: 1000 mcg in 50 mL D_5W by syringe pump at 1 mL/hr.
   Pediatric dosage: 0.05–0.1 mcg/kg/min.
   Drug available: alprostadil 500 mcg/mL.

7. A 7-year-old child with pulmonary embolism.
   Child weighs 20 kg.
   Order: Heparin 25 U/kg/hr.
   Dilute: 10,000 U heparin in 50 mL D_5W at 5 mL/hr.
   Pediatric dosage: 25–50 U/kg.
   Drug available: Heparin 10,000 U/mL.

ANSWERS

1. *Step 1:* Infusion rates for concentration.
Concentration per hour.

$$10.5 \text{ kg} \times 0.85 \text{ mg/kg/hr} = 8.9 \text{ mg/hr}$$

Step 2: Concentration of solution.

$$\frac{8.9 \text{ mg/hr}}{40 \text{ mL/hr}} = 0.22 \text{ mg/mL}$$

Step 3: Accuracy of dilution order.

$$\text{mg} : \text{mL} :: \text{mg} : \text{mL}$$
$$0.22 : 1 :: \text{X} : 500$$
$$\text{X} = 110 \text{ mg}$$

Dilution order is correct.

Preparation of drug dosage:

$$\frac{D}{H} \times V = \frac{110}{250} \times 10 = \frac{1100}{250} = 4.4 \text{ mL}$$

or

$$250 \text{ mg} : 10 \text{ mL} :: 110 \text{ mg} \quad \text{X mL}$$
$$250 \text{ X} = 1100$$
$$\text{X} = 4.4 \text{ mL}$$

2. *Step 1:* Infusion rates for concentration/unit time.
a. Concentration per minute.

$$30 \text{ kg} \times 20 \text{ mcg/kg/min} = 600 \text{ mcg/min}$$

b. Concentration per hour.

$$600 \text{ mcg/min} \times 60 \text{ min/hr} = 36,000 \text{ mcg/hr}$$

Step 2: Concentration of solution.

$$\frac{36,000 \text{ mcg/hr}}{30 \text{ mL/hr}} = 1200 \text{ mcg/mL} \quad \text{or} \quad 1.2 \text{ mg/mL}$$

Step 3: Accuracy of dilution order.

$$1.2 \text{ mg} : 1 \text{ mL} :: \text{X mg} : 250 \text{ mL}$$
$$\text{X} = 300 \text{ mg}$$

Dilution order is correct.

Preparation of drug dosage:

$$\frac{D}{H} \times V = \frac{300}{1000} \times 25 = \frac{7500}{1000} = 7.5 \text{ mL}$$

or

$$1000 \text{ mg} : 25 \text{ mL} :: 300 \text{ mg} : \text{X mL}$$
$$1000 \text{ X} = 7500$$
$$\text{X} = 7.5 \text{ mL}$$

Answer: 7.5 mL of lidocaine added to 250 mL.

3. *Step 1:* Infusion rate for concentration.

   a. Concentration per minute.

$$9 \text{ kg} \times 5 \text{ mcg/kg/min} = 45 \text{ mcg/min}$$

   b. Concentration per hour.

$$45 \text{ mcg/min} \times 60 \text{ min/hr} = 2700 \text{ mcg/hr}$$

Step 2: Concentration of solution.

$$\frac{2700 \text{ mcg/hr}}{6.75 \text{ mL/hr}} = 400 \text{ mcg/mL}$$

Step 3: Accuracy of dilution order.

$$400 \text{ mcg} : 1 \text{ mL} :: \text{X mcg} : 200 \text{ mL}$$
$$\text{X} = 80,000 \text{ mcg} \quad \text{or} \quad 80 \text{ mg in } 200 \text{ mL}$$

Dilution order is incorrect.

4. *Step 1:* Infusion rates for concentration.

   a. Concentration per minute.

$$16 \text{ kg} \times 2 \text{ mcg/kg/min} = 32 \text{ mcg/min}$$

   b. Concentration per hour.

$$32 \text{ mcg/min} \times 60 \text{ min/hr} = 1920 \text{ mcg/hr}$$

Step 2: Concentration of solution.

$$\frac{1920 \text{ mcg/hr}}{19 \text{ mL/hr}} = 101 \text{ mcg/mL}$$

Step 3: Accuracy of order.

$$101 \text{ mcg} : 1 \text{ mL} :: \text{X mcg} : 250 \text{ mL}$$
$$\text{X} = 25,250 \text{ mcg} \quad \text{or} \quad 25.25 \text{ mg}$$

Dilution order is correct.

Preparation of drug dosage:

$$\frac{D}{H} \times V = \frac{25.25}{50} \times 5 = 2.52 \text{ mL}$$

or

$$50 \text{ mg} : 5 \text{ mL} :: 25.25 \text{ mg} : \text{X mL}$$
$$50 \text{ X} = 126.25$$
$$\text{X} = 2.52 \text{ mL}$$

Answer: 2.52 mL of sodium nitropruside added to 250 mL.

5. *Step 1:* Infusion rate for concentration.

   Concentration per hour.

$$32 \text{ kg} \times 0.1 \text{ U/kg/hr} = 3.2 \text{ U/hr}$$

Step 2: Concentration of solution.

$$\frac{3.2 \text{ U/hr}}{32 \text{ mL/hr}} = 0.10 \text{ U/mL}$$

Step 3: Accuracy of dilution order.

$$0.1 \text{ U} : 1 \text{ mL} :: X \text{ U} : 500 \text{ mL}$$
$$X = 50 \text{ U}$$

Dilution order is correct.

Preparation of drug dose:

$$\frac{D}{H} \times V = \frac{50 \text{ U}}{100 \text{ U}} \times 1 = 0.5 \text{ mL}$$

Answer: 50 U/0.5 mL—use a U 100 insulin syringe.

6. *Step 1:* Infusion rates for concentration.
   a. Concentration per minute.

$$3.4 \text{ kg} \times 0.1 \text{ mcg/kg/min} = 0.34 \text{ mcg/min}$$

   b. Concentration per hour.

$$0.34 \text{ mcg/min} \times 60 \text{ min/hr} = 20.4 \text{ mcg/hr}$$

Step 2: Concentration of solution.

$$\frac{20.4 \text{ mcg/hr}}{1 \text{ mL/hr}} = 20.4 \text{ mcg/mL} \quad \text{or} \quad 20 \text{ mcg/mL}$$

Step 3: Accuracy of dilution order.

$$20 \text{ mcg} : 1 \text{ ml} :: X \text{ mcg} : 50 \text{ mL}$$
$$X = 1000 \text{ mcg}$$

Dilution order is correct.

7. *Step 1:* Infusion rates for concentration.
   Concentration per hour.

$$20 \text{ kg} \times 25 \text{ U/kg/hr} = 500 \text{ U/hr}$$

Step 2: Concentration of solution.

$$\frac{500 \text{ U/hr}}{5 \text{ mL/hr}} = 100 \text{ U/mL}$$

Step 3: Determine the accuracy of dilution order.

$$100 \text{ U} : 1 \text{ mL} :: X \text{ U} : 5 \text{ mL}$$
$$1X = 500$$
$$X = 500 \text{ U}$$

Accuracy of dilution order.

$$500 \text{ U} : \text{mL} :: X : 50 \text{ mL}$$
$$X = 25,000 \text{ U/mL}$$

Answer: The dilution order is incorrect. Heparin 10,000 U/mL must be diluted in 100 mL D_5W to deliver 25 U/kg/min.

labor and delivery

objectives

- State the complication related to IV fluid administration in the high-risk mother.
- Recognize the different types of fluid administration used in high-risk labors.
- Determine the infusion rates of a drug in solution when the drug is prescribed by concentration or volume.

outline

Drug calculations for labor and delivery are the same as those used in critical care. Determinations of the concentration of the solution, infusion rates, and titration factors are the primary calculation skills used. Accurate calculations are essential, as is the monitoring of intravenous (IV) fluid intake for medications and anesthetic procedures. Impaired renal filtration in preeclampsia and the antidiuretic effect of tocolytic drugs make the monitoring of fluid intake vital. Accurate measurement of IV fluid intake along with pulmonary assessment can decrease the risk of fluid overload and the sequelae of acute pulmonary edema in the high-risk mother.

Physicians' orders and hospital protocols give specific guidelines for administering IV drugs. The nurse is responsible for managing the IV drug therapy, monitoring the patient's fluid balance, and assessing the client's response to drug therapy.

FACTORS INFLUENCING INTRAVENOUS FLUID AND DRUG MANAGEMENT

The most important concept in labor and delivery is that the drugs given to the mother also affect the unborn baby. Therefore, the response of the patient and the unborn baby must be closely monitored. Vital signs, urine output, reflexes, and contraction patterns are the main indicators of the mother's status. For the fetus, fetal heart rate is the primary guide.

TITRATION OF MEDICATIONS WITH MAINTENANCE INTRAVENOUS FLUIDS

Women in labor receive IV fluids to prevent dehydration when oral intake is contraindicated. IV drugs are given to stimulate labor, treat preeclampsia, or inhibit preterm labor. Normally, the IV fluids, 200 to 500 mL, may be given to initially hydrate the mother, especially in preterm labor or prior to conductive anesthesia. Any IV medications that are given by titration are a part of the hourly IV rate. The client has a primary IV line and a secondary IV line for medications. All IV medications should be delivered by a volumetric pump, which ensures that the specified volume and correct dosage are delivered.

Titration of drugs is frequency done for high-risk mothers with preeclampsia and mothers experiencing preterm labor. The most common use of titration is in the induction or stimulation of labor. In the following example, an oxytocic drug is given, and the primary IV rate is adjusted with the secondary IV drug line to achieve a therapeutic effect and maintain adequate maternal hydration. Note that the drug is ordered to be given by concentration and that the infusion rates for volume per minute and hour must be determined.

Administration by Concentration

. . . .

example

1. Give IV fluids at 100 mL/hr with D_5 ½ NSS.

2. Mix 10 U of oxytocin in 1000 NSS. Start at 5 mU/min, increase by 1 or 2 mU/min, q10min, until uterine contractions are 2 to 3 minutes apart. Do not exceed 40 mU/min.

Note: 1 Unit (U) = 1000 milliunits (mU)

Available: Secondary set:
                oxytocin 10 U/mL
                1000 mL NSS
                microdrop IV set 60 gtt/mL
                infusion pump
            Primary set:
                1000 mL D_5 ½ NSS
                IV set drop factor 60 gtt/mL

For the *secondary* set IV, the following calculations must be made:

1. Concentration of solution.

2. Infusion rates: volume per minute and volume per hour.

3. Titration factor in concentration per minute (mU/min).

For the *primary* IV, the following calculations must be made:

1. Drop rate per minute. If a pump is used, set rate at mL/hr.

2. Balance primary IV flow with secondary IV rate to achieve 100 mL/hr.

Secondary IV (see Chapter 6 for formulas)

1. Concentration of solution:

$$10\ U:100\ mL\ ::\ X:1\ mL$$
$$1000\ X = 10$$
$$X = 0.01\ U\ or\ 10\ mU$$

The concentration of solution is 10 mU/mL.

2. Infusion rates for volume:

$$\frac{concentration/minute}{concentration\ of\ solution} = volume/min \times 60\ minutes = volume/hr$$

Volume per minute   *Volume per hour*

$$\frac{1\ mU/min}{10\ mU/mL} = 0.1\ mL/min \times 60\ minutes = 6\ mL/hr$$

$$\frac{2\ mU/min}{10\ mU/mL} = 0.2\ mL/min \times 60\ minutes = 12\ mL/hr$$

$$\frac{5\ mU/min}{10\ mU/mL} = 0.5\ mL/min \times 60\ minutes = 30\ mL/hr$$

3. Titration factor (see Chapter 8): to increase the concentration by increments of 1 mU/min, the hourly rate on the pump must be increased by 6 mL/hr. The titration factor for this problem is 6 mL/hr. To increase the concentration to a higher rate, multiply the rate of increase times 6 mL/hr. (Example: to increase infusion to 5 mU/min, multiply 5 by 6 mL = 30 mL/hr.)

For the secondary IV line, the concentration of the solution is 10 mU/mL of oxytocin, with the infusion rate of 30 mL/hr to be increased in increments of 6 to 12 mL every 10 minutes until contractions are 2 to 3 minutes apart.

Primary IV

The secondary IV rate will start at 30 mL/hr; therefore, the primary rate will be 70 mL/hr. (A balance is needed to achieve 100 mL/hr.)
    Drop rate using a 60 gtt/mL set will be the mL/hr rate on a pump.

$$\frac{70\ \text{mL/hr} \times 60\ \text{gtt/mL}}{60\ \text{minutes}} = 70\ \text{gtt/min}$$

For every increase in rate from the secondary line, a corresponding decrease must be made with the primary IV line. If the rate of the secondary line exceeds the ordered hourly rate, the primary IV may be shut off completely. The concentration of the solution may be changed by the physician if the mother is receiving too much fluid.

Administration by Volume

In the previous example, the oxytocin was ordered to infuse by concentration (mU/min), which is the recommended method for patient safety. Sometimes in clinical practice, the infusion rate may be ordered by volume (mL/hr).

· ·

example

Mix 10 U of oxytocin in 1000 mL NSS. Start at 30 mL/hr and increase by 6 to 12 mL q10min until uterine contractions are 2 to 3 minutes apart. Do not exceed 40 mU/min.
    To determine the concentration per hour of infusion, multiply concentration of the solution by volume/hr = concentration/hr:

$$10\ \text{mU/mL} \times 30\ \text{mL/hr} = 300\ \text{mU/hr}$$

To determine the concentration of the infusion per minute, divide:

$$\frac{\text{concentration/hr}}{60\ \text{min/hr}} = \text{concentration/min}$$

$$\frac{300\ \text{mU/hr}}{60\ \text{min/hr}} = 5\ \text{mU/min}$$

Therefore, an oxytocin solution with a concentration of 10 mU/mL infused at 30 mL/hr will administer 5 mU/min of the drug.

INTRAVENOUS LOADING DOSE

Some situations require intravenous medications to be infused over a short period to obtain a serum level for a therapeutic effect. This type of IV drug administration is called a *loading dose.*

In the following example, a patient with preeclampsia receives a loading dose of magnesium sulfate, followed by a maintenance dose of magnesium sulfate via the secondary IV line. A primary IV line is also maintained after the loading dose is given. At the end of this example, the total IV intake is determined for an 8-hour period.

example

1. Mix magnesium sulfate 20 g in 1000 mL of D_5W.

2. Infuse 4 g over 20 minutes, then maintain at 1 g/hr.

3. Start D_5 LRS at 75 mL/hr after magnesium sulfate loading dose.

Available: Secondary set:
magnesium sulfate 50% (5 g in 10-mL ampules)
1000 mL D_5W
microdrip IV set 60 gtt/mL
infusion pump
Primary set:
1000 mL D_2 LRS
IV set drop factor 10 gtt/mL

For the *secondary* IV, the following calculations must be made:

1. Dose of magnesium sulfate in IV.

2. Concentration of solution.

3. Volume of loading dose and flow rate for infusion pump (see Chapter 8).

4. Infusion rate: volume per hour of magnesium sulfate infusion.

For the *primary* IV, the following calculation must be made:

1. Drop rate per minute.

For the total IV intake, the following solutions must be added:

1. Volume of loading dose.

2. Volume of secondary IV for 8 hours.

3. Volume of primary IV for 8 hours.

Secondary IV

1. $\dfrac{D}{H} \times V = \dfrac{20\ g}{5\ g} \times 10\ mL = 40\ mL$ of magnesium sulfate or 4 ampules

2. Concentration of solution:

$$20 \text{ g} = 20,000 \text{ mg}$$
$$20,000 \text{ mg} : 1000 \text{ mL} :: X : 1 \text{ mL}$$
$$1000 X = 20,000$$
$$X = 20 \text{ mg}$$

The concentration of solution is 20 mg/mL.

3. Volume of loading dose:

$$4 \text{ g} = 4000 \text{ mg}$$
$$20 \text{ mg} : 1 \text{ mL} :: 4000 \text{ mg} : X \text{ mL}$$
$$20 X = 4000$$
$$X = 200 \text{ mL}$$

Flow rate for the pump:

$$200 \text{ mL} \div \frac{20 \text{ min}}{60 \text{ min/hr}} = 200 \times \frac{\overset{3}{\cancel{60}}}{\underset{1}{\cancel{20}}} = 600 \text{ mL/hr}$$

The rate on the infusion pump for the 4 g infusion of magnesium sulfate over 20 minutes is 600 mL/hr. If the pump cannot be adjusted to that rate, then the infusion rate must be monitored closely and the client observed for response to drug therapy.

4. Infusion rate: volume per hour:

$$\frac{\text{concentration/hr}}{\text{concentration of solution}} = \text{volume/hr}$$

$$1 \text{ g} = 1000 \text{ mg}$$
$$\frac{100 \text{ mg/hr}}{20 \text{ mg/mL}} = 50 \text{ mL/hr}$$

The rate on the pump for the 1 g/hr infusion is 50 mL/hr.

Primary IV

After the loading dose of magnesium sulfate, the primary IV will run at 75 mL/hr.

Drop rate using a 10 gtt/mL set is:

$$\frac{75 \text{ mL/hr} \times 10 \text{ gtt/min}}{60 \text{ min}} = 12.5 \text{ or } 13 \text{ gtt/min}$$

Total IV Intake Over 8 Hours

Volume of loading dose		200 mL
Volume of secondary IV	50 mL × 8 =	400 mL
Volume of primary IV	75 mL × 8 =	+ 600 mL
		1200 mL

Because fluid overload is a potential problem for preeclampsia patients, all IV fluids must be calculated accurately. The use of infusion pumps, if available, when high volumes of fluid need to be infused, will provide accuracy when drops are too fast to count.

INTRAVENOUS FLUID BOLUS

An IV fluid *bolus* is a large volume, 200 to 500 mL, of IV fluid infused over a short time (1 hour or less). A bolus may be given prior to conductive anesthesia or to a preterm patient in labor.

In the next example, calculate the flow rate of an IV bolus from the primary IV followed by an infusion of a tocolytic drug given by titration. At the end of this example, calculate the client's fluid intake for 8 hours.

....

e x a m p l e

1. Start 1000 D_5 LRS at 300 mL/10 min, then reduce to 125 mL/hr.
2. Mix terbutaline 5 mg in 1000 mL of NSS; start at 10 mcg/min; increase 5 mcg/min q10min until contractions subside.

Available: Primary set:
   1000 mL D_5 LRS
   IV set drop factor 10 gtt/mL
 Secondary set:
   terbutaline 1 mg/mL
   500 mL NSS
   microdrip IV set 60 gtt/mL
   infusion pump

For the *secondary* IV, the following calculations must be made:

1. The dose of terbutaline in IV.
2. Concentration of solution.
3. Infusion rates: volume per minute and hour.
4. Titration factor for 5 mcg/mL.

For the *primary* IV, determine the following:

1. Drop rate per minute for 300 mL over 10 minutes and 125 mL/hr.
2. Balance the primary IV with the secondary IV to achieve a rate of 125 mL/hr.

Total the IV fluids for 8 hours.

Secondary IV

1. $\dfrac{D}{H} \times V = \dfrac{5 \text{ mg}}{1 \text{ mg}} \times 1 \text{ mL} = 5 \text{ mL}$ of terbutaline of 5 ampules

2. Concentration of solution:

$$5 \text{ mg} = 5000 \text{ mcg}$$
$$5000 \text{ mcg} : 1000 \text{ mL} :: X \text{ mcg} : 1 \text{ mL}$$
$$1000 X = 5000$$
$$X = 5 \text{ mcg}$$

The concentration of solution is 5 mcg/mL.

3. Infusion rates: volume per minute and volume per hour.

$$\frac{10 \text{ mcg/min}}{5 \text{ mcg/mL}} = 2 \text{ mL/min} \times 60 \text{ min/hr} = 120 \text{ mL/hr}$$

4. Titration factor: to increase the concentration by increments of 5 mcg/min, the volume of the increment of change must be calculated per minute and per hour:

$$\frac{\text{concentration/minute}}{\text{concentration of solution}} = \text{mL/min} \qquad \frac{5 \text{ mcg/min}}{5 \text{ mcg/mL}} = 1 \text{ mL/min}$$

$$\text{volume/min} \times 60 \text{ min/hr} = \text{volume/hr}$$
$$1 \text{ mL/min} \times 60 \text{ min/hr} = 60 \text{ mL/hr}$$

The titration factor is 1 mL/min or 60 mL/hr. Increasing or decreasing the infusion rate by 5 mcg/min will correspond to an increase or decrease in volume by 1 mL/min or 60 mL/hr.

Primary IV

1. Drop rate for 300 mL over 10 minutes:

$$\frac{300 \text{ mL} \times \overset{1}{\cancel{10}} \text{ gtt/mL}}{\underset{1}{\cancel{10}} \text{ min}} = 300 \text{ gtt/min}$$

Because this rate is too fast to count, the flow must be monitored closely. Drop rate for 125 mL/hr:

$$\frac{125 \text{ ml} \times \overset{1}{\cancel{10}} \text{ gtt/mL}}{\underset{6}{\cancel{60}} \text{ min}} = 20.8 \text{ or } 21 \text{ gtt/min}$$

Total IV Intake Over 8 Hours

Volume of loading dose		300 mL
Volume of primary set	125 mL × 8 =	1000 mL
Volume of secondary set	180 mL × 8 =	+ 1440 mL
		2740 mL

Assume that an average of 180 mL/hr was given.

Summary Practice Problems

---

1. Preterm labor.

   a. Give NSS 500 mL over 15 minutes, then infuse at 100 mL/hr.

   b. If contractions are still regular, mix ritodrine 150 mg in 500 mL NSS. Infuse at 50 mcg/min and increase by 50 mcg q10min until contractions cease. Do not infuse more than 350 mcg/min.

   Available: Primary set:
   　　1000 mL NSS
   　　IV set with drop factor of 10 gtt/mL
   　Secondary set:
   　　ritodrine 50 mg in 5-mL ampules
   　　500 mL NSS
   　　microdrip set 60 gtt/mL
   　　infusion pump

Determine the following:

a. Secondary IV:
   (1) Ritodrine dosage.
   (2) Concentration of solution.
   (3) Infusion rate for volume per minute and hour.
   (4) Titration factor.

b. Primary IV: drop rate for 500 mL over 15 minutes and 100 mL/hr.

c. Total fluid intake for 8 hours.

2. Preeclamptic labor.

a. Mix magnesium sulfate 20 g in 1000 mL D$_5$W.

b. Infuse 4 g over 30 minutes, then maintain at 2 g/hr.

c. Start LRS 1000 mL at 50 mL/hr after loading dose of magnesium sulfate.

Available: Secondary set:
               magnesium sulfate 50% (5 g in 10 mL)
               1000 mL D$_5$W
               microdrip IV set 60 gtt/mL
               infusion pump
            Primary set:
               1000 mL LRS
               IV set 10 gtt/mL

Determine the following:

a. Secondary IV:
   (1) Magnesium sulfate dosage.
   (2) Concentration of solution.
   (3) Volume of loading dose and infusion rate for pump.
   (4) Infusion rate per hour of magnesium sulfate.

b. Primary IV: drop rate for 50 mL/hr.

c. Total fluid intake for 8 hours.

ANSWERS

1. a. Secondary IV:
   (1) Ritodrine dosage:

$$\frac{D}{H} \times V = \frac{150 \text{ mg}}{50 \text{ mg}} \times 5 \text{ mL} = 15 \text{ mL}$$

   Add 15 mL or 3 ampules of ritodrine to 500 mL NSS.
   (2) Concentration of solution:

$$150 \text{ mg}:500 \text{ mL} :: X \text{ mg}:1 \text{ mL}$$
$$500 X = 150$$
$$X = 0.3 \text{ mg/mL}$$

or

300 mcg/mL

(3) Infusion rates: volume per minute and per hour:

$$\frac{50 \text{ mcg/min}}{300 \text{ mcg/mL}} = 0.16 \text{ mL/min} \times 60 \text{ min/hr} = 9.6 \text{ or } 10 \text{ mL/hr}$$

(4) Titration factor: because the increment of increase is 50 mcg/min, the volume per hour, 10 mL/hr, is the titration factor, which increases the concentration by 50 mcg.

b. Primary IV:

(1) Drop rate for 500 mL over 15 minutes:

$$\frac{500 \text{ mL} \times 10 \text{ gtt/mL}}{15 \text{ min}} = 333 \text{ gtt/min}$$

This rate is impossible to count. Therefore, the infusion must be monitored closely during infusion time.

(2) Drop rate for 100 mL/hr:

$$\frac{100 \text{ mL} \times 10 \text{ gtt/mL}}{60 \text{ min}} = 16.6 \text{ or } 17 \text{ gtt mL}$$

c. Total IV intake for 8 hours:

IV fluid bolus	500 mL
Primary IV 100 mL × 8 hr	800 mL
Secondary IV 50 mL × 8 hr	+ 400 mL
	1700 mL

Assume that an average of 50 mL/hr was given.

2. a. Secondary IV:

(1) Magnesium sulfate dosage:

$$\frac{D}{H} \times V = \frac{20 \text{ g}}{5 \text{ g}} \times 10 \text{ mL} = 40 \text{ mL or 4 ampules of magnesium sulfate}$$

(2) Concentration of solution:

$$20 \text{ g} = 200,000 \text{ mg}$$
$$20,000 \text{ mg} : 1000 \text{ mL} \ :: \ X \text{ mg} : 1 \text{ mL}$$
$$1000 \text{ X} = 20,000$$
$$X = 20 \text{ mg}$$

The concentration of solution is 20 mg/mL.

(3) Volume of loading dose:

$$4 \text{ g} = 4000 \text{ mg}$$
$$20 \text{ mg} : 1 \text{ mL} \ :: \ 4000 \text{ mg} : X \text{ mL}$$
$$20 \text{ X} = 4000$$
$$X = 200 \text{ mL}$$

Infusion rate for 30 minutes:

$$200 \text{ mL} \div \frac{30 \text{ min}}{60 \text{ min/hr}} = 200 \times \frac{\overset{2}{\cancel{60}}}{\underset{1}{\cancel{30}}} = 400 \text{ mL/hr}$$

(4) Infusion rate: volume per hour:

$$2 \text{ g} = 2000 \text{ mg}$$

$$\frac{2000 \text{ mg/hr}}{20 \text{ mg/mL}} = 100 \text{ mL/hr}$$

b. Primary IV:

After the loading dose:

$$\frac{50 \text{ mL/hr} \times 10 \text{ gtt/min}}{60 \text{ min}} = 8.3 \text{ or } 8 \text{ gtt/min}$$

c. Total IV intake over 8 hours:

Volume of loading dose		200 mL
Volume of secondary IV	100 mL × 8 =	800 mL
Volume of primary IV	50 mL × 8 =	+ 400 mL
		1400 mL

community

Objectives

- Identify the problems with conversion of metric to household measure.
- Name the components of a solution.
- List three methods for preparing a solution.
- Recognize three ways solutions are labeled.
- State the formula used for calculating a solution of a desired concentration.
- State the formula used for calculating a weaker solution from a stronger solution.
- Identify the types of devices used for home infusion therapy.

Outline

METRIC TO HOUSEHOLD CONVERSION
PREPARING A SOLUTION OF A DESIRED
CONCENTRATION
Changing a Ratio to Fractions and Percentage
Calculating a Solution from a Ratio
Calculating a Solution from a Percentage
PREPARING A WEAKER SOLUTION FROM A
STRONGER SOLUTION
GUIDELINES FOR HOME SOLUTIONS
HOME INFUSION THERAPY
Home Infusion Devices

Although the metric system has become widespread in the clinical area, the home setting generally does not have the devices of metric measure. This becomes a problem when liquid medication is prescribed in metric measure for the home patient. The community nurse should be able to assist the client in converting metric to household measure when necessary.

Preparation of solutions in the home setting may involve conversion between the metric and household systems. Solutions used in the home setting can be used for oral fluid replacement, topical application, irrigation, or disinfection. Although the majority of the solutions are commercially available, solutions that can be prepared in the home can be effective and less costly than the premixed items.

When commercially prepared drugs are too concentrated for the client's use and must be diluted, it becomes necessary to calculate the strength of the solution to meet the therapeutic need as prescribed by the physician. Knowledge of solution preparation and metric–household conversion can be a useful skill for the community nurse.

METRIC TO HOUSEHOLD CONVERSION

When changing from metric to household measure, use the ounce from the apothecary system as an intermediary, because there is no clear conversion between the two systems.

The conversion factors for volume are:

Ounces to milliliters: multiply ounces × 29.57
Milliliters to ounces: multiply milliliters × 0.034

The conversion factors for weight are:

Ounces to grams: multiply ounces × 28.35
Grams to ounces: multiply grams × 0.035

Note that weight and volume measures differ in the metric system. The properties of crystals, powders, and other solids account for the differences more so than the liquids. Also, as liquid measures increase in volume, there are greater discrepancies between metric and standard household measure. Table 13–1 shows the current approximate equivalents. Deciliters and liters are also included with the volume measurements. These terms will be seen more commonly as the use of the metric system increases. Although conversion charts are helpful guides, a metric measuring device would be optimal for drug administration. Standard household measuring devices should be used instead of tableware if a metric device is not available.

I Practice Problems: Metric to Household Conversion

Use Table 13–1 to convert metric to household measure.

1. Dimetapp 2.5 mL every 6 hours as necessary.

---

table 13·1
HOUSEHOLD TO METRIC CONVERSIONS

STANDARD HOUSEHOLD MEASURE	APOTHECARY	METRIC VOLUME	METRIC WEIGHT
⅛ teaspoon	7–8 gtt/¹⁄₄₈ oz	0.6 mL	0.6 g
¼ teaspooon	15 gtt/¹⁄₂₄ oz	1.25 mL	1.25 g
½ teaspoon	30 gtt/¹⁄₁₂ oz	2.5 mL	2.5 g
1 teaspoon	60 gtt/⅙ oz	5 mL	5 g
1 tablespoon/3 teaspoons	½ oz	15 mL	15 g
2 tablespoons/6 teaspoons	1 oz	¼ dL/30 mL	30 g
¼ cup/4 tablespoons	2 oz	½ dL/60 mL	55 g
⅓ cup/5 tablespoons	2½ oz	¾ dL/75 mL	75 g
½ cup	4 oz	1 dL/120 mL	110 g
1 cup	8 oz	¼ L/240–250 mL	225 g
1 pint	16 oz	½ L/480–500 mL	
1 quart	32 oz	1 L/1000 mL	
2 quarts/½ gallon	64 oz	2 L/2000 mL	
1 gallon	128 oz	3¾ L/3840–4000 mL	

2. Ceclor 5 mL fours times per day.

_____

3. Tylenol elixir 1.25 mL every 6 hours as necessary for temperature greater than 102°F.

_____

4. Maalox 30 mL after meals and at bedtime.

_____

5. Neo-Calglucon 7.5 mL three times per day.

_____

6. Basaljel 45 mL after each meal.

_____

7. Castor oil 60 mL at bedtime.

_____

8. Metamucil 5 g in 1 glass of water every morning.

_____

9. Dilantin-30 Pediatric suspension 10 mL twice per day.

_____

10. Homemade pediatric electrolyte solution:

H_2O 1 L, boiled _____

Sugar 30 g _____

Salt 1.5 g _____

Lite salt 2.5 g _____

Baking soda 2.5 g _____

11. A nonalcoholic mouthwash:

H_2O 500 mL boiled _____

Table salt 5 mL _____

Baking soda 5 mL _____

12. Magic mouthwash:

Benadryl 50 mg/10 mL _____

Maalox 10 mL _____

PREPARING A SOLUTION OF A DESIRED CONCENTRATION

All solutions contain a solute (drug) and a solvent (liquid). Solutions can be mixed three different ways:

1. *Weight to weight:* Involves mixing the weight of a given solute with the weight of a given liquid.

Example: 5 g sugar with 100 g H_2O

This type of preparation is used in the pharmaceutical setting and is the *most accurate.* Scales for weight to weight preparation are not usually found in the home setting.

2. *Weight to volume:* Uses the weight of a given solute with the volume of an appropriate amount of solvent.

Example: 10 g of salt in 1 L of H_2O

or

2 oz of salt in 1 qt of H_2O

Again, a scale is needed for this preparation.

3. *Volume to volume:* Means that a given volume of solution is mixed with a given volume of solution.

Example: 10 mL of hydrogen peroxide 3% in 1 dL H_2O

or

2 T of hydrogen peroxide 3% in ½ c H_2O

Preparation of solutions volume to volume is commonly used in both the clinical and home settings.

After a solution is prepared, the strength can be expressed numerically in three different ways:

1. A ratio—1:20 acetic acid

2. A fraction—5 g/100 mL acetic acid

3. A percentage—5% acetic acid

With a ratio, the first number is the solute and the second number is the solvent. In a fraction, the numerator is the drug and the denominator is the liquid. A solution labeled by percentage indicates the amount of solute in 100 mL of liquid. All pharmaceutically prepared solutions use the metric system, and the ratio, fraction, and percentages are interpreted in *grams per milliliter.*

Changing a Ratio to Fractions and Percentage

Change a ratio to a percentage or a fraction by setting up a proportion using the following variables:

known drug : known volume : : desired drug : desired volume

A proportion can also be set up like a fraction:

$$\frac{\text{known drug}}{\text{known volume}} = \frac{\text{desired drug}}{\text{desired volume}}$$

Any variable in this formula can be found if the other three variables are known.

REMEMBER

. . . .

e x a m p l e

PROBLEM 1: Change acetic acid 1 : 20 to a percentage

$$1 \text{ g} : 20 \text{ mL} = X \text{ g} : 100\text{mL}$$
$$20 \text{ X} = 100$$
$$X = 5 \text{ g}$$
$$1 \text{ g} : 20 \text{ mL} = 5 \text{ g} : 100 \text{ mL}$$

Note: In percentage, the volume of liquid is 100 mL.

The ratio can be expressed as a fraction, 5 g/100 mL, or as a percentage, 5%. Another method of changing a ratio to a percentage involves finding a multiple of 100 for volume (denominator), then multiplying both terms by that multiple.

II Practice Problems: Preparing a Solution of a Desired Concentration

Change the following ratios to fractions and percentages.

1. 4 : 1

2. 2 : 1

3. 1 : 50

4. 1 : 3

5. 1 : 1000

6. 1 : 10,000

7. 1 : 4

8. 1 : 5000

9. 1 : 200

10. 1 : 10

In the previous problems, grams per milliliter is the unit of measure used for preparing solutions. Scales for measuring grams are rarely found in the clinical area or the home environment. Volume (mL) is the common measurement of drugs for administration. Drugs that are powders, crystals, or liquids are measured in graduated measuring cups with metric, apothecary, or household units. The milliliter, although a volume measure, can be substituted for a gram, a measure of mass, because at 4°C, 1 mL of water weighs 1 g. Mass and volume differ with the type of substance; thus, grams and milliliters are not exact equivalents in all instances, but they can be accepted as approximate values for preparation of solution.

Calculating a Solution from a Ratio

To obtain a solution from a ratio, use the proportion or fraction method.

....

examples

PROBLEM 1: Prepare 500 mL of a 1 : 100 vinegar–water solution for a vaginal douche.

$$\text{known drug} : \text{known volume} : : \text{desired drug} : \text{desired volume}$$
$$1 \text{ mL} \quad : \quad 100 \text{ mL} \quad : : \quad X \text{ mL} \quad : \quad 500 \text{ mL}$$
$$100 \, X = 500$$
$$X = 5 \text{ mL}$$

or

$$\frac{\text{known drug}}{\text{known volume}} = \frac{\text{desired drug}}{\text{desired volume}}$$
$$\frac{1 \text{ mL}}{100 \text{ mL}} = \frac{X}{500 \text{ mL}}$$
$$100 \, X = 500$$
$$X = 5 \text{ mL}$$

Answer: 5 mL of vinegar added to 500 mL of water is a 1 : 100 vinegar-water solution.

Note: Five milliliters did not increase the volume of the solution by a large amount. When mixing volume and volume solutions, the total amount of *desired volume* should not be exceeded. Therefore, it is important to determine the volume of desired drug first, then remove that volume from the appropriate amount of solvent (solution). When mixing the solution, begin with the desired drug and add the premeasured solvent. This process ensures that the solution has an accurate concentration.

PROBLEM 2: Prepare 100 mL of a 1 : 4 hydrogen peroxide 3% and normal saline mouthwash.

$$\text{known drug} : \text{known volume} : : \text{desired drug} : \text{desired volume}$$
$$1 \text{ mL} \quad : \quad 4 \text{ mL} \quad : : \quad X \text{ mL} \quad : \quad 100 \text{ mL}$$
$$4 \, X = 100 \text{ mL}$$
$$X = 25 \text{ mL}$$

25 mL of hydrogen peroxide 3% is the amount of desired

drug. To calculate the amount of normal saline, use the following formula:

$$\text{desired volume} - \text{desired drug} = \text{desired solvent}$$
$$100\ \text{mL} \quad - \quad 25\ \text{mL} \quad = \quad 75\ \text{mL}$$

Answer: *75 mL of saline and 25 mL of hydrogen peroxide 3% make 100 mL of a 1 : 4 mouthwash.*

Calculating a Solution from a Percentage

To obtain a solution from a percentage, use the same formula with either the proportion or fraction method.

. . . .
e x a m p l e

PROBLEM 1: Prepare 1000 mL of a 0.9% NaCl solution.

$$\text{known drug} : \text{known volume} : : \text{desired drug} : \text{desired volume}$$
$$0.9\ \text{g} \quad : \quad 100\ \text{mL} \quad : : \quad X\ \text{g} \quad : \quad 1000\ \text{mL}$$
$$100\ X = 900$$
$$X = 9\ \text{g or 9 mL}$$

Answer: *9 g or 9 mL of NaCl in 1000 mL makes a 0.9% NaCl solution.*

PREPARING A WEAKER SOLUTION FROM A STRONGER SOLUTION

When a situation requires the preparation of a weaker solution from a stronger solution, the amount of desired drug must be determined. The known variables are the desired solution, the available or on-hand solution, and the desired volume. The formula can be set up with the strength of the solutions expressed in either ratio or percentage. The proportion method or the fractional method can be used to solve the problem. The first ratio or fraction, the desired solution (weaker solution), is the numerator, and the available or on-hand solution (stronger solution) is the denominator.

$$\text{desired solution} : \text{available solution} : : \text{desired drug} : \text{desired volume}$$

or

$$\frac{\text{desired solution}}{\text{available solution}} = \frac{\text{desired drug}}{\text{desired volume}}$$

. . . .
e x a m p l e

PROBLEM 1: Prepare 500 mL of a 2.5% aluminum acetate solution from a 5% aluminum acetate solution. Use water as the solvent.

$$2.5\% \ : \ 5\% : : X : 500\ \text{mL}$$
$$2.5\ \text{mL} : 5\ \text{mL} : : X : 500\ \text{mL}$$
$$5\ X = 1250$$
$$X = 250\ \text{mL}$$

Answer: Use 250 mL of 5% aluminum acetate to make 500 mL of 2.5% aluminum acetate solution.

Determine the amount of water needed.

$$\text{desired volume} - \text{desired drug} = \text{desired solvent}$$
$$500 \text{ mL} \quad - \quad 250 \text{ mL} \quad = \quad 250 \text{ mL}$$

or

Same problem using the fractional method:

$$\frac{2.5\%}{5\%} \times \frac{X}{500 \text{ mL}} =$$

$$5 X = 1250$$
$$X = 250 \text{ mL of 5\% aluminum acetate}$$

or

Same problem but stated as a ratio:

Prepare 500 mL of a 1:40 aluminum acetate solution from a 1:20 aluminum acetate solution with water as the solvent.

$$\frac{1}{40} : \frac{1}{20} :: X : 500 \text{ mL}$$

$$\frac{1}{20 \, X} = \frac{500}{40}$$

$$X = \frac{500}{\overset{2}{\cancel{40}}} \times \frac{\overset{1}{\cancel{20}}}{1} = \frac{500}{2}$$

$$X = 250 \text{ mL of 5\% aluminum acetate solution}$$

GUIDELINES FOR HOME SOLUTIONS

For solutions prepared by clients in the home, directions need to be very specific and in written form, if possible. People often think that more is better. Teach the client that solutions can be dangerous if they are too concentrated. Higher concentrations of solutions can irritate tissues and prevent the desired effect. Recommend that standard measuring spoons and cups be used rather than tableware. Level measures rather than heaping measures of dry solutes should be used. Utensils and containers for solution preparation should be *clean or sterilized by boiling* if used for infants. Avoid mixing acidic solutions in aluminum containers, especially if the solution is for oral use. Although there is no evidence of toxicity, a metallic taste is noticeable. Glass, enamel, or plastic containers can be used. Solutions should be made fresh daily or just prior to use. Oral solutions, especially for infants, require refrigeration; topical solutions do not.

When preparing the solution, start with the desired drug and then add the solvent. This helps to disperse the drug and ensures that the desired volume of solution is not exceeded.

Solution problems are best calculated within the metric system. Fractional and percentage dosages are difficult to determine within the household system.

HOME INFUSION THERAPY

Home Infusion Devices

Home infusion therapy is the administration of a wide range of intravenous products by the nurse or family member to the patients in the home setting. The intravenous products include total parental nutrition (TPN) antibiotics, potent vasopressors (dobutamine and milrinone), blood products, chemotherapeutic agents, pain medication, and immunoglobulins. The criteria for home infusion therapy are as follows:

- Patent venous access
- Safe home environment
- A responsible care giver
- A medication that is safe to administer at home

Medication and IV fluids for home infusions are generally premixed by a pharmacy working with the infusion agency. Although most fluids are premixed, TPN may have additives, such as multivitamins, histamine$_2$-blocking agents, and insulin, that may have to be added before infusion. Home infusion therapy has led to innovative technologies for fluid and medication delivery (Table 13–2). The new devices are pump-types that are small, portable, quiet, and lightweight.

Part III Practice Problems: Preparing a Weaker Solution from a Stronger One

---

Identify the known variables and choose the appropriate formula. Calculate the following solutions using the metric system. Use Table 13–1 to obtain the household equivalent.

1. Prepare 250 mL of a 0.6% NaCl and sterile water solution for nose drops.

2. Prepare 250 mL of a 5% glucose and sterile water solution for an infant feeding.

3. Prepare 1000 mL of a 25% Betadine solution with sterile saline for a foot soak.

table 13•2
HOME INFUSION DEVICES

MECHANICAL INFUSION DEVICES

Elastometric balloon	Portable, hard outer shell with a balloon inside that inflates with air. A sterile reservoir inside is filled with medication. Positive pressure in balloon pushes medication through a regulator, which controls flow rate. Used for small volumes of antibiotic or chemotherapeutic agents. Single-use and disposable. Comes in various volumes, 50 to 500 mL. Designed for ambulatory care and used in pediatrics.
Spring-coil container	Pocket-sized round disk contains a spring-loaded pressure plate and a sterile reservoir. Spring plate presses against reservoir, and positive pressure forces fluid from reservoir, through the regulator. Used for small volumes of intermittent IV drugs, analgesics, antibiotics, and chemotherapy. Volume sizes are limited. Designed for ambulatory care.

ELECTRONIC INFUSION DEVICES

Stationary pump	Usually mounted on a pole. Can be used with any type of fluid or medication. Programmable with tamperproof abilities. Used primarily in hospitals. See Chapter 8.
Ambulatory	Small, battery-powered. Used for small or large volumes. Sets up like a stationary pump. Can be used for continuous or bolus infusions. Versatile, can infuse any type of fluid. Small, lightweight, can be carried in a backpack with IV fluid. Used in ambulatory care. Allows for continuous and bolus infusions. Special tubing needed.
Implantable	Small, light, preprogrammed. Can be surgically implanted into a pocket of subcutaneous fat. Titanium pump can hold 10 to 20 mL of medication. Can be refilled with a needle inserted into the filling port of the pump. Used for control of chronic pain. Can infuse antibiotics or chemotherapeutic agents.

4. Prepare 2 L of a 2% Lysol solution for cleaning a changing area.

5. Prepare 20 L of a 2% sodium bicarbonate solution for a bath.

6. Prepare 100 mL of a 50% hydrogen peroxide 3% and water mouthwash.

7. Prepare 500 mL of a modified Dakin solution 0.5% from a 5% sodium hypochlorite solution with sterile water as the solvent.

8. Prepare 1500 mL of a 0.9% NaCl solution for an enema.

9. Prepare 2 L of a 1:1000 Neosporin bladder irrigation with sterile saline. (Omit the household conversion.)

10. Determine how much alcohol is needed for a 3:1 alcohol and white vinegar solution for an external ear irrigation. Vinegar 30 mL is used. Solve using the proportion method.

11. Prepare 1000 mL of a 1:10 sodium hypochlorite and water solution for cleaning.

12. Prepare 1000 mL of a 3% sodium hypochlorite and water solution.

13. Prepare 2000 L of a 1:9 Lysol solution to clean color-fast linens soiled with body fluids. (Omit the household conversion.)

ANSWERS

Part I

1. Dimetapp 2.5 mL = ½ t

2. Ceclor 5 mL = 1 t

3. Tylenol elixir 1.25 mL = ¼ t

4. Maalox 30 mL = 2 T

5. Neo-Calglucon 7.5 mL = 1½ t

6. Basaljel 45 mL = 3 T

7. Castor oil 60 mL = 4 T or ¼ c

8. Metamucil 5 g = 1 t

9. Dilantin-30 Pediatric suspension 10 mL = 2 t

10. H_2O 1 L = 1 qt
    Sugar 30 g = 2 T
    Salt 1.25 g = ¼ t
    Lite salt 2.5 g = ½ t
    Baking soda 2.5 g = ½ t

11. H_2O 500 ml = 1 qt
    Table salt 5 mL = 1 t
    Baking soda 5 mL = 1 t

12. Benadryl 50 mg/10 mL = 2 t
    Maalox 10 mL = 2 t

ANSWERS

Part II

1. $4:1 = X:100$
$\quad X = 400$
$\quad \dfrac{400}{100}, 400\%$

2. $2:1 = X:100$
$\quad X = 200$
$\quad \dfrac{200}{100}, 200\%$

3. $1:50 = X:100$
$\quad 50\,X = 100$
$\quad X = 2$
$\quad \dfrac{2}{100}, 2\%$

4. $1:3 = X:100$
$\quad 3\,X = 100$
$\quad X = 33.3$
$\quad \dfrac{33.3}{100}, 33.3\%$

5. $1:1000 = X:100$
$\quad 1000\,X = 100$
$\quad X = 0.1$
$\quad \dfrac{0.1}{100}, 0.1\%$

6. $1:10,000 = X:100$
$\quad 10,000\,X = 100$
$\quad X = 0.01$
$\quad \dfrac{1}{10,000}, 0.01\%$

7. $1:4 = X:100$
$\quad 4\,X = 100$
$\quad X = 25$
$\quad \dfrac{25}{100}, 25\%$

8. $1:5000 = X:100$
$\quad 5000\,X = 100$
$\quad X = 0.02$
$\quad \dfrac{0.02}{100}, 0.02\%$

9. $1:200 = X:100$
$\quad 200\,X = 100$
$\quad X = 0.5$
$\quad \dfrac{0.5}{100}, 0.5\%$

10. $1:10 = X:100$
$\quad 10\,X = 100$
$\quad X = 10$
$\quad \dfrac{10}{100}, 10\%$

ANSWERS

Part III

1. Known drug: 0.6% NaCl $0.6:100 :: X:250$
   Known volume: 100 mL $100\,X = 150$
   Desired drug: X $X = 1.5$ mL
   Desired volume: 250 mL

1.5 mL of NaCl in 250 mL of water yields a 0.6% NaCl solution. Household equivalents are approximately ¼ teaspoon salt and 1 cup sterile water.

2. Known drug: 5% glucose (sugar) $5:100 :: X:250$
   Known volume: 100 mL $100\,X = 1250$
   Desired drug: X $X = 12.5$ mL
   Desired volume: 250 mL

12.5 mL of sugar in 250 mL of water yields a 5% glucose solution. Household equivalents are approximately 1 tablespoon in 1 cup of sterile water.

3. Known drug: 25% Betadine $25:100 :: X:1000$
   Known volume: 100 mL $100\,X = 25,000$
   Desired drug: X $X = 250$ mL
   Desired volume: 1000 mL $1000 \text{ mL} - 250 \text{ mL} = 750 \text{ mL}$

250 mL of Betadine in 750 mL saline yields a 25% Betadine solution. Household equivalents are 1 cup Betadine in 3 cups sterile saline.

4. Known drug: 2% Lysol   2 : 100 : : X : 2000 mL
   Known volume: 100 mL   100 X = 4000
   Desired drug: X   X = 40 mL
   Desired volume: 2 L = 2000 mL

   40 mL of Lysol in 2 L of water yields a 2% Lysol solution. Household equivalents are 2 tablespoons and 2 teaspoons (40 mL) of Lysol to 2 quarts or ½ gallon of water.

5. Known drug: 2% sodium bicarbonate   2 : 100 : : X : 20,000 mL
   Known volume: 100 mL   X = 40,000
   Desired drug: X   X = 400 mL or 400 g
   Desired volume: 20,000 mL

   400 mL or 400 g of sodium bicarbonate (baking soda) in 20,000 mL of water yields a 2% sodium bicarbonate solution. Household equivalents are 1½ cups and 2 tablespoons baking soda in 5 gallons of water.

6. Known drug: 50% hydrogen peroxide 50 : 100 : : X : 100
   Known volume: 100 mL   100 X = 5000
   Desired drug: X   X = 50 mL
   Desired volume: 100 mL   100 mL − 50 mL = 50 mL

   50 mL of hydrogen peroxide 3% in 50 mL water yields a 50% solution. Household equivalents are approximately 3 tablespoons of hydrogen peroxide 3% in 3 tablespoons of water.

7. Known drug: 0.5%   0.5 : 5 : : X : 500
   Available solution: 5%   5 X = 250
   Desired drug: X   X = 50 mL
   Desired volume: 500 mL   500 mL − 50 mL = 450 mL

   50 mL of sodium hypochlorite in 450 mL sterile water yields a 0.5% modified Dakin's solution. Household equivalents are 3 tablespoons and 1 teaspoon of Dakin's solution in 1 pint minus 3 tablespoons of water.

8. Known drug: 0.9%   0.9 : 100 : : X : 1500
   Known volume: 100 mL   100 X = 1350
   Desired drug: X   X = 13.5 mL
   Desired volume: 1500 mL

   13.5 mL of NaCl in 1500 mL water yields a 0.9% NaCl solution. Household equivalents are 2½ teaspoons of salt in 1½ quarts of water.

9. Known drug: 1 mL   1 : 1000 : : X : 2000
   Known volume: 1000 mL   1000 X = 2000
   Desired drug: X   X = 2 mL
   Desired volume: 2000 mL

   2 mL of Neosporin irrigant in 2000 mL sterile saline yields a 1 : 1000 solution for continuous bladder irrgation. This treatment is done primarily in the clinical setting.

10. Use ratio and proportion to solve this problem.

    3 : 1 : : X : 30 mL
    X = 90 mL

    Add 90 mL of alcohol to 30 mL of vinegar to yield a 3 : 1 solution for an external ear wash. Household equivalents are 6 tablespoons of alcohol and 2 tablespoons of vinegar.

11. Known drug: 1 mL   1 : 10 : : X : 1000
    Known volume: 10 mL   10 X = 1000
    Desired drug: X   X = 100 mL
    Desired volume: 1000 mL   1000 mL − 100 mL = 900 mL

    100 mL of sodium hypochlorite (bleach) in 900 mL water yields a 1 : 10 sodium hypochlorite solution. Household equivalents are ⅓ cup and 2 tablespoons sodium hypochlorite in approximately 1 quart minus ⅓ cup and 2 tablespoons of water.

12. Known drug: 3 mL   3 : 100 : : X : 1000
    Known volume: 100 mL   100 X = 3000
    Desired drug: X   X = 30 mL
    Desired volume: 1000 mL   1000 mL − 30 mL = 970 mL

    30 mL of sodium hypochlorite (bleach) in 970 mL water yields a 3% sodium hypochlorite solution. Household equivalents are 2 tablespoons in 1 quart minus 2 tablespoons of water.

13. Use ratio and proportion to solve this problem.

$$1 : 9 : : x : 2000 \text{ mL}$$
$$9x = 2000 \text{ mL}$$
$$x = 222 \text{ mL}$$

desired volume − desired drug = desired solvent
2000 mL − 222 mL   = 1778 mL

222 mL of Lysol in 1778 mL of H_2O yields a 1 : 9 solution cleansing solution for colorfast linens soiled with body fluids.

post-test: orals, injectables, intravenous, and pediatrics

The post-test is for testing content of Part III, orals, injectables, intravenous, and Chapter 9, pediatrics. The test is divided into four sections. There are 50 drug problems, and the test should take 1 to 1½ hours to complete. You may use a conversion table as needed. Minimum passing score is 44 correct or 88%. If you get more than two drug problems wrong in a section of the test, return to the chapter in the book for that test section and rework the practice problems.

ORAL PREPARATIONS

1. Order: meperidine (Demerol) 100 mg, po, q4h, PRN for pain.
Drug available: (unit packaged doses)

How many tablets of meperidine would you give? _____ 2

2. Order: Coumadin 7.5 mg, po, qd.
Drug available: (tablet is scored)

How many tablets of Coumadin would you give? _____ 1½

3. Order: lorazepam (Ativan) 1.5 mg, po, hs.
Drug available:

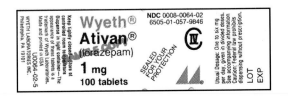

How many tablets should the client receive? _____ 1½

4. Order: nitroglycerin (Nitrostat) gr 1/200, SL, STAT.
   Drug available:

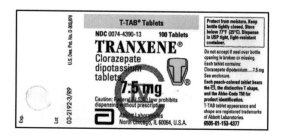

Usual Dosage–0.3 to 0.6 mg sublingually as needed. See package insert for full prescribing information. Keep this and all drugs out of the reach of children. Dispense in original unopened container. Store up to 25°C (77°F). Protect from moisture. See lot number and expiration date on bottom. © 1997-'98, Warner-Lambert Co. **PARKE-DAVIS** Div of Warner-Lambert Co Morris Plains, NJ 07950 USA	**N 0071-0569-24** **Nitrostat®** (Nitroglycerin Tablets, USP) **0.3 mg (1/200 gr)** ℞ only **100 TABLETS** Ⓟ **PARKE-DAVIS**	Usual Dosage–0.3 to 0.6 mg sublingually as needed. See package insert for full prescribing information. Keep this and all drugs out of the reach of children. Dispense in original unopened container. Store up to 25°C (77°F). Protect from moisture. See lot number and expiration date on bottom. © 1997-'98, Warner-Lambert Co. **PARKE-DAVIS** Div of Warner-Lambert Co Morris Plains, NJ 07950 USA	**N 0071-0570-24** **Nitrostat®** (Nitroglycerin Tablets, USP) **0.4 mg (1/150 gr)** ℞ only **100 TABLETS** Ⓟ **PARKE-DAVIS**	Usual Dosage–0.3 to 0.6 mg sublingually as needed. See package insert for full prescribing information. Keep this and all drugs out of the reach of children. Dispense in original unopened container. Store up to 25°C (77°F). Protect from moisture. See lot number and expiration date on bottom. © 1997-'98, Warner-Lambert Co. **PARKE-DAVIS** Div of Warner-Lambert Co Morris Plains, NJ 07950 USA	**N 0071-0571-24** **Nitrostat®** (Nitroglycerin Tablets, USP) **0.6 mg (1/100 gr)** ℞ only **100 TABLETS** Ⓟ **PARKE-DAVIS**

The drug is available in three different strengths. Which drug label would you select? Why? .3mg (1/200 gr), because that is exactly how much we need

5. Order: clorazepate sodium (Tranxene) gr 1/4/d, po, hs.
   Drug available:

	T-TAB® Tablets	Protect from moisture. Keep bottle tightly closed. Store below 77°F (25°C). Dispense in USP tight, light-resistant container.
U.S. Des. Pat. No. D-302,878	**NDC 0074-4390-13 100 Tablets** **TRANXENE®** Clorazepate dipotassium tablets **7.5 mg** ® Caution: Federal U.S.A. law prohibits dispensing without prescription. Abbott Laboratories North Chicago, IL 60064, U.S.A.	Do not accept if seal over bottle opening is broken or missing. Each tablet contains: Clorazepate dipotassium....7.5 mg See enclosure. Each peach-colored tablet bears the ℈, the distinctive T shape, and the Abbo-Code TM for product identification. T-TAB tablet appearance and shape are registered trademarks of Abbott Laboratories. 6505-01-153-4377

.167
1/6 gr = 10 mg
1/4 gr = (15 mg)

a. Change grain ¼ to milligrams. Use conversion table if needed. How many milligrams (mg) is equivalent to grain ¼? _____ 15

b. How many tablets should the client receive? _____ 2

6. Order: clarithromycin (Biaxin) 0.5 g, bid × 10 d, po.
   Drug available:

0.5 g → ?mg

1 g ⟹ 1000 mg

a. 0.5 gram is equivalent to _____500_____ milligram (mg).

b. How many tablets would you give? ____2____

7. Order: acetaminophen (Tylenol) gr x, po, PRN, for headache.
Drug available:

(10 gr)

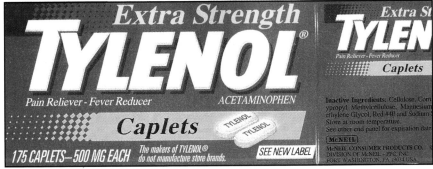

10 gr → ?mg

5 gr → 300 mg

a. Grain x is equivalent to _____600_____ milligrams (mg).

b. Which Tylenol bottle would you select? ____325 mg____

c. How many tablets or caplets should the client receive?

____2____

8. Order: allopurinol (Zyloprim) 0.2 g, po, bid.
Drug available:

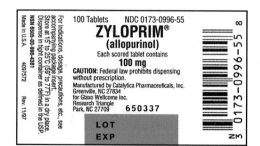

handwritten: .2g → ? mg ; 1g → 1000 mg

a. Gram 0.2 is equivalent to _____*200 mg*_____ milligrams (mg).

b. The client should receive how many tablets of allopurinol per day?

_____*2*_____

9. Order: prochlorperazine (Compazine) 10 mg, po, tid.
Drug available:

A

B

a. Which Compazine bottle would you select? Why? ___*5mg/5mL*___

b. How many milliliters (mL) would you give? ___*20*___

10. Order: cefuroxime axetil (Ceftin) 500 mg, po, q12h.
Drug available:

a. Which Ceftin bottle would you select? Explain. _250_____

b. The client would receive how many grams _____|_____ or
milligrams (mg) ___1000_____ of Ceftin per day?

c. How many milliliters (mL) should the client receive?

_____

11. Order: cefaclor (Ceclor) 250 mg, po, q8h.
Drug available:

a. Which Ceclor bottle would you select? _187 mg_

b. How many milliliters (mL) should the client receive per dose?

_7_

c. Is there another solution to this drug problem? _3.3 ml of 375_

12. Order: simvastatin (Zocor) 40 mg, po, qd. _(everyday)_
Drug available:

a. Which Zocor bottle would you select? Why?

_20 mg_

b. How many tablets should the client receive? _2_

13. Order: etretinate (Tegison) 0.75 mg/kg/day, po, in two divided doses.
Client weighs 150 pounds.
Drug available: Tegison 10 mg and 25 mg capsules.

   a. How many kilograms (kg) does the client weigh? _____68_____

   b. How many milligrams (mg) of Tegison should the client receive per

   day? _(.75)(68)=51g_

   c. How many capsules of Tegison per dose? ___2 for 25 mg capsule___

14. Order: theophylline 5 mg/kg/LD (loading dose), po.
Client weighs 70 kg.
Drug available: Oral solution 80 mg/15 mL and 150 mg/15mL.

   a. Which oral solution bottle would you select? ___150 mg/15mL___

   b. How many milliliters (mL) of theophylline should the client receive

   as a loading dose? ___35 mL___

15. Order: docusate sodium (Colace) 100 mg, po, bid per NG (nasogastric) tube.
Drug available: Colace 50 mg/5 mL.
Osmolality of docusate sodium is 3900 mOsm. The desired osmolality is 500 mOsm.

   a. How many milliliters (mL) of Colace should the client receive?

   _____10_____

   b. How much water dilution is needed to obtain the desired osmolality?

   _____78 mL_____

INJECTABLES

16. Order: hydroxyzine (Vistaril) 25 mg, deep IM, STAT.
Drug available: Vistaril 100 mg/2 mL in a vial.

   How many milliliters (mL) of Vistaril would you give?

   _____.5_____

17. Order: digoxin (Lanoxin) 0.25 mg, IM, qd.
Drug available:

2 mL DOSETTE® Ampul   A-1410F
DIGOXIN
INJECTION, USP
500 mcg/2 mL
0.5 mg/2 mL (250 mcg/mL)
FOR **SLOW IV** OR
DEEP IM USE
ESI ELKINS-SINN, INC.
CHERRY HILL, NJ 08003
SAMPLE COPY

How many milliliters (mL) of digoxin would you give?

_____ 1 ml

18. Order: meperidine (Demerol) 40 mg and atropine sulfate 0.5 mg, IM, STAT.
Drug available:

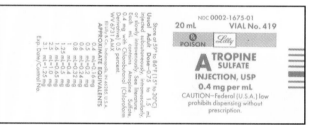

a. How many milliliters (mL) of meperidine and how many milliliters (mL) of atropine would you administer? .8 mL & 1.25 mL

b. Explain how the two drugs would be mixed in the cartridge

_____

19. Order: heparin 2500 units (U), SC, q6h.
Drug available:

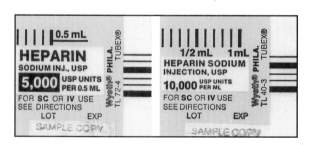

a. Which drug cartridge would you use? 5,000

b. How many milliliters (mL) of heparin should the client receive?

_____ .25 mL

20. Order: naloxone (Narcan) 0.5 mg, IM, STAT.
    Drug available:

    How many milliliters (mL) of naloxone should the client receive?

    _____1.25 mL_____

21. Order: NPH insulin 45 units and Humulin R (regular) 10 units.
    a. Explain the method for mixing the two insulins.

    _____

    b. Mark on the U 100/mL insulin syringe how much regular and NPH
       insulins should be withdrawn.

22. Order: vitamin B_{12} 500 μg, IM, 3 × a week.
    Drug available:

    a. Which cyanocobalamin would you select? Why?

    ___1,000, less Volume to take___

    b. How many milliliters (mL) would you give? ___.5 mL___

23. Order: morphine gr ⅙, IM, STAT.
Drug available:

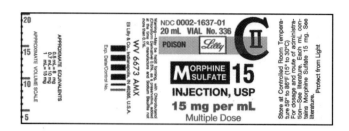

How many milliliters (mL) of morphine would you administer?

.67 mL

Note: Change grains to milligrams. Use conversion table if needed.

24. Order: phytonadione (AquaMEPHYTON) 5 mg, IM, STAT.
Drug available:

How many milliliters (mL) of AquaMEPHYTON would you administer?

½ mL

25. Order: ranitidine HCl (Zantac) 35 mg, IM, q8h.
Drug available:

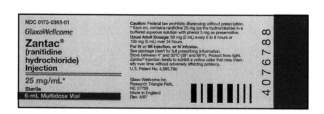

How many milliliters (mL) of Zantac should the client receive?

1.4 mL

26. Order: tobramycin (Nebcin) 3 mg/kg/day, IM, in three divided doses.
Patient weighs 145 pounds.

Drug available:

145 lb → x
2.2 lb → 1 kg

a. How many kilograms (kg) does the patient weigh? _66 kg_

b. How many milligrams (mg) of Nebcin should the client receive per day? _198 mg_

c. How many milligrams (mg) of Nebcin should the client receive per dose? _66 mg_

80 mg → 2 mL
66 mg → x

d. How many milliliters (mL) of Nebcin would you administer per dose? _1.65 mL_

27. Order: bethanechol Cl (Urecholine) 2.5 mg, SC, STAT and may repeat in 1 hour.
    Drug available:

5.15 mg → 1 mL
2.5 mg → x

How many milliliters (mL) of Urecholine would you give?
_____ .49 mL = .50 mL

28. Order: cefamandole (Mandol) 500 mg, IM, q12h.
    Drug available:

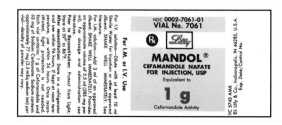

285 mg → 1 mL
500 mg → x

a. How much diluent would you mix with the Mandol powder? (See label for mixing.) _____

b. How many milliliters (mL) should be given? *1.8 mg*

29. Order: cefazolin (Ancef) 0.25 g, IM, q12h.
    Drug available: Mixing: Add 2.0 mL of diluent = 2.2 mL drug solution.

.25g = 250 mg

250 → X

500 → 2.2 mL

Note: Change grams to milligrams; drug label is in milligrams.
How many milliliters (mL) of Ancef should the client receive per dose?

1.1 mL

30. Order: oxacillin sodium 150 mg, IM, q6h.
    Drug available:

250 mg → 1.5 mL

150 mg → X

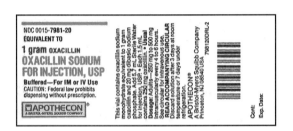

a. Label stated to add _____ mL of diluent to equal

_____ mL per 250 mg.

b. How many milliliters (mL) of oxacillin should the client receive per

dose? *.9 mL*

31. Order: ceftazidime (Fortaz) 750 mg, IM, q12h.
    Drug available: Add 2.5 mL of diluent = 3 mL of drug solution.

.750g → X

1g → 3mL

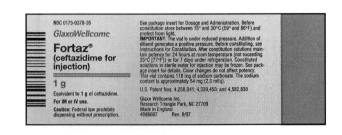

How many milliliters (mL) of ceftazidime would you administer per dose?

_2.25 mL_

32. Order: gentamicin sulfate 4 mg/kg/day, IM, in three divided doses.
Client weighs 165 pounds.
Drug available: gentamicin 10 mg/mL and 40 mg/mL.

165 lbs → X
2.2 lbs → 1 kg

   a. How many kilograms (kg) does the client weigh?

   _75_

   b. How many milligrams (mg) of gentamicin per day should the client

   receive? _300 mg_

   (75 kg)(4 mg/kg/day)

   c. How many milligrams (mg) of gentamicin per dose?

   _100 mg_

   d. Which gentamicin bottle would you select? Explain.

   40 mg/mL → easier

   e. How many milliliters (mL) of gentamicin per dose should the client

   receive? _2.5 mL_

   100 mg → X
   40 mg → 1 mL

INTRAVENOUS

33. Order: 1000 mL of 5% Dextrose/0.45% NaCl in 8 hours.
Available: 1 liter of 5% D/½ NSS; IV set labeled 10 gtt/mL.
How many drops per minute should the client receive?

_____

34. Order: 500 mL of D_5W in 2 hours.
Available: 500 mL of D_5W; IV set labeled 15 gtt/mL.
How many drops per minute should the client receive?

_____

35. Order: ticarcillin disodium (Ticar) 600 mg, IV q6h.
Available: Calibrated cyclinder (Buretrol) set with drop factor 60 gtt/mL;
500 mL D_5W.
Drug available:

Instruction: Dilute drug in 60 mL of D$_5$W and infuse in 30 minutes.

a. *Drug calculation:*

b. *Flow rate calculation:*

36. Order: cefazolin (Kefzol) 500 mg, IV, q6h.
Available: Secondary set: drop factor 15 gtt/mL; 100 mL D$_5$W.
Drug available: Add 2.5 mL of diluent to yield 3 mL of drug solution.

Instruction: Dilute drug in 100 mL and infuse in 45 minutes.

a. *Drug calculation:*

b. *Flow rate calculation:*

37. Order: chlorpromazine HCl (Thorazine) 50 mg, IV, to run for 4 hours.
Available: Secondary set: drop factor 15 gtt/mL; 500 mL of NSS (normal saline *solution*).
Drug available:

Instruction: Dilute Thorazine 50 mg in 500 mL of 0.9% NaCl (NSS) to run for 4 hours.

a. *Drug calculation:*

b. *Flow rate calculation:*

38. Order: cefepime HCl (Maxipime) 0.5 g, IV, q12h.
Available: Infusion pump.
Drug available: Add 2.0 mL diluent = 2.5 mL.

Instruction: Dilute in 50 mL of D$_5$W and infuse over 20 minutes.

a. *Drug calculation:*

_____

b. *Infusion pump rate:*

_____

39. Order: diltiazem (Cardizem) 10 mg/h, IV for 5 h.
Available: Infusion pump; 500 mL of D$_5$W.
Drug available:

Instruction: Infuse diltiazem 10 mg/h over 5 hours.

a. *Drug calculation:*

_____

   (1) How many milligrams (mg) of Cardizem should the client receive over 5 hours? _____

   (2) How many milliliters (mL) of Cardizem should be mixed in the 500 mL of D$_5$W? _____

b. *Infusion pump rate:*

_____

40. Order: ifosfamide (Ifex) 1.2 g/m²/d for 5 consecutive days.
Client: Weight 158 pounds; Height: 70 inches = 1.98 m².
Available: Infusion pump; 5% dextrose solution.
Drug available: Add 20 mL of diluent to 1 g of Ifex.

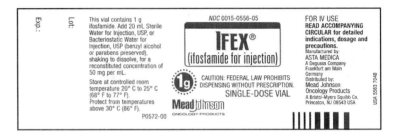

Instruction: Dilute Ifex in 50 mL of D₅W; infuse over 30 minutes.

a. *Drug calculation:*

How many grams or milligrams of Ifex should the client receive?

b. How much diluent would you add to 2.4 g of Ifex?

c. *Infusion pump rate:*

PEDIATRICS

41. Child with cardiac disorder.
Order: Lanoxin pediatric elixir 0.5 mg, po, qd.
Drug available: Lanoxin 0.05 mg/mL.
Child's age and weight: 3 years, 15 kg.
Pediatric dose: 0.040−0.060 mg/kg.

by mouth / every day

a. Is this drug dose within safe parameters? *no, it is < pediatr. dose*

b. How many milliliters (mL) would you administer?
10 mL

42. Child with high fever.
Order: ibuprofen (Motrin) 0.1 g, PRN temperature > 102°F.
Child's age and weight: 3 years, 15 kg.
Pediatric dose range: 100 mg, q6−8h, not to exceed 400 mg/day.

Drug available:

a. Is this drug dose within safe parameters? _yes if ≥ 100mg._   *100mg → 5mL*

b. How many milliliters (mL) should the child receive per dose?

_5mL_

43. Child with strep throat.
Order: penicillin V potassium (Veetids) 400,000 units, po, q6h.   *(4mouth every 6hours)*
Child's age and weight: 8 years, 53 pounds. — *÷ 24.1kg*
Pediatric dose range: 25,000–90,000 units/kg/day in three to six divided   *400,000 × 4 = 1600000*
doses.

24kg   24kg

600000   2160000

Drug available:

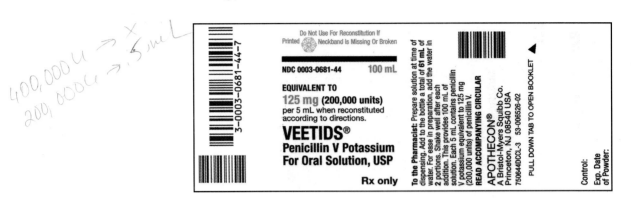

(handwritten, left margin)
400,000 U → X
200,000 U → 5 mL

a. Is the drug dose within the safe parameters? *Yes*

b. How many milliliters (mL) of penicillin V would you give?

10 mL

44. Child with otitis media.
Order: amoxicillin (Amoxil) 250 mg, po, q6h. *(per mouth every 6h)*
Child's age and weight: 5 years, 19 kg.
Pediatric dose range: 20–40 mg/kg/day in three divided doses.
Drug available:

(handwritten, left margin)
250 mg · 4 = 1000 mg/day

(handwritten, above label)
X   X
19   19
380 mg/day   760

a. Is the drug dose within the safe parameters? *No, it overexceeds*

b. How many milliliters (mL) would you give? *none, due to overexces*

45. Child with asthma.
Order: theophylline elixir 100 mg, po, q6h.
Child's age and weight: 7 years, 22 kg.
Pediatric dose range: 400 mg/24 h in four doses.
Drug available: theophylline elixir 80 mg/15 mL.

(handwritten, left margin)
100 × 4 = 400 mg/dos
80 mg → 15 mL
100 mg → X

a. Is the drug dose within the safe parameters? *Yes*

b. How many milliliters (mL) would you give? *18.75 mL*

25 × 3 = 75 mg/day
5 × 16 = 80 mg/day
12.5 mg → 5 mL
→ ?
→ 25 mg

46. Child with pruritus.
    Order: diphenhydramine HCl (Benadryl) 25 mg, po, tid. *(×3)*
    Child's age and weight: 2 years, 16 kg.
    Pediatric dose range: 5 mg/kg/day.
    Drug available: Benadryl 12.5 mg/5 mL.

    a. Is the drug dose within the safe parameters? *Yes*

    b. How many milliliters (mL) would you give? *10 mL*

47. Child with a lower respiratory infection.
    Order: cefaclor (Ceclor) 100 mg, q8h.
    Child's age and weight: 4 years, 44 pounds.
    Pediatric dose range: 20–40 mg/kg/day in three divided doses. *(3)*
    Drug available:

    100 mg × 3 = 300

    min 20 × 20 = 400 mg/day
    max 40 × 20 = 800 mg/day

440/22, 40/20

44 lb → ?
2.2 lb → 1 kg

    a. How many kilograms (kg) does the child weigh?

    20 kg

    b. Is the drug dose within the safe parameters? *No*

    c. How many milliliters (mL) should the child receive?

    2.6 mL

    187 mg → 5 mL
    100 mg → X

    374 | 2.6
    260
    1122

48. Child with severe systemic infection.
    Order: tobramycin (Nebcin) 15 mg, IV, q8h. *(every 8 hours)*
    Child's age and weight: 18 months, 10 kg.
    Pediatric dose range: 3–5 mg/kg/day in three divided doses.

    30 – 50 mg/day   *15 × 3 = 45*

Drug available:

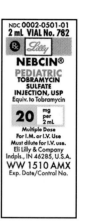

(handwritten calculations in margin:
30 | 20 | 1.5
20
100

20 mg → 2 mL
15 mg → x *)*

a. Is the drug dose within the safe parameters? _Yes_

b. How many milliliters (mL) of tobramycin would you give?

_1.5 mL_

49. Child with a severe central nervous system (CNS) infection.
    Order: ceftazidime (Fortaz) 250 mg, IV, q6h. (every 6 hrs)
    Child's age and weight: 6 years, 27 kg.
    Pediatric dose range: 30–50 mg/kg/day in three divided doses.
    Drug available: Add 2.0 mL of diluent = 2.4 mL of drug solution.

(handwritten margin calculations:
x 27 / 30 / 8 10   x 50 / 30

810–1500 mg/day

250 × 4 = 1000

→ 2.4 mL
→ 1.2 mL
500 mg
250 mg *)*

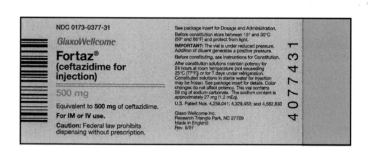

a. Is the drug dose within the safe parameters? _Yes_

b. How many milliliters (mL) of Fortaz would be given?

_1.2 mL_

50. Child with a severe respiratory infection.
    Order: kanamycin (Kantrex) 60 mg, IV, q8h. (every 8 hr)
    Child's age and weight: 1 year, 26 pounds.
    Pediatric dose range: 15 mg/kg/day, q8–12h.

(handwritten margin calculations:
26 lb → x
2.2 lb → 1 kg
26 / 2.2
22 / 40
22 / 80

12 lb / x 1.5 / 60   x3   390   11.8 lb / x 15 / 180 mg *)*

Drug available:

a. How many milligrams (mg) of kanamycin will the child receive per day? Per dose? _____ *80mg/day, 60mg/dose*

b. How many milliliters (mL) of kanamycin will the child receive per dose?

_____ *1.6mL*

c. Is the drug dose within safe parameters? _____ *yes*

ANSWERS

Orals

1. 2 tablets

2. 1½ tablets

3. 1½ tablets

4. Nitrostat 0.3 mg (use conversion table as needed)

5. a. grain ¼ = 15 mg

   b. 2 tablets

6. a. 0.5 gram = 500 mg

   b. 2 tablets

7. a. 600 to 650 mg = gr x

   b. 325 mg bottle

   c. 2 tablets from the 325 mg bottle

8. a. 0.2 g = 200 mg

   b. 2 tablets

9. a. Compazine 5 mg/5 mL; Compazine 5 mg/mL is for injection.

   b. 10 mL

10. a. Select 250 mg/5 mL bottle. However, either bottle could be used; 125 mg/5 mL = 20 mL.

   b. 1 gram; 1000 mg

   c. 500 mg = 10 mL

11. a. Either 187 mg/5 mL or 375 mg/5 mL.

   b. With (preferred) 187 mg/5 mL bottle:

$$\frac{250 \text{ mg}}{187 \text{ mg}} \times 5 \text{ mL} = \frac{1250}{187} = 6.67 \text{ or } 7 \text{ mL per dose}$$

With the 375 mg/5 mL, 3.3 mL per dose.

12. a. Zocor bottle 20 mg. Either bottle; however, with 10 mg Zocor bottle, more tablets would be taken (Zocor 10 mg bottle = 4 tablets).

    b. 2 tablets (Zocor 20 mg bottle)

13. a. 150 pounds = 68 kg

    b. 0.75 × 68 = 51 mg or 50 mg

    c. Select 25 mg capsule bottle. Two capsules.

14. a. 5 mg × 70 kg = 350 mg loading dose

    b. Select the 150 mg/15 mL bottle.

    c. 35 mL theophylline

15. a. 10 mL = 100 mg Colace

    b. *known mOsm (3900)* × Vol of drug (10) = $\dfrac{39,000}{500}$ = 78 mL drug solution and water desired mOsm (500)

        78 mL of drug solution and water − 10 mL of drug sol
                            = 68 mL of water to dilute the osmolality of the drug

Injectables

16. ½ mL or 0.5 mL

17. 1 mL

18. a. Meperidine 0.8 mL; atropine 1.25 mL

    b. (1) Expel 0.2 mL meperidine; (2) draw 1.25 mL air and insert into the atropine bottle; (3) withdraw 1.25 mL atropine into the meperidine cartridge.

19. a. Could use either cartridge: U 5000/0.5 mL; U 10,000/1 mL.

    b. 0.25 mL

20. 1.25 mL

21. a. Withdraw the regular Humulin insulin first and then the NPH insulin.

    b. Total of 55 units of regular and NPH insulin.

22. a. Select 1000 mcg/mL. If you choose the 100 mcg/mL cartridge, you would need 5 cartridges to give 500 μg (mcg).

    b. ½ mL or 0.5 mL

23. grain ⅙ = 10 mg (use conversion table as needed)
0.66 mL or 0.7 mL

24. ½ mL or 0.5 mL

25. 1.4 mL

26. a. 145 ÷ 2.2 = 65.9 kg or 66 kg

    b. 3 mg × 66 kg = 198 mg/day

c. $198 \div 3 = 66$ mg per dose

d. $\dfrac{66 \text{ mg}}{80} \times 2 \text{ mL} = \dfrac{132}{80} = 1.65$ or 1.7 mL per dose

27. 0.5 mL

28. a. Add 3 mL diluent = 3.5 mL drug solution; 1 g = 1000 mg.

b. $\dfrac{500 \text{ mg}}{1000 \text{ mg}} \times 3.5 \text{ mL} = \dfrac{1750}{1000} = 1.75$ mL or 1.8 mL per dose

29. 0.25 g = 250 mg

$$\frac{250 \text{ mg}}{500} \times 2.2 \text{ mL} = \frac{550}{500} = 1.1 \text{ mL per dose}$$

30. a. Add 5.7 mL diluent = 6.0 mL per 1 gram of oxacillin; 250 mg = 1.5 mL

b. 0.9 mL per dose

31. 2.25 mL Fortaz

32. a. 165 lbs $\div$ 2.2 = 75 kg

b. 4 mg $\times$ 75 kg = 300 mg/day

c. 100 mg per dose

d. Select 40 mg/mL bottle of gentamicin sulfate. (Normally less than 3 mL, IM, should be given at one site.)

e. 2.5 mL of gentamicin per dose

Intravenous

33. 125 mL per hour

$$\frac{125 \text{ mL} \times 10 \text{ gtt/min}}{60 \text{ min/hr}} = \frac{1250}{60} = 20.8 \text{ gtt/min or 21 gtt/min}$$

34. 62–63 gtt/min

35. Add 2.0 mL diluent = 2.6 mL drug solution; 1 g = 1000 mg.

a. $\dfrac{6\cancel{0}0 \text{ mg}}{10\cancel{0}0 \text{ mg}} \times 2.6 \text{ mL} = \dfrac{15.6}{10} = 1.56$ mL or 1.6 mL Ticar per dose

b. $\dfrac{\text{amount of solution} \times \text{gtt/mL}}{\text{minutes}} = \dfrac{60 \text{ mg} \times \overset{2}{\cancel{60}} \text{ gtt/mL}}{\underset{1}{\cancel{30}} \text{ minutes}} = 120 \text{ gtt/min}$

36. a. 1.5 mL

b. $\dfrac{100 \text{ mL} \times \overset{1}{\cancel{15}} \text{ gtt/mL}}{\underset{3}{\cancel{45}} \text{ min}} = \dfrac{100}{3} = 33.3 \text{ or } 33 \text{ gtt/min}$

37. a. Add 2 mL Thorazine to 500 mL. For 4 hours: 500 mL $\div$ 4 = 125 mL per hour.

b. $\dfrac{125 \text{ mL} \times \overset{1}{\cancel{15}} \text{ gtt/mL}}{\underset{4}{\cancel{60}} \text{ min/1 h}} = \dfrac{125}{4} = 31 \text{ gtt/min for 4 hours}$

38. a. 0.5 g = 500 mg; add 2.0 mL of diluent = 2.5 mL of drug solution; 500 mg = 2.5 mL

b. Amount of solution $\div \dfrac{\text{min to admin}}{60 \text{ min/h}}$ = mL /hr

$$2.5 \text{ mL drug} + 50 \text{ mL} \div \frac{20 \text{ min}}{60 \text{ min/h}} = 52.5 \text{ mL} \times \frac{\overset{3}{\cancel{60}}}{\underset{1}{\cancel{20}}} = 157.5 \text{ mL/hr}$$

Set pump to deliver in 20 minutes.

39. a. 10 mg/h × 5 h = 50 mg Cardizem

b. $\dfrac{50 \text{ mg}}{5} \times 1 \text{ mL} = 10 \text{ mL Cardizem to add to 500 mL}$

c. 10 mL drug solution + 500 mL $\div \dfrac{300 \text{ min}}{60 \text{ min/hr}}$

$$= 510 \text{ mL} \times \frac{\overset{1}{\cancel{60}} \text{ min}}{\underset{5}{\cancel{300}} \text{ min (5 h)}} = \frac{510}{5} = 102 \text{ mL/hr}$$

40. a. 1.2 g × 1.98 m² = 2.37 g or 2.4 g or 2400 mg

b. 2.4 g × 20 mL/1 g = 48 mL dilulent added to Ifex vials to yield 54 mL of drug solution

c. 54 mL of drug sol + 50 mL $\div \dfrac{30 \text{ min}}{60 \text{ min}} = 104 \text{ mL} \times \dfrac{\overset{2}{\cancel{60}} \text{ min}}{\underset{1}{\cancel{30}} \text{ min}} = 208 \text{ mL/hr}$

Set pump to deliver in 30 minutes.

Pediatrics

41. a. Drug dose is within safe parameters.

b. 10 mL

42. a. Drug dose is within safe parameters.

b. 5 mL or 1 tsp

43. a. Drug dose is within safe parameters; 53 pounds ÷ 2.2 = 24 kg. 25,000 × 24 = 600,000 units; 90,000 × 24 = 2,160,000 units/day. Child receives 400,000 units × 4 (q6h) = 1,600,000 units/day.

b. U 400,000 = 10 mL per dose

44. a. No; the drug dose is *NOT* within safe parameters. Do *NOT* give. Contact the physician or health care provider.
Drug parameters: 380–760 mg/day
Order 250 mg × 4 (q6h) = 1000 mg/day; *TOO MUCH*

b. Would not give medication.

45. a. Drug dose is within safe parameters.

b. 18.75 mL or 19 mL theophylline elixir.

46. a. Drug dose is within safe parameters.

       5 mg × 16 kg = 80 mg; child receives 25 mg × 3 (tid) = 75 mg; *SAFE*

   b. 10 mL

47. a. 44 lb ÷ 2.2 = 20 kg

   b. Drug dose is less than pediatric drug range. Check with the health care provider.
20 mg × 20 kg = 400 mg/day; 40 mg × 20 kg = 800 mg/day. Child to receive 100 mg × 3 (q8h) = 300 mg/day: less than 400−800 mg/day.

   c. 2.67 mL or 2.7 mL per dose = 100 mg

48. a. Drug dose is within safe parameters.
3 mg × 10 kg = 30 mg/day; 5 mg × 10 kg = 50 mg/day. Child to receive 15 mg × 3 (q8h) = 45 mg/day.

   b. 1.5 mL per dose

49. a. Drug dose is within the safe parameters.
30 mg × 27 kg = 810 mg/day; 50 mg × 27 kg = 1350 mg/day. Child to receive 250 mg × 4 (q6h) = 1000 mg/day.

   b. 1.2 mL per dose

50. a. 180 mg/d; 60 mg/dose

   b. $\dfrac{60}{75} \times 2 \text{ mL} = \dfrac{120}{75} = 1.6 \text{ mL per dose}$

   c. Drug dose is within safe parameters.
Child's weight: 26 lbs ÷ 2.2 = 11.8 or 12 kg
15 mg × 12 kg = 180 mg/day; child to receive 180 mg/day or 60 mg per dose.

references

Akers, M. J. (1987). Considerations in using the IV route for drug delivery. *American Journal of Hospital Pharmacy, 44,* 2528–2530.

Axton, S. E., and Fugate, T. (1987). A protocol for pediatric IV meds. *American Journal of Nursing, 7,* 943–945.

Barnhart, E. R. (1998). *Physician's Desk Reference* (52nd ed.). Oradell, NJ: Medical Economics.

Behrman, R. E., and Vaughan, V. C. (1987). *Nelson Textbook of Pediatrics* (13th ed.). Philadelphia: W.B. Saunders.

Body-surface area as a basic for dosing of anticancer agents: Science, myth, or habit? (1998). *Journal of Clinical Oncology, 16,* 2297–2298.

Briars, G. L., and Bailey, B. J. (1994). Surface area estimation: Pocket calculator vs. nomogram. *Archives of Disease in Childhood, 70,* 246–247.

Carey, B. (1982). Microdrop calculations of neonates in converting micrograms/kilograms/minute to microdrops. *Dimensions of Critical Care Nursing, 6,* 338–339.

Colangelo, A. (1987). Drug preparation techniques for IV drug delivery systems. *American Journal of Hospital Pharmacy, 44,* 2550–2553.

Comer, J. (1981). *Pharmacology in Critical Care.* Bethany, CT: Fleschner Publishing.

Daniels, J. M., and Smith L. M. (1990). *Clinical Calculations* (2nd ed.). Albany, NY: Delmar Publishers.

Deglin, J. H. (1988). *Dosage Calculations Manual.* Springhouse, PA: Springhouse.

Deglin, J. H., Vallerand, A. H., and Russin, M. M. (1991). *Davis's Drug Guide for Nurses* (2nd ed.). Philadelphia: F.A. Davis.

Edmunds, M. W. (1991). *Introduction to Clinical Pharmacology.* St. Louis: C.V. Mosby.

Estoup, M. (1994). Approaches and limitations of medication delivery in patients with enteral feeding tubes. *Critical Care Nurse, 14,* 68–79.

Gilman, A. G., Goodman, L. S., and Gilman, A. (Eds.). (1991). *Goodman and Gilman's The Pharmacological Basis of Therapeutics* (8th ed.). New York: Pergamon Press.

Gurney, H. P., Ackland, S., Gebski, V., and Farrell, G. (1998). Factors affecting epirubicin pharmacokinetics and toxicity: Evidence against using body-surface areas for dose calculation. *Journal of Clinical Oncology, 16,* 2299–2304.

Hodgson, B. B., and Kizior, R. J. (2000). *Saunders Nursing Drug Handbook 2000.* Philadelphia: W.B. Saunders.

Howry, L. B., Bindler, R. M., and Tso, Y. (1981). *Pediatric Medications.* Philadelphia: J. B. Lippincott.

Katzung, B. G. (1992). *Basic and Clinical Pharmacology* (5th ed.) Norwalk, CT: Appleton & Lange.

Kee, J. L., and Hayes, E. R. (2000). *Pharmacology: A Nursing Process Approach.* (3rd ed.). Philadelphia: W.B. Saunders.

Kee, J. L., and Paulanka, B. J. (1998). *Fluids and Electrolytes with Clinical Applications* (6th ed.). Albany, NY: Delmar Publishers.

Keenan, P. (1982). The "key number" conversion method in converting micrograms/kilograms/minute to microdrops. *Dimensions of Critical Care Nursing, 6,* 332–333.

Lack, J. A., and Stuart-Taylor, M. E. (1997). Calculation of drug dosage and body surface area of children. *British Journal of Anaesthesia, 78,* 601–605.

Leff, R. D. (1987). Features of IV devices and equipment that affect IV drug delivery. *American Journal of Hospital Pharmacy, 44,* 2530–2533.

Lilley, L. L., and Guanci, R. (1994). Getting back to basics. *American Journal of Nursing, 9,* 15–16.

Merenstein, G., and Gardner, S. (1998). *Handbook of Neonatal Intensive Care.* St. Louis: Mosby–Year Book.

Miyagawa, C. I. (1993). Drug-nutrient interactions in critically ill patients. *Critical Care Nurse, 13,* 69–87.

Norton, B. A., and Miller, A. M. (1986). *Skills for Professional Nursing Practice.* Norwalk, CT: Appleton-Century-Crofts.

Phillips, L. (1997). *Manuel of IV Therapeutics.* Philadelphia: F.A. Davis.

Piecoro, J. J. (1987). Development of an institutional IV drug delivery policy. *American Journal of Hospital Pharmacy, 44,* 2557–2559.

Rapp, R. P. (1987). Considering product features and costs in selecting a system for intermittent IV drug delivery. *American Journal of Hospital Pharmacy, 44,* 2533–2538.

Reilly, K. M. (1987). Problems in administration techniques and dose measurement that influence accuracy of IV drug delivery. *American Journal of Hospital Pharmacy, 44,* 2545–2550.

Rimar, J. M. (1987). Guidelines for the intravenous administration of medications used in pediatrics. *Maternal Child Nursing, 12,* 322–340.

Rosenthal, K. (1982). Charts vs. formula method in converting micrograms/kilograms/minute to microdrops. *Dimensions of Critical Care Nursing, 6,* 326–331.

Russell, H. (1980). *Pediatric Drugs and Nursing Interventions.* New York: McGraw-Hill.

Savinetti-Rose, B., and Bolmer, L. (1997). Understanding continuous subcutaneous insulin infusion therapy. *American Journal of Nursing, 97,* 42–49.

Skokal, W. (1997). Infusion pump update. *RN, 60,* 35–38.

Smith, A. J. (1989). *Dosage and Solutions Calculations.* St. Louis: C.V. Mosby.

Spratto, G. R., and Woods, A. L. (1998). *Nurse's Drug Reference (NDR 98)*. Albany, NY: Delmar Publishers.

Terry, J., Baranowski, L., Lonsway, R., and Hedrick, C. (1995). *Intravenous Therapy: Clinical Principles and Practice*. Philadelphia: W.B. Saunders.

Vallerand, A. H., and Deglin, J. H. (1991). *Nurse's Guide for IV Medications*. Philadelphia: F.A. Davis.

Weyant, H. (1984). Utilization of an intravenous drug guide. *Focus on Critical Care, 2,* 58–62.

Wong, D. L. (1995). *Nursing Care of Infants* (6th ed.). St. Louis: C.V. Mosby.

Wyeth Laboratories (1988). *Intramuscular Injections*. Philadelphia: Wyeth Laboratories.

Zenk, K. E. (1980). Dosage calculations for drugs administered by infusion. *American Journal of Hospital Pharmacy, 37,* 1304–1305.

Zenk, K. E. (1987). Intravenous drug delivery in infants with limited IV access and fluid restriction. *American Journal of Hospital Pharmacy, 44,* 2542–2545.

guidelines for administration of medications

● u t l i n e

ADMINISTRATION
ORAL MEDICATIONS
INJECTABLE MEDICATIONS
INTRAVENOUS FLOW AND MEDICATIONS

GENERAL DRUG ADMINISTRATION

1. Check medication order with doctor's orders, MAR (i.e., medication administration record), medicine card (if available), and/or other methods, such as computerized records.
2. Check label of drug container three times.
3. Check drug label for expiration date of *all* drugs. Return drugs that are outdated to the pharmacy.
4. Identify the client by identification bracelet and by asking client his or her name.
5. Stay with the client until the medication is taken.
6. Give medications last to clients who need more assistance.
7. Report any drug error immediately to the head nurse and physician. An incident report must be made.
8. Record drug given, including the name of the drug, dosage, date, time, and your initials.
9. Record drugs soon after they are given, especially STAT medications. Also indicate on the drug sheet if the drug was not given.
10. Record the amount of fluid taken orally with medication if client's intake (I) and output (O) are being recorded.
11. Be aware that nurses have the right to question drug orders. Physicians are responsible for medication order, dosage, and route of drug administration. Nurses are responsible for administering medications.
12. Administer drug within 30 minutes of its prescribed time (30 minutes before or 30 minutes after prescribed time).
13. Do not guess when preparing medications. Check the order sheet if the drug order is not clear. Call the pharmacist, physician, and/or nursing supervisor if in doubt.
14. Do not give drugs poured by others.
15. Do not leave drug tray or cart out of your sight.
16. Know that clients have the right to refuse medication. If possible, ascertain why a client refuses the medication. Report refusal to take medications.
17. Check if client states that he or she has an allergy to a drug or a drug group.
18. Know the five *rights:* right drug, right dose, right route, right time, and right client.

ORAL MEDICATIONS

1. Wash hands before preparing oral medications.
2. Pour tablet or capsule into drug container's cap (top) and *not* into your hand. Drugs prepared for unit dose can be opened at the time of administration in the client's room. Discard drugs that are dropped on the floor.

3. Pour liquids on a flat surface at eye level with your thumbnail at medicine cup line indicating the desired amount.

4. Do not mix liquids with tablets or liquids with liquids in the same container. Tablets and capsules can be put in the same container *except* for oral narcotics, digoxin, and PRN and STAT medications.

5. Do not pour drugs from containers with labels that are difficult to read.

6. Do not return poured medication to its container. Properly discard poured medication if not used.

7. Do not transfer medication from one container to another.

8. Pour liquid medications from the side opposite the bottle's label to avoid spilling medicine on the label.

9. Dilute liquid medications that irritate gastric mucosa, e.g., potassium products, or that could discolor or damage tooth enamel, e.g., SSKI, or have client take the drug with meals.

10. Offer ice chips prior to distasteful medications in order to numb the client's taste buds.

11. Assist the client into upright position when administering oral medications. Stay with the client until medication is taken.

12. Give at least 50 to 100 mL of oral fluids with medications unless the client has a fluid restriction. Doing so helps to ensure that medication reaches the stomach.

13. For clients having difficulty in swallowing or for clients receiving nutrients through a nasogastric or gastric tube, crush tablets (*not* spansules) and dissolve in juice or applesauce for oral ingestion or in water for tube administration. Give oral medication in small amounts to prevent choking. For the client who has difficulty swallowing, gently stroke the throat in a downward motion to enhance swallowing.

14. For drugs given by oral syringe, direct the syringe across the tongue and toward the side of the mouth.

15. If a client or a child spits out *all* of the liquid medication, repeat the dose. If a client or a child spits out more than one half of the liquid medication, repeat one half of the dose. If the client or the child spits out less than one half of the liquid medication or if there is a question regarding repeating the dose, the physician must be notified and another route of administration chosen.

INJECTABLE MEDICATIONS

1. Wash hands before preparing injectable medications.

2. Select the proper syringe and needle size for the type of medication to be administered.

3. Assess the amount of subcutaneous fat at the injection site before choosing the needle length for an intramuscular injection.

4. Select the injection site according to the drug.

5. Check for drug compatibility before mixing drugs in the same syringe.

6. Check the expiration date on the drug label before preparing medication. If in doubt, check with the pharmacist.

7. Check the label on the drug container to determine method(s) for drug administration, i.e., IM, IV, SC.

8. Do not give parenteral medications that are cloudy, are discolored, or have precipitated.

9. Aspirate the plunger before injecting medication. If blood returns, *stop,* withdraw the needle, and prepare a new solution. Check the policy of your institution.

10. Do not massage the injection site if using the Z-track method, intradermal injection, heparin, or any anticoagulant solution.

11. Do not administer injections into inflamed and edematous tissues or into lesion (moles, birthmarks, scar) sites.

12. Recognize that individuals experiencing edema, shock, or poor circulation have a very slow tissue absorption rate following intramuscular injection.

13. Discard liquid drugs into the sink or toilet, *not* into the trash can.

14. Discard needles safely into the proper container.

15. Refrigerate unused reconstituted powdered medication in a vial. Write date, time, and your initials on the vial.

16. Discard unused solution in ampules. After they are opened, ampules cannot be reused.

17. Do not administer IM medications subcutaneously. Sloughing of the subcutaneous tissue could occur.

INTRAVENOUS FLOW AND MEDICATIONS

1. Wash hands before changing IV fluids and tubing and before preparing IV drugs.

2. Use aseptic technique when inserting IV catheters and changing IV tubing and bags. Be able to recognize symptoms of septicemia, such as chills, fever, tachycardia.

3. Select appropriate IV tubing sets for continuous IV infusion. For IV fluids to infuse in 10 hours or *more,* use a microdrip set (60 gtt/min); for IV fluids to infuse in 10 hours or *less, use* a macrodrip set (10, 15, 20 gtt/min).

4. Add IV drugs such as vitamins and potassium chloride to the IV fluid before connecting the IV fluid to the IV tubing. Invert the IV bag or bottle several times to ensure drug distribution. If the IV fluid is running and IV medication needs to be added, temporarily stop the IV fluid by clamping the tubing, Invert the IV bag or bottle several times, then unclamp the tubing and maintain the ordered IV flow rate.

5. Check for patency of the IV catheter (heparin lock) before administering drugs by inserting 2 mL of saline solution. Flush IV line with 15 mL of saline solution to empty the IV line of drug solution, if necessary.

6. Use the proper diluent to reconstitute a powdered drug, and use the proper IV solution for infusion. Drug labels and drug information inserts usually indicate the types of diluents to use.

7. Record on the vial containing unused drug the date of reconstitution and your initials.

8. Monitor all IV flow rates (conventional tubing or electronic IV regulators) hourly as needed. IV flow rates can alter owing to the client's position or to a kink in the tubing.

9. Check for air bubbles in the IV tubing. Remove air from the tubing by clamping below the air bubbles and aspirating with a syringe, or use the method indicated by your institution.

10. Assess for allergic reactions to the IV drug. If reactions are seen, stop the flow of IV drug immediately.

11. Avoid administering drugs rapidly in IV solutions. Speed shock could occur as a result of drug concentration and accumulation. Symptoms of speed shock include tachycardia, syncope, and drop in blood pressure.

12. Observe the infusion site for signs and symptoms of infiltration, such as swelling, coolness, and pain. If these signs and symptoms are observed, discontinue IV and restart at another site.

13. Assess for signs and symptoms of phlebitis, such as redness, warmth, swelling, and pain. Redness may be seen above the infusion site along the vein.

14. Do not forcefully irrigate IV catheters. A clot could be dislodged from the catheter site and become an embolus.

15. Avoid using leg veins, elbow (antecubital) site, and affected limbs for IV therapy.

16. Change the IV site every 3 days or as indicated. Certain IV catheters, such as polyethylene catheters, can cause phlebitis.

17. Change IV tubing every 24–48 hours, and change IV bags every 24 hours.

18. Apply cold compresses followed later by warm compresses to any hematoma site, according to the physician's orders.

nomograms

● u t l i n e

BODY SURFACE AREA FOR ADULTS – NOMOGRAM

HEIGHT	BODY SURFACE AREA (BSA)	WEIGHT
cm 200 — 79 inch	2.80 m²	kg 150 — 330 lb
78	2.70	145 — 320
195 — 77		140 — 310
76	2.60	135 — 300
190 — 75		130 — 290
74	2.50	125 — 280
185 — 73		120 — 270
72	2.40	115 — 260
180 — 71	2.30	250
70		110 — 240
175 — 69	2.20	105 — 230
68		100 — 220
170 — 67	2.10	
66		95 — 210
165 — 65	2.00	90 — 200
64	1.95	
160 — 63	1.90	85 — 190
62	1.85	80 — 180
155 — 61	1.80	
60	1.75	170
150 — 59	1.70	75 — 160
58	1.65	
145 — 57	1.60	70 — 150
56	1.55	
140 — 55	1.50	65 — 140
54	1.45	60 — 130
135 — 53	1.40	
52		55 — 120
130 — 51	1.35	
50	1.30	
125 — 49	1.25	50 — 110
48	1.20	105
120 — 47	1.15	45 — 100
46	1.10	95
115 — 45		90
44	1.05	40 — 85
110 — 43	1.00	80
42		35 — 75
105 — 41	0.95	
	0.90	70
cm 100 — 40	0.86 m²	kg 30 — 66 lb
39 in		

Body Surface Area (BSA) Nomogram for Adultsd

Directions: (1) find height; (2) find weight; (3) draw a straight line connecting the height and weight. Where the line intersects on the BSA column is the body surface area (m²). From Deglin, J. H., Vallerand, A. H., and Russin, M. M. (1991). *Davis's Drug Guide for Nurses.* (2nd ed.). Philadelphia: F. A. Davis, p. 1218. Used with permission from Lentner C. (ed.). (1981). *Geigy Scientific Tables.* (8th ed.). Vol. 1. Basel, Switzerland: Ciba-Geigy, pp. 226–227.

West Nomogram for Infants and Children

Directions: (1) find height; (2) find weight; (3) draw a straight line connecting the height and weight. Where the line intersects on the SA column is the body surface area (m²). Modified from data of E. Boyd and C. D. West, in Behrman, R. E. and Vaughan, V. C. (1996). *Nelson Textbook of Pediatrics* (15th ed.). Philadelphia: W.B. Saunders.

index

Note: Page numbers followed by "t" refer to tables.